Arpad Kelemen, Ajith Abraham, Yulan Liang (Eds.)

Computational Intelligence in Medical Informatics

Studies in Computational Intelligence, Volume 85

Editor-in-chief
Prof. Janusz Kacprzyk
Systems Research Institute
Polish Academy of Sciences
ul. Newelska 6
01-447 Warsaw
Poland
E-mail: kacprzyk@ibspan.waw.pl

Further volumes of this series can be found on our homepage: springer.com

Vol. 62. Lakhmi C. Jain, Raymond A. Tedman and Debra K. Tedman (Eds.)
Evolution of Teaching and Learning Paradigms in Intelligent Environment, 2007
ISBN 978-3-540-71973-1

Vol. 63. Wlodzislaw Duch and Jacek Mańdziuk (Eds.)
Challenges for Computational Intelligence, 2007
ISBN 978-3-540-71983-0

Vol. 64. Lorenzo Magnani and Ping Li (Eds.)
Model-Based Reasoning in Science, Technology, and Medicine, 2007
ISBN 978-3-540-71985-4

Vol. 65. S. Vaidya, L.C. Jain and H. Yoshida (Eds.)
Advanced Computational Intelligence Paradigms in Healthcare-2, 2007
ISBN 978-3-540-72374-5

Vol. 66. Lakhmi C. Jain, Vasile Palade and Dipti Srinivasan (Eds.)
Advances in Evolutionary Computing for System Design, 2007
ISBN 978-3-540-72376-9

Vol. 67. Vassilis G. Kaburlasos and Gerhard X. Ritter (Eds.)
Computational Intelligence Based on Lattice Theory, 2007
ISBN 978-3-540-72686-9

Vol. 68. Cipriano Galindo, Juan-Antonio Fernández-Madrigal and Javier Gonzalez
A Multi-Hierarchical Symbolic Model of the Environment for Improving Mobile Robot Operation, 2007
ISBN 978-3-540-72688-3

Vol. 69. Falko Dressler and Iacopo Carreras (Eds.)
Advances in Biologically Inspired Information Systems: Models, Methods, and Tools, 2007
ISBN 978-3-540-72692-0

Vol. 70. Javaan Singh Chahl, Lakhmi C. Jain, Akiko Mizutani and Mika Sato-Ilic (Eds.)
Innovations in Intelligent Machines-1, 2007
ISBN 978-3-540-72695-1

Vol. 71. Norio Baba, Lakhmi C. Jain and Hisashi Handa (Eds.)
Advanced Intelligent Paradigms in Computer Games, 2007
ISBN 978-3-540-72704-0

Vol. 72. Raymond S.T. Lee and Vincenzo Loia (Eds.)
Computation Intelligence for Agent-based Systems, 2007
ISBN 978-3-540-73175-7

Vol. 73. Petra Perner (Ed.)
Case-Based Reasoning on Images and Signals, 2008
ISBN 978-3-540-73178-8

Vol. 74. Robert Schaefer
Foundation of Global Genetic Optimization, 2007
ISBN 978-3-540-73191-7

Vol. 75. Crina Grosan, Ajith Abraham and Hisao Ishibuchi (Eds.)
Hybrid Evolutionary Algorithms, 2007
ISBN 978-3-540-73296-9

Vol. 76. Subhas Chandra Mukhopadhyay and Gourab Sen Gupta (Eds.)
Autonomous Robots and Agents, 2007
ISBN 978-3-540-73423-9

Vol. 77. Barbara Hammer and Pascal Hitzler (Eds.)
Perspectives of Neural-Symbolic Integration, 2007
ISBN 978-3-540-73953-1

Vol. 78. Costin Badica and Marcin Paprzycki (Eds.)
Intelligent and Distributed Computing, 2008
ISBN 978-3-540-74929-5

Vol. 79. Xing Cai and T.-C. Jim Yeh (Eds.)
Quantitative Information Fusion for Hydrological Sciences, 2008
ISBN 978-3-540-75383-4

Vol. 80. Joachim Diederich
Rule Extraction from Support Vector Machines, 2008
ISBN 978-3-540-75389-6

Vol. 81. K. Sridharan
Robotic Exploration and Landmark Determination, 2008
ISBN 978-3-540-75393-3

Vol. 82. Ajith Abraham, Crina Grosan and Witold Pedrycz (Eds.)
Engineering Evolutionary Intelligent Systems, 2008
ISBN 978-3-540-75395-7

Vol. 83. Bhanu Prasad and S.R.M. Prasanna (Eds.)
Speech, Audio, Image and Biomedical Signal Processing using Neural Networks, 2008
ISBN 978-3-540-75397-1

Vol. 84. Marek R. Ogiela and Ryszard Tadeusiewicz
Modern Computational Intelligence Methods for the Interpretation of Medical Images, 2008
ISBN 978-3-540-75399-5

Vol. 85. Arpad Kelemen, Ajith Abraham and Yulan Liang (Eds.)
Computational Intelligence in Medical Informatics, 2008
ISBN 978-3-540-75766-5

Arpad Kelemen
Ajith Abraham
Yulan Liang
(Eds.)

Computational Intelligence in Medical Informatics

With 137 Figures and 27 Tables

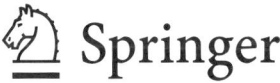

Prof. Arpad Kelemen
Buffalo Neuroimaging Analysis Center
The Jacobs Neurological Institute
University at Buffalo
The State University of New York
100 High Street
Buffalo, NY 14203
U.S.A
akelemen@buffalo.edu

Prof. Yulan Liang
Biostatistics Dept.
University at Buffalo
The State University of New York
252A2 Farber Hall, 3435 Main st.
Buffalo, NY 14214
U.S.A
yliang@buffalo.edu

Prof. Ajith Abraham
Centre for Quantifiable Quality of Service
in Communication Systems (Q2S)
Centre of Excellence
Norwegian University of Science
and Technology
O.S. Bragstads plass 2E
N-7491 Trondheim
Norway
ajith.abraham@ieee.org

ISBN 978-3-540-75766-5   e-ISBN 978-3-540-75767-2

Studies in Computational Intelligence ISSN 1860-949X

Library of Congress Control Number: 2007937181

© 2008 Springer-Verlag Berlin Heidelberg

This work is subject to copyright. All rights are reserved, whether the whole or part of the material is concerned, specifically the rights of translation, reprinting, reuse of illustrations, recitation, broadcasting, reproduction on microfilm or in any other way, and storage in data banks. Duplication of this publication or parts thereof is permitted only under the provisions of the German Copyright Law of September 9, 1965, in its current version, and permission for use must always be obtained from Springer-Verlag. Violations are liable to prosecution under the German Copyright Law.

The use of general descriptive names, registered names, trademarks, etc. in this publication does not imply, even in the absence of a specific statement, that such names are exempt from the relevant protective laws and regulations and therefore free for general use.

Cover design: Deblik, Berlin, Germany

Printed on acid-free paper

9 8 7 6 5 4 3 2 1

springer.com

Preface

Medical informatics is an emerging interdisciplinary science that deals with clinical health-related information, its structure, acquisition and use. Medical Informatics (MI) is grounded in the principles of computer science, artificial intelligence, as well as the clinical and basic sciences. MI includes scientific endeavors ranging from building theoretical models and evaluation of applied systems.

Computational intelligence is a well-established paradigm, where new theories with a sound biological understanding have been evolving. Defining computational intelligence is not an easy task. In a nutshell, which becomes quite apparent in light of the current research pursuits, the area is heterogeneous with a combination of such technologies as neural networks, fuzzy systems, rough set, evolutionary computation, swarm intelligence, probabilistic reasoning, multi-agent systems etc. The recent trend is to integrate different components to take advantage of complementary features and to develop a synergistic system.

This book deals with the application of computational intelligence in medical informatics. Addressing the various issues of medical informatics using different computational intelligence approaches is the novelty of this edited volume. This volume comprises of 15 chapters' including an introductory chapter giving the fundamental definitions and some important research challenges. Chapters were selected on the basis of fundamental ideas/concepts rather than the thoroughness of techniques deployed. The fifteen chapters are organized as follows.

In the introductory Chapter, *Kelemen et al.* provide a review of recently developed theories and applications in computational intelligence for gene-gene and gene-environment interactions in complex diseases in genetic association study.

Chapter 2 by *Burns et al.* is designed to act as an introduction to the field of biomedical text-mining for computer scientists who are unfamiliar with the way that biomedical research uses the literature. Authors describe how creating knowledge bases from the primary biomedical literature is formally equivalent to the process of performing a literature review or a 'research synthesis'. The main body of the chapter is concerned with the use of text mining approaches to populate knowledge representations for different types of experiment. Authors provide a detailed example from neuroscience and describe a detailed description of the methodology used to perform the text mining based on the conditional random fields model.

Tamalika Chaira and *Tridib Chaira* in Chapter 3 propose a new image segmentation technique using intuitionistic fuzzy set and is applied for brain images and blood cell for edge detection. The proposed method works well even on poor quality images.

In Chapter 4, *Kreinovich* and *Shpak* illustrate that in general, detecting aggregability is NP-hard even for linear systems, and thus (unless P=NP), there is only hope to find efficient detection algorithms for specific classes of systems. Authors illustrate that in the linear case, once the blocks are known, it is possible to efficiently find appropriate linear combinations.

Siebel et al. in the fifth Chapter propose the automatic design of neural networks as a controller in a visuo-motor control scenario. Evolutionary Acquisition of Neural Topologies (EANT) uses evolutionary search methods on two levels: In an outer optimization loop called structural exploration new networks are developed by gradually adding new structures to an initially minimal network. In an inner optimization loop called structural exploitation the parameters of current networks are optimized. EANT was used with a complete simulation of a visuo-motor control scenario to learn neural networks by reinforcement learning.

In Chapter 6, *Lee at al.* propose Block Principal Components Analysis (PCA) and a variable selection method based on principal component loadings for dimension reduction. The main focus of this is how to deal with large number of variables (gene expressions) in microarray data sets. Authors also investigate the effect ill-conditioning has on the Mahalanobis distance between clusters using the well-known Hilbert matrix.

De Roberto Jr et al. in the seventh Chapter describes the development of a new tool for genome interpretation. The software recognizes coding regions with a user-friendly interface. The system is based on a gene model and combines the weight-position matrix technique with the flexibility of artificial neural networks in classification problems.

In Chapter 8, *Bogan-Marta et al.* discuss about the diversity of language engineering techniques and those involving information theoretic principles in analyzing protein sequences from similarity perspective. Authors also present a survey of the different approaches identified with a focus on two methods, which the they experimented.

Sehgal et al. in Chapter 9, investigate the impact of missing values on post genomic knowledge discovery methods like, gene selection and Gene Regulatory Network (GRN) reconstruction. A framework for robust subsequent biological knowledge inference is proposed, which has shown significant improvements in the outcomes of gene selection and GRN reconstruction methods.

In Chapter 10, *Sehgal et al.* provide a comprehensive comparative study on GRN reconstruction algorithms. The methods discussed are diverse and vary from simple similarity based methods to state of the art hybrid and probabilistic methods. The Chapter also emphasizes the need of strategies, which should be able to model the stochastic behavior of gene regulation in the presence of limited number of samples, noisy data, multi-collinearity for high number of genes.

Kasabov et al. in Chapter 11 present some preliminary results on the Brain-Gene Ontology project that is concerned with the collection, presentation and use of knowledge in the form of ontology equipped with the knowledge discovery means of computational intelligence. Brain-Gene Ontology system includes various concepts, facts, data, graphs, visualizations, animations, and other information forms, related to brain functions, brain diseases, their genetic basis and the relationship between all of them, and various software simulators.

In Chapter 12, *Dohnal et al.* present the metric space approach and its applications in the field of Bioinformatics. Authors describe some of the most popular centralized disk-based metric indexes with a focus on parallel and distributed access methods, which can deal with data collections that for practical purposes can be arbitrary large. An experimental evaluation of the presented distributed approaches on real-life data sets is also presented.

Kroc in Chapter 13 illustrates that the development of an adequate mechanical model of living tissues provides the morphological model with sufficient flexibility necessary to achieve expected morphological development. Author focuses on the development of mesenchymal and epithelial tissues, which creates the basic mechanism of tooth development.

In Chapter 14, *Bobrik et al.* describe two simplified models of Darwinian evolution at the molecular level by applying the methods of artificial chemistry. A metaphor of a chemical reactor (chemostat) is considered and then a simplified formal system *Typogenetics*, is discussed.

In the last Chapter *Bobrik et al.* present the third simplified model of Darwinian evolution at the molecular level, following the two presented in Chapter 14. An artificial-life application is designed as a modification of the metaphor of chemostat, where the secondary structure of binary strings specifies instructions for replication of binary strings.

We are very much grateful to the authors of this volume and to the reviewers for their tremendous service by critically reviewing the chapters. The editors would like to thank Dr. Thomas Ditzinger (Springer Engineering Inhouse Editor) and Professor Janusz Kacprzyk (Editor-in-Chief, Springer Studies in Computational Intelligence Series) and Ms. Heather King (Springer Verlag, Heidelberg) for the editorial assistance and excellent cooperative collaboration to produce this important scientific work. We hope that the reader will share our excitement to present this volume on '*Computational Intelligence in Medical Informatics*' and will find it useful.

Arpad Kelemen, Ajith Abraham and Yulan Liang (Editors)
August 2007

Contents

1 Review of Computational Intelligence for Gene-Gene and Gene-Environment Interactions in Disease Mapping
Arpad Kelemen, Yulan Liang and Athanasios Vasilakos 1
1.1 Introduction 1
1.2 Computational challenges in genomic association study of common complex diseases 3
1.3 The promise of computational intelligence 3
1.4 Computational intelligence approaches for SNP-disease associations ... 7
1.5 Conclusions 11
References 11

2 Intelligent Approaches to Mining the Primary Research Literature: Techniques, Systems, and Examples
Gully A.P.C. Burns, Donghui Feng, Eduard Hovy 17
2.1 Introduction 17
2.2 A framework for conceptual biology 19
2.3 Partitioning the literature - the notion of 'experimental type' 23
2.4 Related Work: Biomedical Knowledge Bases based on published studies 25
2.5 Practical applications: 'Research Synthesis' 28
2.6 An Example Experiment Type: 'Tract-Tracing Experiments' 30
2.7 Methodology 33
        The overall challenge, from text to knowledge 33
        Information extraction techniques: from Patterns to Conditional Random Fields 34
        Stage 1: Corpus Processing 37
        Stage 2: The basic text processing and feature definition 38
        Stage 3: Evaluating the results 39
2.8 Results 40
2.9 Conclusions 42
2.10 Acknowledgements 43
References 43

3 Intuitionistic Fuzzy Set: Application to Medical Image Segmentation
Tamalika Chaira, Tridib Chaira 51
- 3.1 Introduction 52
- 3.2 Related work in medical informatics 54
- 3.3 Prelimineries on intuitionistic fuzzy set 56
- 3.4 Use of intuitionistic fuzzy set theory in medical informatics - segmentation 57
  - 3.4.1 Edge detection 57
  - 3.4.2 Calculation of membership, non-membership degree and intuitionistic fuzzy index 60
  - 3.4.3 Application of intuitionistic fuzzy set theory in image thresholding 61
- 3.5 The proposed method 63
- 3.6 Results and Discussion 65
- 3.7 Conclusions 67
- References 67

4 Decomposable Aggregability in Population Genetics and Evolutionary Computations: Algorithms and Computational Complexity
Vladik Kreinovich, Max Shpak 69
- 4.1 What is Aggregability 69
  - *Comment.* 71
- 4.2 Exact Aggregability: A Simple Example 71
- 4.3 Detecting Aggregability is Important 73
- 4.4 What We Do in This Chapter 74
  - *Comment.* 74
  - 75
- 4.5 First Theoretical Result: Detecting Decomposable Aggregability Is NP-Hard 76
  - *Comment.* 76
  - 76
  - *Comment.* 77
  - *Comments.* 77
- 4.6 Approximate Aggregability: Possible Definitions 78
  - *Comment.* 80
- 4.7 Second Theoretical Result: Detecting Approximate Decomposable Aggregability Is Also NP-Hard 80
  - *Comment.* 81
- 4.8 Once We Find the Partition, Finding the Combinations is Feasible 81
  - 4.8.1 Algorithm 81
    - *Comment.* 81
  - 4.8.2 Calculating aggregate dynamics 82
  - 4.8.3 Example 82
  - 4.8.4 What to Do in the Case of Approximate Aggregation 82
- 4.9 Proofs 83

	4.9.1	Proof of Theorem 1	83
		"If" part.	84
		"Only if" part.	84
	4.9.2	Proof of Theorem 2	86
4.10	Conclusions	90
References	91

5 Evolutionary Learning of Neural Structures for Visuo-Motor Control
Nils T Siebel, Gerald Sommer, Yohannes Kassahun 93

5.1	Introduction	93
	5.1.1	Current Practice	94
	5.1.2	Problems and Biology-inspired Solutions	94
5.2	Problem Formulation and Related Work	96
	5.2.1	Visuo-Motor Control	96
	5.2.2	Related Work: Visuo-Motor Control	98
5.3	Developing Neural Networks with EANT	99
	5.3.1	EANT's Encoding of Neural Networks: The Linear Genome ..	99
	5.3.2	Initialisation of the EANT Population of Networks	101
	5.3.3	Structural Exploration: Search for Optimal Structures ..	101
	5.3.4	Structural Exploitation: Search for Optimal Parameters .	103
	5.3.5	Related Work: Evolving Neural Networks	104
5.4	Combining EANT with CMA-ES	105
	5.4.1	Motivation	105
	5.4.2	Improving the convergence with CMA-ES	105
5.5	Experimental Evaluation	108
	5.5.1	Experimental Setup	108
	5.5.2	Parameter Sets	108
		Original EANT	109
		CMA-ES EANT, many fevals	109
		CMA-ES EANT, few fevals	109
	5.5.3	Training and Testing	110
	5.5.4	Results	110
	5.5.5	Discussion	111
5.6	Conclusions	112
References	113

6 Dimension reduction for performing discriminant analysis for microarrays
Sang Hee Lee, A. K. Singh, and Laxmi P Gewali 117

6.1	Introduction	117
6.2	Methodology	118
6.3	Results	123
6.4	Conclusion and Recommendations	127
References	129

7 Auxiliary tool for the identification of genetic coding sequences in eukaryotic organisms

Vincenzo De Roberto Junior Nelson F. F. Ebecken, Elias Restum Antonio 133
7.1 Introduction 133
7.2 The main gene finding programs 134
7.3 Data characteristics 137
    7.3.1 Data volume 137
    7.3.2 Information consistency 138
    7.3.3 Stored information 138
    7.3.4 Database format 138
7.4 Accuracy measures 139
    7.4.1 Nucleotide level 139
    7.4.2 Exon level 139
7.5 Gene model 141
    7.5.1 Data selection 142
    7.5.2 The model for the discovery of coding areas 142
7.6 ExonBR system 144
7.7 Results and conclusion 147
References 148

8 Language engineering and information theoretic methods in protein sequence similarity studies

A. Bogan-Marta, A. Hategan, I. Pitas 151
8.1 Introduction 151
8.2 A survey of language engineering and information theoretic methods for protein sequence similarity 154
    8.2.1 Protein sequence similarity based on linguistic techniques 155
        Similarity due to regions as index terms in information retrieval 155
        Semantic similarity measures 156
        Language techniques for protein sequence relations 158
    8.2.2 Sequence similarity based on information theoretic methods 160
8.3 Statistical language modeling method for sequence similarity 163
    8.3.1 Theoretical concepts 163
    8.3.2 Method description 165
    8.3.3 Protein similarity search 165
        165
        166
    8.3.4 Experimental results 166
    8.3.5 Discussions 168
8.4 Protein similarity detection based on lossless compression of protein sequences 168
    8.4.1 Theoretical concepts 169
    8.4.2 ProtComp algorithm and its use in sequence comparison 169
    8.4.3 Experimental results 173
    8.4.4 Discussions 175

8.5	Conclusions		176
References			178

9 Gene Expression Imputation Techniques for Robust Post Genomic Knowledge Discovery
Muhammad Shoaib Sehgal, Iqbal Gondal and Laurence Dooley 185

9.1	Introduction		185
9.2	Missing Values Estimation Methods		187
	9.2.1	Imputation Nomenclature	187
	9.2.2	Zero and Average Based Imputation [17]	189
	9.2.3	Singular Value Decomposition Based Imputation (SVDImpute) [12]	189
	9.2.4	K-Nearest Neighbour (KNN) Estimation [12]	190
	9.2.5	Least Square Impute (LSImpute) [13]	191
	9.2.6	Local Least Square Impute (LLSImpute) [10]	191
	9.2.7	Bayesian Principal Component Analysis based Estimation (BPCA) [6]	192
	9.2.8	Collateral Missing Value Estimation (CMVE) [14]	192
9.3	Post Genomic Knowledge Discovery Methods		194
	9.3.1	Gene Selection	195
	9.3.2	Gene Regulatory Network Reconstruction	195
	9.3.3	Statistical Significance Test	196
9.4	Analysis and Discussion of Results		196
9.5	Software Availability		203
9.6	Conclusions		203
References			203

10 Computational Modelling Strategies for Gene Regulatory Network Reconstruction
Muhammad Shoaib Sehgal, Iqbal Gondal and Laurence Dooley 207

10.1	Introduction	207
10.2	Pair Wise GRN Reconstruction Methods	210
	Correlation and Distance Functions	211
	Mutual Information	211
	Local Shape Based Similarity	212
10.3	Deterministic Methods for GRN Inference	213
	Differential Equations	213
	Boolean GRN Modelling Methods	213
10.4	Probabilistic GRN Reconstructed Strategies	214
10.5	Hybrid GRN Inference Methods	215
10.6	Conclusions	217
References		218

11 Integration of Brain-Gene Ontology and Simulation Systems for Learning, Modelling and Discovery
Nik Kasabov, Vishal Jain, Lubica Benuskova, Paulo C. M. Gottgtroy and Frances Joseph 221
11.1 Introduction 221
11.2 Evolving Implementation of BGO in Protégé 223
11.3 New Discoveries with BGO 225
11.4 BGO for Teaching 231
11.5 Conclusions and Future Directions 231
11.6 Acknowledgments 233
References 233

12 Efficiency and Scalability Issues in Metric Access Methods
Vlastislav Dohnal, Claudio Gennaro, Pavel Zezula 235
12.1 The Metric Space Approach 236
    12.1.1 Metric Spaces in Bioinformatics 236
    12.1.2 Software Tools 238
12.2 Centralized Metric Access Methods 239
    12.2.1 Metric Tree Family 239
    12.2.2 Hash-based Similarity Indexing 241
    12.2.3 Performance Trials 241
12.3 Exploiting Multiple Computational Resources 243
    12.3.1 Parallel Similarity Searching 244
    12.3.2 Centralized Coordination 244
            Metric Grid 244
    12.3.3 Scalable and Distributed Search Structures 245
            Native Metric Search Structures 246
            Metric Content Addressable Network 248
            Metric Chord 250
12.4 Experience from Performance Trials 251
    12.4.1 Performance Tuning 254
12.5 Conclusions 257
References 259

13 Computational Modelling of the Biomechanics of Epithelial and Mesenchymal Cell Interactions During Morphological Development
Jiří Kroc 265
13.1 Introduction 265
13.2 Introduction to Cell and Tissue Biology 268
13.3 Overview of Morphological Development of Tooth Resulting from Interaction of Epithelium and Mesenchyme 269
13.4 Simplifications used in model of morphological growth 271
13.5 Model 273
    13.5.1 Three inter-dependent parts of the model 273
    13.5.2 Mechanical interaction of epithelium and mesenchyme 274

	13.5.3	Tissue growth	278

	13.5.3	Tissue growth	278
	13.5.4	Implementation of diffusion by two computational sub-steps	279
	13.5.5	Signalling, switching and cell differentiation	280
13.6	Results and Discussions		281
13.7	Future development		291
13.8	Conclusions		292
References			293

14 Artificial Chemistry and Molecular Darwinian Evolution of DNA/RNA-Like Systems I - Typogenetics and Chemostat

Marian Bobrik, Vladimir Kvasnicka, Jiri Pospichal 295

14.1	Introduction		295
14.2	Eigen Theory of Molecular Replicators		298
	14.2.1	Replicators and Molecular Darwinian Evolution	301
	14.2.2	Artificial Chemistry and a Metaphor of Chemostat	303
	14.2.3	Summary	306
14.3	Hofstadter's Theory of DNA-Like Molecules, Typogenetics		307
	14.3.1	Basic Principles of Typogenetics	309
	14.3.2	An Expression of Strands by Enzymes	310
	14.3.3	Replicators	314
	14.3.4	Hypercycles	319
	14.3.5	Summary	321
14.4	Folding of RNA-Like Molecules that are Represented by Binary Strings		321
	14.4.1	Chemostat Simulation of Molecular Darwinian Evolution	330
	14.4.2	Summary	332
References			334

15 Artificial Chemistry and Molecular Darwinian Evolution of DNA/RNA-Like Systems II – Programmable folding

Marian Bobrik, Vladimir Kvasnicka, Jiri Pospichal 337

15.1	Programmable Folding of RNA-Like Molecules		337
15.2	Source of the Instruction Set		338
15.3	Architecture of Programmable RNA System		342
15.4	Comparison with the Instruction Based System		347
15.5	Replicator Evolution by Artificial Selection		348
	15.5.1	The behavior of the System	350
	15.5.2	String Splitting	354
15.6	The Chemostat		358
	15.6.1	Perfectly Mixed Chemostat	360
	15.6.2	Chemostat with Spatial Structure	360
	15.6.3	Replicator Spatial Structures	362
	15.6.4	The Mechanism of Resistance against Parasites	366
15.7	Conclusions		371
References			372

Index 375

1

Review of Computational Intelligence for Gene-Gene and Gene-Environment Interactions in Disease Mapping

Arpad Kelemen[1]*, Yulan Liang[2] and Athanasios Vasilakos[3]

[1] Buffalo Neuroimaging Analysis Center, The Jacobs Neurological Institute, University at Buffalo, the State University of New York, 100 High Street Buffalo, NY 14203, USA
akelemen@buffalo.edu
[2] Department of Biostatistics University at Buffalo, the State University of New York Buffalo NY 14214, USA
[3] Dept. of Computer and Telecommunications Engineering University of Western Macedonia 50100 Kozani, Greece

Summary. Comprehensive evaluation of common genetic variations through association of SNP structure with common complex disease in the genome-wide scale is currently a hot area in human genome research. Computational science, which includes computational intelligence, has recently become the third method of scientific enquiry besides theory and experimentation. Interest grew fast in developing and applying computational intelligence techniques to disease mapping using SNP and haplotype data. This review provides a coverage of recently developed theories and applications in computational intelligence for gene-gene and gene-environment interactions in complex diseases in genetic association study.

Key words: Computational intelligence, SNP, Haplotype, Complex common diseases, Gene-gene interactions, Gene-environment interactions

1.1 Introduction

Correlating variations in DNA sequence with phenotypic differences has been one of the grand challenges in biomedical research. Substantial effort has been made to obtain all common genetic variations in humans, including single nucleotide polymorphisms (SNPs), deletions and insertions. A SNP occurs when a single nucleotide is altered, i.e. when (usually two) different sequence alternatives exist at a single base pair position. To distinguish a SNP from a mutation, the less frequent variant has to occur in at least 1% of the population [1]. The HapMap Project [2-4] has collected genotypes of millions of SNPs from populations with ancestry from Africa, Asia and Europe and makes this information freely available in the public domain. Haplotype is a set of single nucleotide polymorphisms (SNPs) on a single chromatid (one of two identical strands into which a chromosome splits during mitosis) that are statistically associated [5]. While millions of SNPs have been identified, with an estimated two common missense variants per gene, there is a great need, conceptually as well as computationally, to develop advanced robust models and analytical methods for characterizing genetic variations that are non-redundant and identify the target SNPs or haplotypes that are most likely to affect the phenotypes and ultimately contribute to disease development. The recent extensive interest in genome polymorphism signifies a development in human genetics research that will have a major impact on population genetics, drug development, forensics, cancer and genetic disease research [6-9].

Knowledge of the interplay between genetic and environmental factors is central to the understanding of multifactorial disease processes [10-15]. The biological interest is in how polymorphic genes interact with each other and with environmental factors to influence susceptibility and outcome in common, complex diseases. The risks of major common diseases, such as cancer, cardiovascular disease, mental illness, auto- immune states, and diabetes are expected to be heavily influenced by the patterns of SNPs one possesses in certain key susceptibility genes and are yet to be identified. The term 'complex disease' refers to the scenario in which these diseases are contributed to the susceptibility by many genes, many environmental factors that interact in a hierarchical fashion with nonlinear, polygenic, epistasis effects. By disregarding these interactions, effect sizes of relative risk for individual genetic variants are expected to be small. Disregarding gene-environment interaction also weakens exposure-disease and gene-disease associations.

During the last few years, there have been fast growing interests in developing and applying computational and statistical approaches in disease mapping in genetic association study using SNPs and haplotype data [16-63]. These computing approaches can be roughly categorized into several groups: (1) statistical testing or modeling based approaches [16, 29-48]; (2) data mining approaches [54-59, 61-62]; (3) machine learning and statistical learning approaches [50-53]; (4) Computational intelligence approaches [51-52, 63-68]. There are some overlaps between these categories such as semi-supervised learning can be either data mining or machine learning or computational intelligence approaches and neural network approaches can be either machine learning or computational intelligence approaches. Several surveys relating these approaches to disease mapping have been provided [77-81]. For instance, Onkamo, et al. provided a survey of data mining approaches of disease mapping in bioinformatics [77]; McKinney, et al. reviewed a number of different machine learning methods that have been applied to detecting gene-gene interactions [81]. Although the amount of publications of SNP-disease association study using computational intelligence approaches is fewer compared to statistical modeling based approaches and is relative new, some recent studies have demonstrated promises and future impacts of this fields, especially when applied to complex disease association analysis [51-52, 63-68]. This review focuses on recent developments in computational intelligence for diseases mapping in genetic association study, especially in modeling gene-gene and gene-environment interactions in common complex diseases.

1.2 Computational challenges in genomic association study of common complex diseases

An important challenge that faces molecular association study in the post genomic era is to understand the inter-connections from a network of genes and their products that are mediated by a variety of environmental changes. Non-reproducibility of many reported significant associations in subsequent studies has led to criticism of association studies.

For SNP and haplotype data in common complex diseases, in addition to being large, redundant, diverse and distributed, there are three important characteristics that pose challenges for data analysis and modeling: 1. heterogeneity, 2. a constantly evolving nature, and 3. complexity. They are heterogeneous, in the sense that they involve a wide array of data types, including categorical, continuous, sequence data, as well as temporal data, incomplete and missing data. They are large with a lot of redundancy in SNP and haplotype databases. They are is very dynamic and continuously evolving-both the data and the schema, which means that they require special knowledge when designing the modeling techniques. Finally, but most importantly, SNP and haplotype data are complex with intrinsic features and subtle patterns, in the sense that they are very rich in associated complex phenotype traits for common multifactor diseases.

In complex diseases, it is likely that a combination of genes predisposing for the disease and environmental factors aggravate the impact of these genes and are jointly responsible for disease development in populations (known as epistasis or epistatic effect). In addition, environmental factors, which seem to have only a moderate impact at the population level might have larger relative risks in subpopulations with certain genetic predispositions. There are major methodological challenges in the study of gene-gene and gene-environment interactions. There is a need for useful and expeditious methods for analyzing massive SNP data in common complex diseases beyond that of traditional statistical approaches.

1.3 The promise of computational intelligence

The theoretical framework considered in the context of this review is Computational Intelligence (CI) [69-70]. CI is a well-established paradigm that seamlessly combines three main technologies aimed at the development of intelligent systems, named granular computing, neural networks and biologically-inspired (evolutionary) optimization. In the design of such systems, we have to address various challenging issues, such as knowledge representation, adaptive properties, learning abilities and structural developments, CI has to a cope with each one of them. Regarding the properties of intelligent systems being supported by the paradigm of CI, we envision two general points of view. These properties can be sought as intrinsic to any intelligent system or they can be extrinsic to them. In the first case, we are concerned with the features that are crucial to the design of the systems, which usually do not manifest externally so by analyzing the performance of the systems we cannot say whether a specific technology has been utilized. Essentially, we are not concerned about that. The extrinsic properties are dominant and become of a paramount relevance when dealing with communication of intelligent systems with others or facilitating an effective interaction with human users. This aspect is extremely relevant in providing the user a sense of intelligent and user-friendly and user-centric capabilities of the systems. Here we can stress that these capabilities are much diversified and could cover a vast territory. For instance, one can envision several interesting scenarios:

- Coping with heterogeneous information. Quite often, in intelligent systems we may encounter information coming not only from sensors (in which case these are numeric readings) but also from users (in the form of linguistic evaluations) or being a result of some initial aggregation or summarization. Interestingly, these inputs are essential to the functioning of a system and cannot be ignored or downplayed. The heterogeneity of information requires special attention in the sense of the use of more advanced mechanisms of processing and representing such a mix of various pieces of evidence.
- Establishing an effective, transparent, and customized communication with the end user when presenting the results of processing completed by a system. Here the notion of generality (abstraction) or granulation of information plays a pivotal role. A suitable level of granulation of information is essential to the effective communication and acceptance of a system (in whichever role we can envision the system to be utilized). This immediately leads us to the concept of adaptive and user-driven interfaces which gradually becomes an essence to most interactive and human centric systems including tutoring architectures, decision-support systems, and knowledge-based architectures (including expert-like systems and their more advanced topologies).

Computational intelligence is generally accepted to include evolutionary computation, fuzzy systems, neural networks, and combinations thereof. One might also extend this definition to include reaction speeds and error rates approaching human performance as an answer to Turing's comment "we may hope that machines will eventually compete with men in all purely intellectual fields" [71].

The term of CI being coined in the 1990s (quite commonly viewed as a synonym of soft computing) helps us establish a sound mapping between the technologies and their dominant role in meeting some specific requests of the domain. What is also very characteristic for CI today is a broad array of hybrid systems (called neuro-fuzzy systems, neuro-evolutionary systems, genetic fuzzy systems). They emerge as a result of an in-depth understanding of the benefits of individual technologies and their genuine complementarity.

In what follows, we briefly highlight the essence of the contributing technologies of CI, discuss their synergies and elaborate on the resulting architectures:

<u>Granular Computing.</u> Granular information is everywhere. We granulate information all the time. We rarely reason on the basis of numbers. Our judgment is often triggered by some aggregates, which in a nutshell are a result of abstraction: a process which leads to human-like decision making. CI embraced fuzzy sets as the key vehicle of information granulation. It is worth stressing that the other fundamental

environments for describing granular information are readily available and a suitable choice depends on the specific problem at hand. Figure 1.1 visualizes the main developments in granular computing; it could help gain a better view as to their possible linkages.

Neurocomputing is inherently associated with adaptive and highly flexible systems - neural networks. The learning abilities of the networks (either through supervised or unsupervised learning) are in the heart of networks. The learning is exploited when building systems that can learn from data, adapt to the nonstationary environment (including preferences of users) and help generalize to new, unknown situations. The spectrum of learning models and network architectures is impressive. Neural networks are highly distributed that makes them fault tolerant and what has been said so far, it is definitely very encouraging. The drawback is with the lack of transparency of the networks. The distributed character of processing can be pointed at as the most prominent reason of this deficiency. Similarly, as no prior domain knowledge could be "downloaded" onto the network, its learning is carried out from scratch, which by itself is not the most encouraging.

Evolutionary Computing. The principle of evolutionary computing cast in the setting of CI becomes a synonym of structural optimization, reconfigurability, combinatorial optimization, and variant selection usually completed in large and complex search spaces. From its inception in the 1970s, evolutionary computing with all its variations of genetic algorithms, evolutionary strategies, genetic programming, etc is aimed at the global, structural system optimization that is carried out in presence of very limited and general information about the optimality criterion.

From the above summary, it becomes apparent that the main agendas of these technologies are different yet highly complementary leading to the scenarios in which the advantages and limitations of each one of them could be strengthened and compensated, respectively. This compensation effect is in essence a crux of the resulting synergy and helps develop interesting and useful linkages. Figure 1.2 highlights the leading tendencies and identifies the ways in which the synergies have been invoked.

As stressed, there are a significant number of possible interactions between the contributing technologies in the realm of CI. Bearing in mind the main objectives of granular computing and neural networks, we can envision a general layered type of the model in which any interaction with the external world (including users) is done through the granular interface (external layers) whereas the core computing part is implemented as a neural network or a neurofuzzy structure (in which case we may be emphasizing the logic facet of ongoing processing faculties).

Success in computational intelligence has been forthcoming. These methods have been widely used in networking, ambient intelligence [72], and engineering for optimization of plant control, scheduling, for the design of small robots for locomotion and for the evolution of an expert-level checkers player all without human expertise. As suggested at the dawn of this era "the old phrase 'the computer never knows more than the programmer' is simply no longer true". These same methods are now being applied to problems in molecular biology and bioinformatics [73].

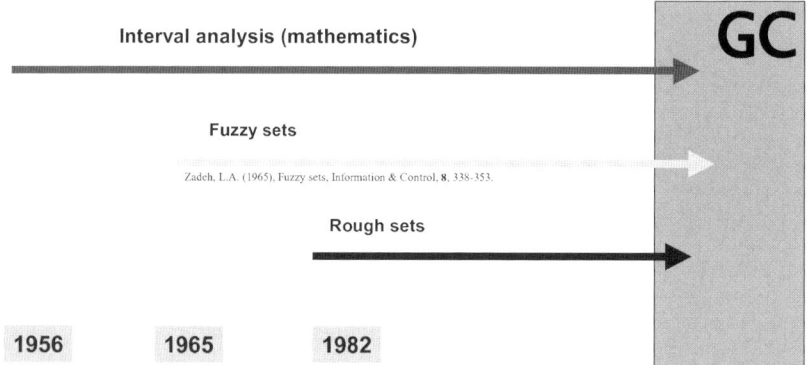

Fig. 1.1. Main developments of granular computing

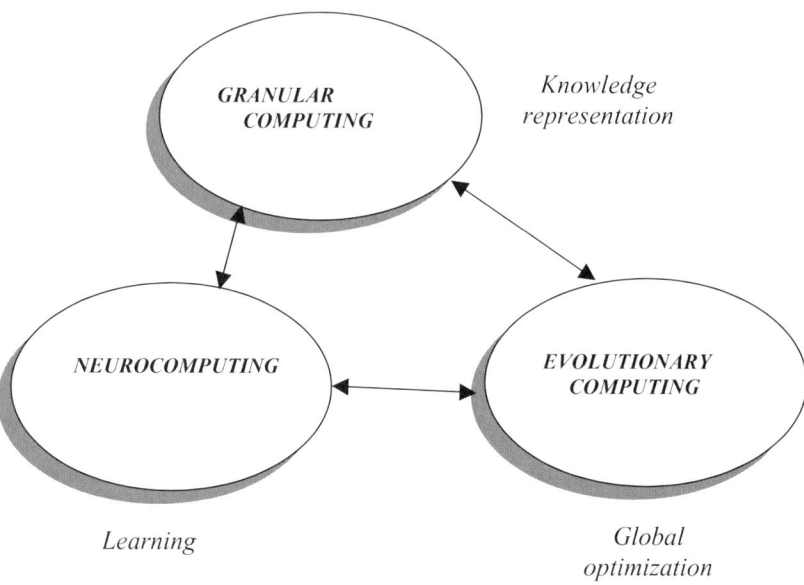

Fig. 1.2. Main synergistic links in Computational Intelligence

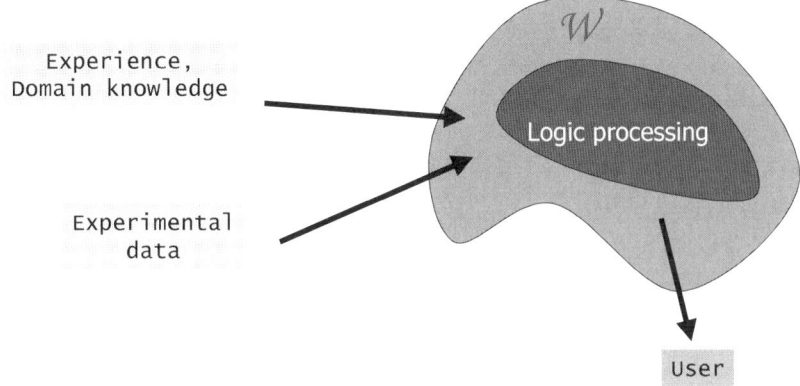

Fig. 1.3. A layered style of CI constructs

No technological advancement has been more directly responsible for the success of molecular biology over the last 50 years than the computer. Computers have become so important in biology that it is difficult to think of any significant advancement in the last 10 years that did not have direct assistance from a computer, whether this is as a viewer for three-dimensional structures, a controller for automated robot maneuvering of 96-well plates for PCR, a means to interpret DNA sequencing gels, microarray data, etc. The revolution of the last 50 years has resulted in such a wealth of data that our understanding of the underlying processes would be significantly reduced if computers were not at hand as our assistants with respect to "bioinformatics". The scale of the biological problems of interest and our understanding of those problems has closely paralleled Moore's Law. Realistically, it was not until the 1970s and 1980s when computers became truly relevant for biological information processing at a rate commensurate with the data being generated. The 1980s and 1990s heralded the Internet, which has become an invaluable resource for sharing biological information. However, in parallel with molecular biology, methods of computational intelligence also share their origins in the 1950s, with refinement over time into a wide array of algorithms useful for data mining, pattern recognition, optimization, and simulation. Today, many of these same algorithms can be said to offer "computational intelligence" something that can handle the large size of experimental output from modern biology.

1.4 Computational intelligence approaches for SNP-disease associations

Recently developed computational intelligence approaches for SNP-disease associations include genetic algorithms [51, 80], neural networks [50, 67, 68], genetic programming [65], evolutionary trees [52], evolutionary algorithms [75] and various hybrid approaches, such as neural networks with genetic programming [63], genetic programming with multifactor dimensionality reduction [74], and so on.

Clark et al. [51] developed a Genetic Algorithm (GA) to construct logic trees consisting of Boolean expressions involving blocks or strings of SNPs and applied to a candidate gene study of quantitative genetic variation. The blocks or strings of the logic trees consist of SNPs in high Linkage Disequilibrium (LD). LD refers to the SNPs that are highly correlated with each other due to evolutionary processes. Studies showed that if high level LD occurred in the population and they are selected by the classification models, only one or two SNPs, respectively, would be enough to obtain a good predictive capacity with no or only a modest reduction in power relative to direct assays of all common SNPs. In contrast, in population, where lower levels of LD are observed at given loci, a larger number of SNPs are required to predict phenotype. Therefore, capturing such block structure of the SNPs offers the possibility to significantly reduce the number of SNPs required to completely genotype a sample with no information loss. In Clark's methods, at each generation of the GA, a population of logic tree models is modified using selection, cross-over and mutation moves. Logic trees are selected for the next generation using a fitness function based on the marginal likelihood in a Bayesian regression framework. Mutation and crossover moves use LD measures to propose changes to the trees, and facilitate the movement through the model space.

Pen et al. studied genetic algorithms that are randomized, evolutionary, population-based search algorithms for capturing the relationships among the SNPs and diseases. They developed estimation procedures of Bayesian Network Algorithm (EBNA) that combines evolutionary computation and probabilistic graphical models as a search engine to discover high-order genetic interactions and genetic interaction networks associated with the disease. The proposed methods for genome-wide association studies were applied to two real data sets and results show that the proposed methods may open a new avenue for network based approaches to genome-wide association studies.

Genetic Programming (GP) is closely related to genetic algorithms. It makes use of genetic algorithms in that it is a stochastic, population based, evolutionary approach for search and optimization. GP uses tree based strategies to represent a solution of a problem instead of a string of variables. Recent studies has shown that GP outperforms many traditional data mining and machine learning methods, such as linear regression and support vector machines. Ritchie et al. introduced a genetic programming optimized neural network (GPNN) as a method for optimizing the architecture of a neural network to improve the identification of gene combinations associated with disease risk [63]. The strength of this approach is the ability to discover the optimal NN architecture as part of the modeling process. Motsinger et al. applied a GPNN approach for detecting epistasis in case-control studies for SNPs data. They evaluated the power of GPNN for identifying high-order gene-gene interactions and applied GPNN to a real data analysis on Parkinson's disease [67].

Motsinger et al. developed a Grammatical Evolution Neural Network (GENN), a machine-learning approach to detect gene-gene or gene-environment interactions in high dimensional genetic epidemiological data [68].

GENN has been shown to be highly successful on a range of simulated data. Regarding the power of GENN to detect interesting interactions in the presence of noise due to genotyping error, missing data, phenocopy, and genetic heterogeneity and it was found that the GENN method is relatively robust to all error types, including genetic heterogeneity.

Motsinger et al. further proposed an Ensemble Learning Approach for Set-association (ELAS) to detect a set of interacting loci that predicts the complex trait. In ELAS, they first search "base-learners" and then combine the effects of the base learners. ELAS can jointly analyze single-marker effects and two order interaction effects for many markers including genome-wide association studies. Simulation studies demonstrated that ELAS is more powerful than single-marker test. ELAS also outperformed the other three existing multi-locus methods in almost all cases. They also applied an application to a large-scale case-control study for Type 2 diabetes. ELAS identified eleven SNPs that have a significant multi-locus effect, while none of the SNPs showed significant marginal effect and none of the two-locus combinations showed significant two-locus interaction effect.

Hubley et al. [75] presented an evolutionary algorithm for multi-objective SNP selection, which approximates the set of optimal trade-off solutions for large problems with semi-supervised learning. This set is very useful for the design of large studies, including those oriented towards disease identification, genetic mapping, population studies, and haplotype-block elucidation. They implemented a modified version of the Strength-Pareto Evolutionary Algorithm in Java and concluded that evolutionary algorithms are particularly suited for optimization problems that involve multiple objectives and a complex search space on which exact methods, such as exhaustive enumeration cannot be applied. This method provides flexibility with respect to the problem formulation if a problem description evolves or changes. Results are produced as a trade-off front, allowing the user to make informed decisions when prioritizing factors. Evolutionary algorithms are well suited for many other applications in genomics.

Haplotype fine mapping by evolutionary trees describe a method that seeks to refine location by analysis of "disease" and "normal" haplotypes, thereby using multivariate information about linkage disequilibrium. Under the assumption that the disease mutation occurs in a specific gap between adjacent markers, the method first combines parsimony and likelihood to build an evolutionary tree of disease haplotypes, with each node (haplotype) separated, by a single mutational or recombinational step, from its parent. If required, latent nodes (unobserved haplotypes) are incorporated to complete the tree. Once the tree is built, its likelihood is computed from probabilities of mutation and recombination. When each gap between adjacent markers is evaluated in this fashion and these results are combined with prior information, they yield a posterior probability distribution to guide the search for the disease mutation. They showed, by evolutionary simulations, that an implementation of these methods, called "FineMap", yields substantial refinement and excellent coverage for the true location of the disease mutation.

The detection of epistasis is an important priority in the genetic analysis of complex human diseases. Epistasis is defined as the masking of the expression of a gene at one position in a chromosome, by one or more genes at other positions. The most challenging epistatic effects to model are those that do not exhibit statistically significant marginal effects. Identifying these types of nonlinear interactions in the context of genome-wide association studies is considered a needle in a haystack problem [74]. Given this complexity, it is unrealistic to expect that stochastic search algorithms will do any better than a simple random search. Hybrid computational intelligence approaches have been investigated for finding epistatic needles with the assistance of expert knowledge [63, 74]. Banzhaf et al. also employed a variety of evolutionary computing methods, such as genetic algorithms for modeling epistasis. Ritchie et al. proposed a neural network with stochastic genetic programming for studying SNP and SNP interaction and used expert knowledge to guide the genome-wide analysis of epistasis [63]. They first developed and evaluated a genetic programming approach with one-objective fitness function of classification accuracy and showed that GP is no better than a simple random search when classification accuracy is used as the fitness function. Then they further included pre-processed estimates of attribute quality (i.e. expert knowledge) using Tuned ReliefF (TuRF) in a multi-objective fitness function which significantly improved the performance of GP over that of random search. Results showed that using expert knowledge to select trees performs as well as a multi-objective fitness function and can not only improve the accuracy of prediction, but also can achieve the same power at one tenth of the population size.

Moore et al. [74] developed a hybrid genetic programming with multifactor dimensionality reduction (MDR) method to pick SNPs for epistasis. They also found no evidence to suggest that GP-MDR performed better than random search on the simulated genome-wide data sets. They further modified GP-MDR to select SNP combinations for virtual recombination, mutation, and reproduction by using ReliefF filter algorithm. ReliefF filter provided statistical measures and prior information about the quality of each SNP as assessed during a pre-processing analysis on which the GP-MDR is based on. They found that the expert knowledge provided by ReliefF about which SNPs might be interacting can significantly improve the ability of GP-MDR to identify epistatic SNPs in the absence of marginal effects over that of a simple random search. An important advantage of this hybrid approach is that any form of expert knowledge could be used to guide the stochastic search algorithm. For example, information about biochemical pathways, protein-protein interactions, Gene Ontology, or even evidence from the literature could be used in addition to statistical measures.

Moore et al. introduced cellular automata (CA) as a novel computational approach for identifying combinations of single-nucleotide polymorphisms (SNPs) associated with clinical endpoints [76]. This alternative approach is nonparametric (i.e. no hypothesis about the value of a statistical parameter is made), is model-free (i.e. assumes no particular inheritance model), and is directly applicable to case-control and discordant sib-pair study designs. They also demonstrated using simulated data that the approach has good power for identifying high-order nonlinear interactions (i.e. epistasis) among four SNPs in the absence of independent main effects.

1.5 Conclusions

Designing, developing and implementing computational intelligence methods for identifying genetic triggers and components responsible for common complex diseases, such as diabetes, cancer, cardiovascular disease, etc. is one of the new and challenging areas of human genetics. Computational intelligence, a side branch of artificial intelligence where well-crafted algorithms are being developed that solve complex, computationally expensive problems that are believed to require intelligence is perhaps the most promoising tool today to approach this problem. CI and its hybrids explore areas, such as learning, fuzzy systems, global optimization, adaptive systems, agents, human-like decision making, and more. This introductory chapter covered some theories and applications of computational intelligence for SNP-disease association study, especially for identifying gene-gene and gene-environment interactions. We demonstrated the promise and the importance of computational intelligence for common complex diseases using SNP-haplotype data and tackled some of the important challenges, including gene-gene and gene-environment interactions, and the notorious "curse of dimensionality" problem. Success in identifying SNPs and haplotypes conferring susceptibility or resistance to common complex diseases will provide a deeper understanding of the architecture of the disease, the risks and offer a more powerful diagnostic tool and predictive treatment.

References

[1] Brookes AJ (1999) Review: The essence of SNPs. Gene (234) 177-186.
[2] The International HapMap Consortium (2003) The International HapMap Project. Nature 426:789-796.
[3] The International HapMap Consortium (2004) Integrating ethics and science in the International HapMap Project. Nat Rev Genet 5:467-475.
[4] The International HapMap Consortium (2005) A haplotype map of the human genome. Nature, 437:1299-1320.
[5] Daly MJ, Rioux JD, Schaffner SF, Hudson TJ, and Lander ES (2001) High-resolution haplotype structure in the human genome. Nat. Genet., 29, 229-232.
[6] Cardon LR, Bell JI (2001) Association study designs for complex diseases. Nat Rev Genet 2:91-99.
[7] Risch NJ (2000) Searching for genetic determinants in the new millennium. Nature 405:847-856.
[8] Risch N, Merikangas K (1996) The future of genetics studies of complex human diseases. Science 273:1516-1517.
[9] Stephens M and Donnelly P (2000) Inference in molecular population genetics. J R Stat Soc B 62:605-655.
[10] Ioannidis JP, Gwinn M, Little J, Higgins JP, Bernstein JL, Boffetta P, Bondy M, Bray MS, Brenchley PE, Buffler PA, Casas JP, Chokkalingam A, Danesh J, Smith GD, Dolan S, Duncan R, Gruis NA, Hartge P, Hashibe M, Hunter DJ, Jarvelin MR, Malmer B, Maraganore DM, Newton-Bishop JA, O'Brien

TR, Petersen G, Riboli E, Salanti G, Seminara D, Smeeth L, Taioli E, Timpson N, Uitterlinden AG, Vineis P, Wareham N, Winn DM, Zimmern R, and Khoury MJ (2006) Human Genome Epidemiology Network and the Network of Investigator Networks, A road map for efficient and reliable human genome epidemiology, Nature Genetics, 38(1):3-5.
[11] Chatterjee N, Kalaylioglu Z, Moslehi R, Peters U, and Wacholder S (2006) Powerful multilocus tests of genetic association in the presence of gene-gene and gene-environment interactions. American Journal of Human Genetics, 79(6):1002-1016.
[12] Cordell HJ, Barratt BJ, and Clayton DG (2004) Case/pseudocontrol analysis in genetic association studies: a unified framework for detection of genotype and haplotype associations, gene-gene and gene-environment interactions, and parent-of-origin effects. Genetic Epidemiology, 26(3):167-185.
[13] Hunter DJ (2005) Gene-environment interactions in human diseases. Nature Reviews Genetics, 6:287-298.
[14] Zondervan KT and Cardon LR (2004) The complex interplay among factors that influence allelic association. Nature Reviews Genetics, 5(2):89-100.
[15] Azevedo L, Suriano G, van Asch B, Harding RM, and Amorim A (2006) Epistatic interactions: how strong in disease and evolution? Trends Genet.
[16] Chapman, JM, Cooper JD, Todd JA, and Clayton DG (2003) Detecting disease associations due to linkage disequilibrium using haplotype tags: a class of tests and the determinants of statistical power. Hum. Hered. 56, 18-31.
[17] Liu Z and Lin S (2005) Multilocus LD measure and tagging SNP selection with generalized mutual information. Genet Epidemiol. 29, 353-364.
[18] Halldrsson BV, Bafna V, Lippert R, Schwartz R, De La Vega FM, Clark AG, and Istraili S (2004) Optimal Haplotype Block-Free Selection of Tagging SNPs for Genome-Wide Association Studies Genome Res. 14, 1633-1640.
[19] Howie BN, Carlson CS, Rieder MJ, and Nickerson DA (2006) Efficient selection of tagging single-nucleotide polymorphisms in multiple populations. Human Genetics, 120(1):58-68.
[20] Gopalakrishnan S and Qin ZS (2006) TagSNP Selection Based on Pairwise LD Criterion and Power Analysis in Association Studies. Pacific Sym. Biocomputing, 11:511-522.
[21] Ke X. and Cardon LR (2003) Efficient selective screening of haplotypes tag SNPs. Bioinformatics, 19, 287-288.
[22] Halperin E, Kimmel G, and Shamir R (2005) Tag SNP Selection in Genotype Data for Maximizing SNP Prediction Accuracy. Bioinformatics, 21(suppl 1): i195-i203, 2005.
[23] Akey J, Jin L, and Xiong M (2001) Haplotypes vs single marker linkage disequilibrium tests: what do we gain? Eur J Hum Genet 9 (4), 291-300.
[24] Zhu X, Zhang S, Kan D, and Cooper R (2004) Haplotype block definition and its application. Pacic Symposium on Biocomputing 9:152-163.
[25] Gabriel SB, Schaffner SF, Nguyen H, Moore JM, Roy J, Blumenstiel B, Higgins J, DeFelice M, Lochner A, Faggart M, Liu-Cordero SN, Rotimi C, Adeyemo A, Cooper R, Ward R, Lander ES, Daly MJ, and Altshuler D (2002)

The structure of haplotype blocks in the human genome. Science 296 (5576), 2225-2229.
[26] Daly MJ, Rioux JD, Schaffner SF, Hudson TJ, Lander ES, Phillips MS, et al. (2003) Chromosome-wide distribution of haplotype blocks and the role of recombination hot spots. Nature Genet. 33, 382-387.
[27] Zhang K, Calabrese P, Nordborg M, and Sun F (2002) Haplotype block structure and its applications to association studies: power and study designs. Am. J. Hum. Genet., 71, 1386-1394.
[28] Meng Z, Zaykin DV, Xu CF, Wagner M, and Ehm MG (2004) Selection of genetic markers for association analyses, using linkage disequilibrium and haplotypes. Am. J. Hum. Genet., 73:115-130.
[29] Anderson EC, and Novembre J (2003) Finding haplotype block boundaries by using the minimum-description-length principle. American Journal of Human Genetics, 73:336-354.
[30] Mannila H, Koivisto M, Perola M, Varilo T, Hennah W, Ekelund J, Lukk M, Peltonen L, and Ukkonen E (2003) Minimum description length block finder, a method to identify haplotype blocks and to compare the strength of block boundaries. Am. J. Hum. Genet., 73, 86-94.
[31] Zhang K, Deng M, Chen T, Waterman MS, and Sun F (2002) A dynamic programming algorithm for haplotype block partitioning. Proc. Natl Acad. Sci. USA, 99, 7335-7339.
[32] Beckmann L, Thomas DC, Fischer C, and Chang-Claude J (2005) Haplotype sharing analysis using Mantel statistics, Human Heredity, 59:67-78.
[33] Levin AM, Ghosh D, et al. (2005) A model-based scan statistics for identifying extreme chromosomal regions of gene expression in human tumors. Bioinformatics 21:2867-2874.
[34] Schaid DJ, Rowland CM, Tines DE, Jacobson RM, and Poland GA (2002) Score test for association between traits and haplotypes when linkage phase is ambiguous. Am J Hum Genet 70:425-443.
[35] Nothnagel M, Furst R, and Rohde K (2002) Entropy as a measure for linkage disequilibrium over multilocus haplotype blocks. Hum Hered, 54:186-198.
[36] Hampe J, Schreiber S, and Krawczak M (2003) Entropy-based SNP selection for genetic association studies. Hum Genet. 114:36-43.
[37] Zhao J, Boerwinkle E, and Xiong M (2005) An entropy-based statistic for genomewide association studies. American Journal of Human Genetics, 77:27-40.
[38] Zaykin DV, Zhivotovsky LA, et al. (2002) Truncated product method for combining P-values. Genet Epidemio 122:170-185.
[39] Ott J (2004) Issues in association analysis: error control in case-control association studies for disease gene discovery. Human Heredity, 58:171-174.
[40] He J and Zelikovsky A (2006) MLR-tagging informative SNP selection for unphased genotypes based on multiple linear regression, Bioinformatics, 22(20):2558-2561.

[41] Durrant C, Zondervan KT, Lon R, Cardon L, Hunt S, Deloukas P, and Morris AP (2004) Linkage Disequilibrium Mapping via Cladistic Analysis of Single-Nucleotide Polymorphism Haplotypes. Am. J. Hum. Genet. 75, 35-43.
[42] Baker SG (2005) A simple loglinear model for haplotype effects in a case-control study involving two unphased genotypes, Statistical Applications in Genetics and Molecular Biology, 4(1):14.
[43] Tzeng J, Wang C, Kao J, and Hsiao CK (2006) Regression-based association analysis with clustered haplotypes through use of genotypes. American Journal of Human Genetics, 78(2):231-242.
[44] Burkett K, McNeney B, and Graham J (2004) A note on inference of trait associations with SNP haplotypes and other attributes in generalized linear models. Human Heredity, 57:200-206.
[45] Greenspan G and Geiger D (2004) Model-based inference of haplotype block variation. J. Comp. Biol. 11, 493-504.
[46] Greenspan G and Geiger D (2006) Modeling Haplotype Block Variation Using Markov Chains, Genetics, 172(4): 2583-2599.
[47] Thomas DC, Stram DO, Conti D, Molitor J, and Marjoram P (2003) Bayesian spatial modeling of haplotype associations, Human Heredity, 56:32-40.
[48] Schwender H and Ickstadt K (2006) Identification of SNP Interactions Using Logic Regression. http://www.sfb475.uni-dortmund.de/berichte/tr31-06.pdf (preprint)
[49] Verzilli CJ, Stallard N, and Whittaker JC (2006) Bayesian graphical models for genomewide association studies. American Journal of Human Genetics, 79(1):100-112.
[50] Ott J (2001) Neural networks and disease association studies. American Journal of Medical Genetics, Volume 105, Issue 1, 60-61.
[51] Clark TG, De Iorio M, Griffiths RC, and Farrall M (2005) Finding associations in dense genetic maps: a genetic algorithm approach. Human Heredity, 60:97-108.
[52] Lam JC, Roeder K, and Devlin B (2000) Haplotype fine mapping by evolutionary trees. Am. J. Hum. Genet. 66 (2), 659-673.
[53] Chang C, Huang Y, and Chao K (2006) A greedier approach for finding tag SNPs, Bioinformatics, 22(6):685-691.
[54] Li J and Jiang T (2005) Haplotype-based linkage disequilibrium mapping via direct data mining, Bioinformatics, 21:4384-4393.
[55] Lin Z and Altman RB (2004) Finding haplotype tagging SNPs by use of principal components analysis. Am. J. Hum. Genet. 75: 850-861.
[56] Horne BD and Camp NJ (2004) Principal component analysis for selection of optimal SNP-sets that capture intragenic genetic variation. Genetic Epidemiology, 26(1):11-21.
[57] Ao S, Yip K, Ng M, Cheung D, Fong PY, Melhado I, and Sham PC (2005) CLUSTAG: hierarchical clustering and graph methods for selecting tag SNPs. Bioinformatics, 21(8):1735-1736.
[58] Kooperberg C, Ruczinski I, LeBlanc M, and Hsu L (2001) Sequence Analysis Using Logic Regression. Genetic Epidemiology, 21:626-631.

[59] Moore JH (2004) Genome-wide analysis of epistasis using multifactor dimensionality reduction: feature selection and construction in the domain of human genetics. In: Zhu, D. (eds.) Knowledge Discovery and Data Mining: Challenges and Realities with Real World Data, IGI.
[60] Liu JS, Sabatti C, Teng J, Keats BJ, and Risch N (2001) Bayesian analysis of haplotypes for linkage disequilibrium mapping. Genome Research 11 (10), 1716-1724.
[79] Molitor J, Marjoram P, and Thomas D (2003) Fine-Scale Mapping of Disease Genes with Multiple Mutations via Spatial Clustering Techniques. Am. J. Hum. Genet. 73, 1368-1384.
[62] Toivonen HT, Onkamo P, Vasko K, Ollikainen V, Sevon P, Mannila H, Herr M, and Kere J (2000) Data mining applied to linkage disequilibrium mapping. Am. J. Hum. Genet. 67 (1), 133-145.
[63] Ritchie MD, White BC, Parker JS, Hahn LW, and Moore JH (2003) PMID Optimization of neural network architecture using genetic programming improves detection and modeling of gene-gene interactions in studies of human diseases. BMC Bioinformatics 4:28.
[64] Banzhaf W, Beslon G, Christensen S, Foster JA, Kepes F, Lefort V, Miller JF, Radman M, and Ramsden JJ (2006) Guidelines: From artificial evolution to computational evolution: a research agenda. Nat Rev Genet. Sep;7(9):729-35.
[65] Moore JH and White BC (2006a) Exploiting expert knowledge for genome-wide genetic analysis using genetic programming. In: Runarsson et al. (eds.) Parallel Problem Solving from Nature - PPSN IX, Lecture Notes in Computer Science 4193, 969-977.
[66] Foster JA. (2001) Evolutionary computation. Nat Rev Genet. 2(6):428-36.
[67] Motsinger AA, Lee SL, Mellick G, and Ritchie MD (2006) GPNN: Power studies and applications of a neural network method for detecting gene-gene interactions in studies of human disease. BMC Bioinformatics. 25;7(1):39.
[68] Motsinger AA, Fanelli TJ, and Ritchie MD (2006) Power of Grammatical Evolution Neural Networks to Detect Gene-Gene Interactions in the Presence of Error Common to Genetic Epidemiological Studies. International Genetic Epidemiology Society 15th Annual Meeting.
[69] Pedrycz W (1997) Computational Intelligence: An Introduction. Boca Raton, FL, CRC
[70] (2000) Pedrycz W and Vasilakos A (2000) Computational Intelligence in Telecommunications Networks. Boca Raton, FL, CRC.
[71] Turing AM (1956) Can a machine think? In: Newman, J.R. (Ed.), The World of Mathematics, vol. 4. Simon and Schuster, New York, 2122.
[72] Vasilakos A and Pedrycz W (2006) Ambient Intelligence, Wireless Networking, Ubiquitous Computing. ArtecHouse, MA, USA.
[73] Fogel GB and Corne DW (2002) Evolutionary Computation in Bioinformatics. Morgan Kaufmann, San Francisco.
[74] Moore JH and White BC (2006b) Detecting Epistatic Needles in Genome-Wide Haystacks. American human genetics conferences.

[75] Hubley RM, Zitzler E, Roach JC (2003) Evolutionary algorithms for the selection of single nucleotide polymorphisms. BMC Bioinformatics 4:30.
[76] Moore JH and Hahn LW (2002) A cellular automata approach to detecting interactions among single-nucleotide polymorphisms in complex multifactorial diseases. Pac Symp Biocomput. 53-64.
[77] Onkamo P and Toivonen H (2006) A survey of data mining methods for linkage disequilibrium mapping. Human Genomics, Vol 2(1), 336-340(5).
[78] Salem, RM, Wessel J, and Schork, NJ (2005) A comprehensive literature review of haplotyping software and methods for use with unrelated individuals. Human Genomics, Vol 2(1) pp. 39-66(28).
[79] Molitor J, Marjoram P, Conti D, and Thomas D (2004) A survey of current Bayesian gene mapping methods. Human Genomics, Vol 1(5) pp. 371-374(4).
[80] Shah SC and Kusiak A (2004) Data mining and genetic algorithm based gene/SNP selection. Artif Intell Med. (3):183-96.
[81] McKinney BA, Reif DM, Ritchie MD, and Moore JH (2006) Machine Learning for Detecting Gene-Gene Interactions: A Review. Applied Bioinformatics. 5(2):77-88.

2

Intelligent Approaches to Mining the Primary Research Literature: Techniques, Systems, and Examples

Gully A.P.C. Burns, Donghui Feng, and Eduard Hovy

Information Sciences Institute / USC, 4676 Admiralty Way Suite 1001 Marina del Rey, CA 90292 {burns,donghui,hovy}@isi.edu

Summary In this chapter, we describe how creating knowledge bases from the primary biomedical literature is formally equivalent to the process of performing a literature review or a 'research synthesis'. We describe a principled approach to partitioning the research literature according to the different types of experiments performed by researchers and how knowledge engineering approaches must be carefully employed to model knowledge from different types of experiment. The main body of the chapter is concerned with the use of text mining approaches to populate knowledge representations for different types of experiment. We provide a detailed example from neuroscience (based on anatomical tract-tracing experiments) and provide a detailed description of the methodology used to perform the text mining itself (based on the Conditional Random Fields model). Finally, we present data from text-mining experiments that illustrate the use of these methods in a real example. This chapter is designed to act as an introduction to the field of biomedical text-mining for computer scientists who are unfamiliar with the way that biomedical research uses the literature.

2.1 Introduction

The overwhelming amount of information available to the biomedical researcher makes the use of intelligent computational tools a necessity. These tools would help the researcher locate information appropriate to his or her goal, identify/extract the precise fragments of information required for each specific task, correlate and sort the extracted information as needed, and summarize or otherwise synthesize it in ways suitable for the task at hand. Such tools are not easy to build, by and large, and require expertise in a variety of computer science specialties, including database management, data analysis, natural language processing, and text mining.

Naturally, the organization and nature of the information to be so manipulated has a great influence on the nature and level of performance of the tools used. For example, the bioinformatics systems most widely used by biomedical researchers, those hosted by the National Center for Biotechnology Information (NCBI) [1], include two types of database: (a) molecular and genetic databases and (b) bibliographic databases (notably PubMed and PubMed Central). The structure of information contained in the bioinformatics databases is precisely defined, tabulated, standardized, homogeneous, and concerned mainly with molecular/genetic data and their derivations. In contrast, the information contained in bibliographic databases, defined as it is in natural language, is non-standardized, massively heterogeneous, and concerned with all aspects of biomedical knowledge (physiology and anatomy at all levels of behavior, the body, its constituent organ systems and subdivisions).

The differences between these two types of system provide the central theme of this chapter: while it is relatively straightforward with current computational techniques to master the former, well-organized material, the latter requires sophisticated natural language processing (NLP) techniques. Additionally, the process of using the literature confirms to rigorous scholarly standards that necessitate careful citation of known data, the accurate representation of complex concepts and (in the case of formal meta-analysis) rigorous statistical analysis [2]. The development of Knowledge Bases (KBs) by manual curation of the literature is being used in a great many fields, including neuroanatomy [3–5], and yeast protein interaction networks [6]. The use of NLP techniques has generated large-scale systems such as Textspresso (for fly genetics [7]) and Geneways (for signal transduction [8]), amongst others.

In many sub-disciplines of the life-sciences (such as non-molecular neuroscience, physiology and endocrinology), there are no large scale databases that tabulate experimental findings for researchers to browse and view. In these subjects, the vast amount of scientific information *is only available to the community in the form of natural language*. The impact of this can be seen in the world of difference that exists between neuroinformatics and bioinformatics databases. The CoCoMac system ('Collations of Connectivity data on the Macaque brain', [4, 9]) is a successful neuroinformatics database project concerned with inter-area connections in the cerebral cortex of the Macaque. It is a mature solution for a problem that was under consideration by national committees concerned as far back as 1989 (L.W. Swanson, personal communication). CoCoMac currently contains roughly 4×10^4 connection reports from 395 papers and is the product of years of painstaking data curation by its development team. By way of contrast, the National Library of Medicine announced in Aug 2005 that the total quantity of publicly available genetic data was 10^{10} individual base pairs from over 165,000 organisms.

Why is there such a massive disparity (six orders of magnitude) between the two types of system? Two key components are present in molecular bioinformatics systems and absent in the other domains: high-throughput Knowledge Acquisition (KA) methods, and appropriately expressive target Knowledge Representation (KR) systems to hold the experimental findings in a coherent structure. High-throughput data acquisition methods have been developed for molecular work and their outputs are relatively quantitative and simple (in comparison to the heterogeneous complexity of neuroscience data). Databases such as NCBI [1], UniProt [10] and the Kyoto Encyclopedia of Genes and Genomes (KEGG [11]) are the products of the use of this technology for over a decade or more. If high throughput knowledge acquisition methods could be used on the published literature to populate a representation that captures the essential details and linkage of experiments, the size of databases such as CoCoMac could increase significantly.

In this chapter, our objective is to describe high-throughput methods to construct KBs based on the application of NLP to the primary experimental literature. A major point of discussion for this work is the ontology engineering methodolgy used to design the target KR that we are attempting to populate. Scientifically speaking, the process of generating a KB in this way is equivalent to the task of compiling a literature review, or more formally: 'research synthesis' [12]. Given the large quantities of effort expended by biomedical scientists studying the literature, we suggest that study tools could have a large impact on the field [13, 14].

Ontology engineering and development is attracting much interest within the Biomedical Informatics community. A National Center for Biomedical Ontology (NCBO) has been established at Stanford University [15], with support from several similar research teams. Ontologies may be defined as 'specifications of conceptualizations' [16], and work in this field is mature, supported by thirty years of research into Artifial Intelligence (AI), widely used data standards (OWL and RDF, Common Logic, *etc.*), codes of best practice (*e.g.,* the Open Biomedical Ontology foundry: http://obofoundry.org/), and an increasing number of reliable open-source software systems [17–19].

This chapter is therefore designed to serve a dual purpose: to provide a philosophical context of text mining work and to describe the process in concrete, experimental terms. We begin by introducing the idea of 'conceptual biology' in section 2, and how this relates to text mining in general. In section 3, we then describe the rationale for partitioning the primary experimental literature based on 'experimental type' and how this provides structure for text-mining work. We discuss existing biomedical knowledge bases that have been derived from the literature in section 4, and then describe how the process of preparing a review article can define the underlying context of the knowledge-intensive task that we are addressing in section 5. In the latter half of the chapter, we show an example from neuroscience by elaborating the theory (section 6), methodology (section 7) and results (section 8) of text-mining experimental work for a specific example taken from neuroscience that we introduced in earlier sections. Finally we synthesize this work as a vision for the development of the next generation of biomedical informatics systems.

2.2 A framework for conceptual biology

The term 'conceptual biology' denotes a computational approach that is based on synthesizing new knowledge from data found in existing, already-published work [20, 21]. Although, this approach lies at the heart of all literature-driven bioinformatics systems, the term is itself rarely used explicitly. The originators of the idea of conceptual biology developed the ARROWSMITH tool [22].

Biology is intrinsically concept-driven and is massively heterogeneous with respect to the representations used for different concepts. This heterogeneity is simply an emergent property of the way that biological experiments are performed and synthesized into facts. The Gene Ontology illustrates this by describing over 21,000 separate terms describing biological processes, cellular components and molecular functions [23].

Let us begin by asking the following question: *How do experiments contribute to new knowledge that may be used by other researchers?*

In Chapter 3 of [24], a non-biologist describes this process from 1962 to 1969 for a Nobel-Prize-winning discovery: the chemical structure of the hormone Thyrotropin Releasing Factor (TRF). This process was multi-stage, iterative and evolutionary. Firstly, it was recognized that the discovery of a new fact (the structure of TRF) would provide an important breakthrough, and then a research community went about solving the problem through a range of experimental techniques. The members of this community were competing fiercely with each other, so that the discoveries of one group were immediately used by the others. Finally, in 1969, the discovery was made that the chemical formula of TRF is 'Pyro-Glu-His-Pro-NH2'. It is important to note that up until that point, publications from the members of the community were concerned with arriving at the definition of the chemical formula. When the formula was derived, all of the previous work was summarized by this single piece of information, which was then available for use by other scientists without any reference to the research that had lead to its discovery.

The research process therefore generates a plethora of different complex representations, arguments and data to supports the discovery of 'scientific facts'. Such facts are rarely as cut and dried as a chemical formula (as was the case with TRF). They must usually be qualified in terms of supporting evidence and may evolve as more research is conducted.

Knowledge engineering approaches to ontology development seek to formalize this information within a compuatable framework to make it more tractable by the scientific community. The fields of biomedical informatics and computational biology depend on this process of formalization and a number of structured representations are being constructed for this purpose. The OBO foundry lists a number of these ontologies defined at various levels. In typical 'top-level' ontologies, concepts are completely generic (*e.g.,* 'Thing', 'Organism', 'Continuant'). These may be used to inform high-level biomedical concepts such as 'disease', 'stress', 'fear', or 'cancer'. In order to investigate these high-level biomedical concepts, specific **experimental models** are used by scientists to provide a framework to investigate phenomena of interest. These experiments provide a rigorous, logical framework for reasoning about biological phenomena. Principles of experimental design provide the building blocks for this framework and we refer interested computer scientists to [25] for an excellent introduction.

Put simply, biomedical experiments generally consist of the demonstration of statistically significant differences between measurements of a *dependent variable* under conditions imposed by the choice of different values of *independent variables*. This is illustrated schematically in Figure 2.1. Thus, reasoning within biology depends on human expertise, experimental design, statistical inference and

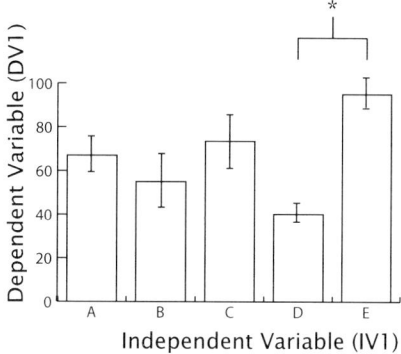

Fig. 2.1. A schematic representation of a hypothetical 'effect' in a biological experiment. The graph shows a statistically significant difference in the dependent variable between conditions D and E.

significance-testing rather than other forms of mathematical logic (which may provide formal methods to model this specialized process).

The values of both independent and dependent variables can be classified based on the four scales of measurement [26]. These scales are (a) ratio measurements (fully numerical with a defined zero point, such as the Kelvin scale of temperature); (b) interval measurements (fully numerical without a defined zero point, such as the Celsius scale); (c) ordinal measurements (ranked data where only relative order is available); (d) nominal measurements (simple enumerated categories). This approach differs from knowledge-engineering approaches where inference rules must be based on boolean values and constructed only from enumerated values.

Thus, a basic individual 'unit' of scientific reasoning is an **experiment**, consisting of a set of independent variables (including the experimental protocol), dependent variables, data and statistics [27]. Typically, conclusions are inferred from this data and then presented as factual statements that are supported by experimental evidence. These facts may then be summarized into a 'model'. This model may then be used as the basis of forming new hypotheses and designing new experiments. This conceptual workflow forms the basis of our approach to text-mining and is illustrated in Figure 2.2.

Within Figure 2.2, we illustrate the construction of knowledge bases from the published literature, raw data files such as images, electronic laboratory notebooks, general multimedia files and online data sources. Any KB would need to store and manage these resources prior to constructing any representation of their content. Descriptions of experimental observations could then be derived either by manual curation, information extraction or other methods. In some cases, facts are also likely to be mined directly from the literature (as is the case with systems that describe protein-protein interactions for example [8]) as well as being inferred from experimental observations.

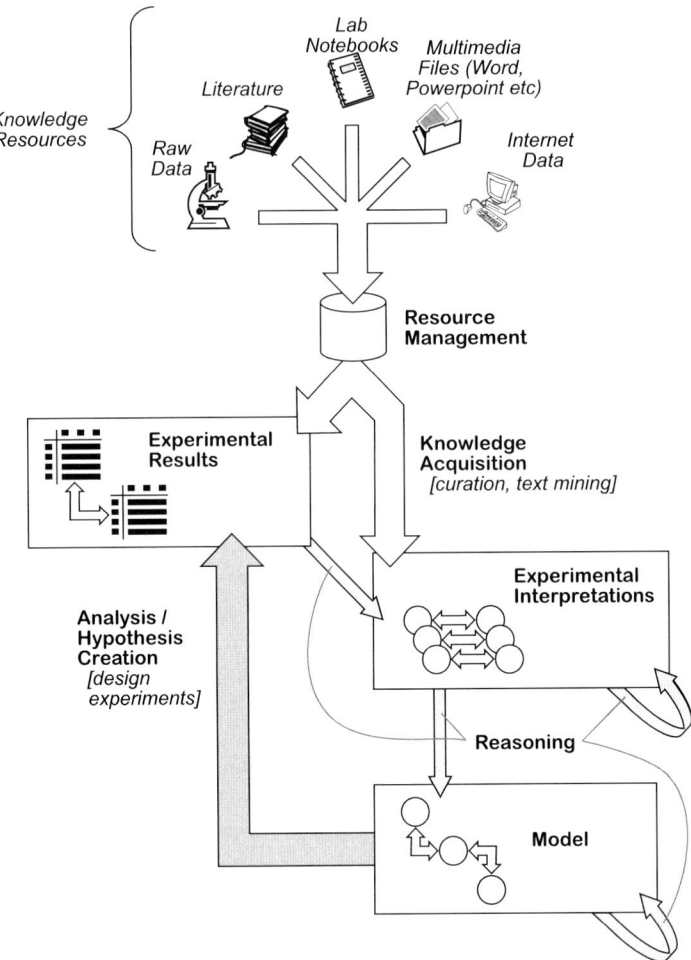

Fig. 2.2. High-level schematic representation for knowledge-base development for conceptual biology based on common knowledge resources. Within this chapter, we emphasize text-mining approaches based on the peer-reviewed published literature, but this framework could conceivably apply to KRs based on any knowledge source.

Standardization is a crucial component of this work. Standards arise from either *de-facto* standard approaches and technology (such as the Gene Ontology [23], or the Protégé system [28]) or from work performed by committees and consortia to agree on appropriate semantics to place on nomenclature and models (such as the Microarray Gene Expression Data Society, or 'MGED' or the International Union of Basic and Clinical Pharmacology or 'IUPHAR'). One viewpoint is that ontologies, data exchange formats, and database schemata constitute 'computational symbolic theories' [29]. Certainly, these are the components where the explicit semantics of biology are embedded into technology for use by the community.

In our attempts to construct a framework for conceptual biology, we emphasize the primary experimental observations as the components that are the most portable between different subject domains. For example, descriptions of histological labeling within tract-tracing experiments are almost indistinguishable from descriptions of histological labeling in *in-situ* hybridization experiments; a single represetation could be used for both types of experiment. Experimental observations typically provide accurate assertions, whereas interpretations are dependent on the evidence that support them. We suggest that observations may therefore be more accurate than interpretations within a KB. The drawback of emphasizing observations over interpretations is that additional inference is required to reconstruct the conclusions of a study.

In order to satisfy conditions of exemplary scholarly practise, it is crucial that the KB provide a fully-annotated link to the original phrase, sentence, figure or article section of the mined or curated information (rather than just the citation). These explicit links to text within the source documents and original experimental data enable users to trace the logic that supports the claim that the interpretations are correct. Without these features in place, users of a KB would have to read the paper in its entirety in order to validate its claims.

Given this general architecture, we now examine how we can segment the prohibitively large literature into more manageable domains upon which we may then operate with NLP-based approaches.

2.3 Partitioning the literature - the notion of 'experimental type'

There are two main types of scientific article: primary experimental reports and reviews. The structure of experimental reports is quite regular and typically has the following sections: abstract, introduction, materials and methods, results, discussion/conclusion and references (as well as figures and tables scattered throughout). In comparison, the structure of review articles is freeform, and is based mainly on citations linking to knowledge found in experimental reports (or other reviews). We focus on the originating source of new scientific knowledge by only considering primary research articles and disregarding reviews.

Computationally, the literature itself is difficult to partition cleanly, since it is primarily a resource designed with human readability and retrieval in mind. Papers are not separated into information-specific categories that then may be collated into appropriate knowledge bases. To assist with this, we define the notion of **experimental-type** based on the design of an experiment. Although there is variability within the design of any given experiment, we adopt a simplistic approach. All of the seemingly complex choices made by an experimentalist to select a model system, methodology, assaying technique, time-points and type of experimental subject are concerned with the independent variables and their values. All measurements made within the experiment are just dependent variables and their values.

If we wish to construct a database for scientific data for a specific experimental-type, we first construct the database schema based on the experimentalists' choice of independent and dependent variables. More specifically, we would want our database design to be widely applicable across a large number of individual experiments and we might ignore the less significant choices made by experimenters. This is typified by the idea of 'minimum information required by an experiment' which denotes the level of detail required in the experimental data to be able to make correct high-level interpretations. This idea has formed the basis of standardized object models for specific experiment types to enable collaboration and data sharing [30–33].

There is a natural parallel between the design of experiments and the design of schemas in bioinformatics systems. Experimental-type is, therefore, a classification of the *knowledge representation schema that can adequately capture the minimum required information for a set of experiments that share the same experimental design and interpretation*. Less formally, if two experiments' data can be entered into a single database in the same set of tables and attributes without needing to alter the database schema, then the two experiments share the same experimental-type.

Another dimension of representation within scientific experiments that we use to partition the literature is the 'depth of representation'. These four categories consist of high-level interpretations and primary experimental observations (shown in Figure 2.2) as well as the complete details of the experimental methods and results (for researchers attempting to replicate the experiment) and a nuanced evaluation of the reliability of the paper. Curation efforts (such as efforts within the GO project [23] and CoCoMac [4]) use codes to denote the source and likely reliability of a specific data entry.

This partition of the primary literature along two orthogonal axes of representation ('experimental-type' and 'depth of representation') is illustrated schematically in Figure 2.3. Within our example described later, we specifically target the shaded 'cell' of this figure: the primary experimental observations of tract-tracing experiments. We will describe tract-tracing experiments later in the chapter. For now, we state that the high-level interpretations of these experiments describe neuronal projections between brain regions and that this information is inferred from experiments where injections of tracer chemicals are made into the brains of experimental animals and then processed to find histological labeling produced by these injections.

It is immediately apparent from Figure 2.3 that two types of text-mining endeavor are possible: 'horizontal' studies that classify papers across experimental type and 'vertical' studies that drill down into the specific literature pertaining to one experimental type. The definition of appropriate knowledge representations and ontologies for each experimental type at each of the different depths of representation is itself a research topic attracting significant interest [31, 34]. Text mining projects that have used unsupervised approaches in biomedicine have been used to index and cluster abstracts in the Medline database [22, 35] provide examples of 'horizontal' studies.

It is possible to identify subtypes and specializations of experiments. Specialized versions of tract-tracing experiments could conceivably include 'double-labeling tract-tracing-experiments', where two (or more) histological labeling methods are used to interactions between neuron populations involved in a projection revealed by the co-localization of labeling. Other examples include ultrastructure experiments (where electron microscopy is used to view the ultrastructure of labeled neurons) and

	e.g. lesion experiments	*e.g.* tract-tracing experiments	*e.g.* activation experiments
high-level interpretations ('punchline')		'brain region A projects to brain region B'	
primary experimental observations		'tracer A was injected into region B and labeling of type C was observed in regions D, E & F	
complete details of experimental methods & results		number of rats, type of injection, handling protocol, methods of data analysis, etc.	
nuanced representation of reliability		quality of histology, reputation of authors, etc.	

Experimental Type →

Depth of Representation ↓

Fig. 2.3. A two-dimensional partition of the published scientific literature.

transneuronal labeling (where tracers may be transmitted between neurons to view multi-synaptic connections) [36]. Each of these experimental types would require a different schema to represent their semantics.

2.4 Related Work: Biomedical Knowledge Bases based on published studies

Thousands of biomedical databases are available to researchers (for a review of the current global state of databases available for molecular biology, see the Molecular Biology Database collection in the 'Database issue' of Nucleic Acids Research [37]). Within the neuroscience community, the 'Neuroscience Database Gateway', provides an online overview of current systems [38]. These systems are often derived from laboratories' primary data (with external links to their publications), rather than synthesizing information found within the literature. Notable systems from within molecular biology that are based on the literature are the BioCyc family of databases (EcoCyc, MetaCyc, *etc.*) [39–41], the BioGRID [42], Textpresso [7], KEGG [43] and GeneWays [8]. The Generic Model Organism Database (GMOD) is a large consortium of organism-specific systems. These include 'dictybase' [44], 'EcoCyc' [39], 'FlyBase' [45], 'MGI' [46], 'RGD' [47], 'SGD' [48], 'TAIR' [49], 'TIGR' [50], 'Wormbase' [51], and 'ZFIN' [52].

A new emerging profession within this field deserves mention: the 'biocurator'. These individuals who populate and maintain large-scale database systems with information in a readable, computable form [53]. As an emerging discipline, biocuration occupies a uniquely important position within biomedical research and this responsibility is often undertaken by teams of Ph.D. level biologists (the Jackson Laboratory has over thirty biocuration staff [54]). Even with this level of commitment and support, most teams are still overwhelmed by the volume of information present in the literature. Crucially, as both databases and ontologies evolve, these large scale efforts will find it increasingly difficult to change the representations they use or update previously curated data to new emerging representations. There is an emerging organized community of biocurators, and the first 'International Biocurator Meeting' was organized in 2005, arising from the collaboration between different databases in the GMOD consortium (http://www.biocurator.org/).

Both Textpresso and GeneWays utilize NLP approaches for knowledge acquisition. Within neuroscience, there are several manually-curated systems: CoCoMac [4] and BAMS [5] describe connections in the Macaque and Rat brain. Also worthy of mention is the work performed within the Tsuji group at the University of Tokyo. Their development of the GENIA text corpus is specifically geared towards the biomedical domain and provides a general reference for Biomedical NLP research [55]. They are also actively engaged in addressed specific research questions concerning information extraction in biomedicine [56].

The BioCyc collection has multiple databases that have undergone extensive manual curation by members of the scientific community [39]. These systems contain knowledge describing signaling pathways derived from (and in conjunction with) genetic data. It has a well-defined ontology [57]. The collection provides model-organism-specific databases (such as EcoCyc for E-Coli [41]) and databases across organisms (such as MetaCyc for metabolism [40]). The EcoCyc database derives information from 8862 publications in the literature (involving extensive manual curation by experts).

The BioGRID system is a large-scale manual curation effort that provides a direct comparison between high-throughput experimental methods for knowledge acquisition and literature curation [6]. It is primarily concerned with protein-protein and protein-gene interactions in yeast (*Saccharomyces cerevisisae*). Within this system, workers have curated information from 31,793 separate abstracts and 6,148 full-text papers [6]. Within this study, the researchers found that the protein interaction datasets taken from high-throughput and literature-curated sources were of roughly equivalent size but only had 14% overlap between them. This suggests that modern, high-throughput techniques augment existing work, but also that the wealth of information reported in the literature cannot easily be reproduced by these methods.

The Textpresso system was originally designed for information retrieval and extraction purposes for the *Caenorhabditis elegans* literature [7]. It involved processing 3,800 full-text articles and 16,000 abstracts and uses regular expression patterns to perform the information extraction step. It also employs entries from the Gene Ontology [23] as entries in its lexicon and used combinatorial rules to build patterns from within programs which could then be applied to its corpus. Systems such as KEGG [43] and the Signal-Transduction Knowledge Environment [58] involves the manual construction of representations of pathways by knowledge engineers.

The GeneWays system is a system for extracting, analyzing, visualizing and integrating molecular pathway data [59]. In 2004, the systems' developers reported that they have downloaded approximately 150,000 articles into the present system. This corpus has yielded roughly 3 million redundant statements that may then be processed with NLP-based approaches [8]. As with the BioCyc systems, GeneWays uses a well defined ontology to describe signaling pathways [59]. Its information extraction system was derived from a mature existing medical Information Extraction (IE) system that is currently used within a production setting in hospitals [60].

It seems clear from this partial review of existing work that the likely coverage of data contained within manually-curated systems is a small percentage of the total that is available. The total size of the published biomedical literature may be estimated from the size of the complete MEDLINE corpus of biomedical citations (available for download as compressed XML from the National Library of Medicine): approximately 1.6×10^7 citations (dating from the mid-fifties to the present day) [61]. Naturally the coverage of each knowledge base may be estimated by the proportion of abstracts available on Medline via a keyword search. If the example presented by the BioGrid is representative, the total number of yeast-specific abstracts was 31,793 and 9,145 were available as full text. Of these, 6,148 papers were curated into the system [6].

Naturally, if the full-text articles are not available, then they simply cannot be included in the contents of a knowledge base. For this reason, licensing and copyright issues become crucial to the development of these systems. Legally, the content of research papers is usually owned by journal publishers. A notable exception to this is the so-called 'open-access' publication model. The federal U.S. government has also issued a request that researchers deposit papers that were supported under federal funding into its open-access repository, PubMedCentral [62]. Under normal licensing conditions for most well-funded universities, researchers have access to large numbers of journals as a matter of course. After examining the online availability of journals relevant to the field of neuroendocrinology available at the authors' home institution (the University of Southern California), we found that from 65 relevant journal titles, we were permitted to access 1886 journal-years worth of text. Thus, even under current conditions of restrictive copyright, it is possible to obtain moderately large quantities of text. Note that, to computer scientists, working in the field of Natural Language Processing, such corpora sizes are not considered large since much work is currently done on terascale crawls of the world wide web [63].

Finally, our own work in this area consists of the NeuroScholar system, which is a knowledge management platform for treatment of the neuroscience literature [13]. This system is designed to be a desktop application that provides direct support for scientists' interaction with the primary research literature (rather than a single large-scale centralized web-based database system). It provides a means to add both unstructured and structured annotations to full-text articles as PDF files [14], an Electronic Laboratory Notebook component [64] and a system to provide support for visualization plugins based on components such as neuroanatomical atlases [65]. NeuroScholar is open-source and provides a platform for development of knowledge-engineering technology for biomedicine. The system is available for download from http://www.neuroscholar.org/.

In the next section, we examine how the interaction between biologists and computer scientists designing such a system would take into account practices and methods from within the preexisting scholarly process.

2.5 Practical applications: 'Research Synthesis'

The terms 'meta-analysis' and 'research synthesis' refer to formalized approaches to reviewing the literature [12]. Within the clinical, social and behavioral sciences such approaches are widely used to attempt to minimize problems of variance and bias across studies. Due perhaps to the concept-driven nature of the subject, experimental biology does not often rely on these formal approaches directly; instead workers in the field use expert narrative reviews to summarize the knowledge contained in specific subfields of the literature. Thus, we propose that the development of formalized approaches to constructing knowledge bases from the published literature is actually a form of research synthesis or meta-analysis for experimental biology. By leveraging a very large number of studies into this process we seek to (a) increase the possible scope of published reviews and (b) provide tools that make writing conventional reviews easier.

Following [66], the process of constructing a literature review may be broken into stages, where researchers perform specific sets of tasks. We illustrate this workflow in Figure 2.4. Using this approach will involve challenges at each stage which may, or may not, be supported by computational tools.

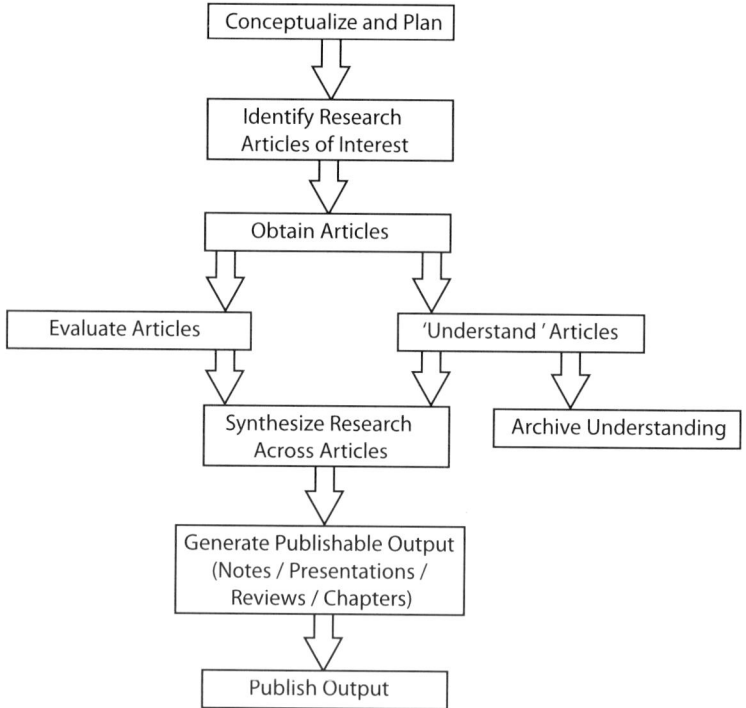

Fig. 2.4. A schematic representation of the process of performing a literature review.

The CommmonKADS framework is a practical methodology of generating solutions for knowledge-intensive tasks [67]. Within this methodology, knowledge engineers are guided through a design process involving a detailed analysis of the task under consideration, the organizational context of the task and the agents performing various roles in relation to it (in addition to issues of representing and acquiring the knowledge necessary to address the task itself). Thus, it is both relevant and necessary to consider the whole task under investigation and to develop models for the contextual and procedural components of the task in question.

At the start of the process of reviewing the literature in a given field, a scientist must first **conceptualize and plan** their study. This currently involves only the researchers' own expertise without support from knowledge tools. Once the researcher has settled on a subject for their review, they must then **identify articles of interest** by searching either Medline or Google Scholar portal. Research is ongoing to improve the performance of these tools (see [68] for an example of adding functionality to Medline). Selecting relevant papers is also called 'literature triage' which has been addressed in community based evaluations such as the KDD challenge cup [69], and TREC 2004 and 2005 [70, 71].

The greatest computationally advances for scientific scholarly work is the ease with which one may now **obtain full-text articles**. This process is determined by copyright issues within the publishing process, and the vast majority of scholarly journals have online access to full-text papers.

The processes of **understanding and evaluating the article** are performed iteratively in parallel depending on how many times and how deeply the researcher reads the paper. Understanding the article may involve reading it several times, taking notes and even discussing the contents of the article with colleagues. Evaluation is based on the quality of the research within the paper (and its relevance to the reviewers). There is not much (if any) computational support for the individual reviewer at this stage, and this work is also the most time consuming and difficult.

Once the researcher has understood the article, he/she may **archive their understanding** by recording notes on file cards, keeping notes, or even storing a structured representation in a local knowledge base [14]. This is an essential component of the process since it is likely that they will forget the details of the article within a few months unless they re-read it. Development within the NeuroScholar system specifically targets this task by providing annotation tools for neuroscientists to be able to store their opinions and accounts as a network of interrelated statements [64]. This is similar to the development of argumentation networks [72, 73]. An important stage of constructing a review is being able to **synthesize research across articles**. This is also the role played by formal meta-analysis when applied across studies with a common set of research criteria (such as with randomized clinical trials [74]). This is a difficult problem, requiring deep knowledge of the subject to create conceptual connections between papers.

Computationally, this is equivalent to data-mining and knowledge discovery. These are analytical techniques that are used extensively within molecular biology to search for correlations and patterns within data stored in databases (see [75–77] for reviews). These are applicable and useful whenever data may be compiled in sufficient quantity, and have also been used in the field of systems-level neuroanatomy to look for patterns in neural connections between brain regions [78, 79].

The final tasks facing the reviewer are to **generate a physical instantiation of the research synthesis** (as the finished review, a presentation or a set of notes) and then **publish or disseminate it**. Given a computational representation, it is relatively simple to generate tabulated or graphical output to represent the knowledge. In addition, Natural Language Generation systems may also be used to create human readable text that summarizes the contents of complex knowledge representations [80].

2.6 An Example Experiment Type: 'Tract-Tracing Experiments'

We describe our approach for a single, specific experiment type: tract-tracing experiments. The methods we describe could be used for any experiment type defined at any depth of representation (see Figure 2.3). This could be accomplished by simply substituting the relevant schema, markup and data into the appropriate place within the methodology.

Tract-tracing experiments were first performed in the early 1970s when tiny amounts of radioactive (tritiated) amino acids were placed into targeted regions of brain tissue [81]. This 'tracer chemical' was taken up by the cells located within the 'injection site' and then transported along the long axonal processes of these neurons. The experimental animal was then sacrificed and its brain processed for radioactivity revealing patches of 'labeling' that revealed the spatial location of the transported tracer. Since these early experiments, the basic design of tract-tracing experiments has remained consistent within the field (see [82] for a treatment of newer methods). The types of tracers used in modern experiments are easier to use, are more precise, suffer less from tissue-specific problems (such as uptake of the tracer by fibers passing through the injection site but not terminating there), and they produce clear histological labeling of cells and their processes. The consistency and relative simplicity of this experimental design, coupled with the number of studies performed and the relative importance and complexity of the resulting data (connections in the brain), sparked the development of several databases of neural connectivity over the last 15 years where the information from these experiments has been partially stored [4, 5, 83, 84]. None of these systems use text mining approaches and all have partial coverage of the literature.

An object-oriented model that captures the logic of this schema is expressed in UML in Figure 2.5, (see also [14, 34]). The logical design of a tract tracing experiment is relatively simple consisting of three sets of entities that may be defined as part of a schema. The first is the `chemical` used as a tracer in the experiments since anterograde tracers (such as Phaseolus Leuco-Agglutinin or 'PHAL' [85]) reveal the outputs of the neurons in the injection site, and retrograde tracers (such as Fluoro Gold or 'FG' [86]) reveal the inputs. Thus the uptake properties of each tracer determine how we should interpret the results. The second is the `injection-site`, which captures the details of where the tracer injection was made and is a child of the **neuroanatomical-location** entity. The third entity in question pertains to the location and description of transported labelling (**labeled-location** entities) which include both the location of the label and salient characteristics, such as **density** and **type** ('cellular', 'fiber', 'varicose', *etc.*).

The <<DV>> stereotypes for **labeled-location** class and the **density** and **type** attributes denote that they are considered dependent variables (and may be processed accordingly when required within our knowledge modeling process). The structure of other entities, such as the **neuroanatomical-location** involves potentially several named structures from an atlas (**atlas-volume** objects) since a single location or site may conceivably involve multiple named structures. The **abbr** attribute denotes the abbreviation commonly used to describe the **atlas-volume**, and the **addr** attribute denotes the 'address' of the region (a construct used to denote the position of the region in the hierarchy).

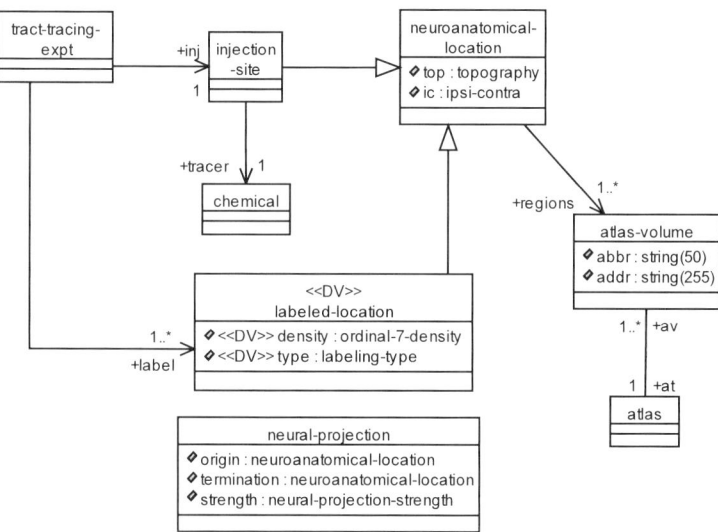

Fig. 2.5. Schema for tract-tracing studies used in the text-mining examples described in this chapter.

In Figure 2.5, note the presence of the **neural-projection** which represents an interpreted 'fact' that takes the form location A projects to location B with strength C. A large number of these facts could be summarized into a large connection matrix and then analyzed mathematically in a form of a model (see Figures 2.2 and 2.3, [78]). The logic required to construct these facts is simple: if the **chemical** is a retrograde tracer, then construct a **neural-projection** originating from the **labeled-location** and terminating in the **injection-site** and vice-versa if the **chemical** is anterograde. This experiment-type therefore provides a suitably simple example for investigating our method's feasibility.

UML is not considered particularly effective as knowledge representation. It is a widely-used inudstrial standard for software engineering and provides an effective way of expressing class/attribute/role relationships diagrammatically. We automatically converted the above schema to OWL format and show the equivalent schema rendered for viewing within the OntoViz plugin of the Protégé ontology editing tool (see Figure 2.6). Using UML presents a low 'barrier to entry' for non-specialists who are familiar with concepts from object-oriented programming.

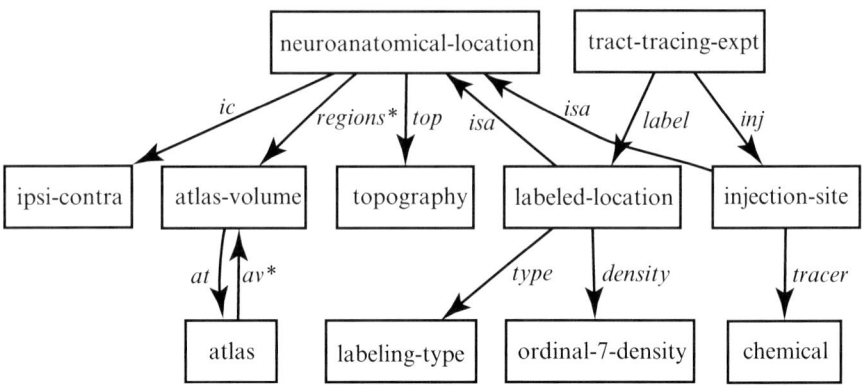

Fig. 2.6. Translation of the UML schema into an OWL ontology, (rendered by OntoViz within Protégé/OWL).

The main challenge is to populate this representation from the textual narrative of published papers. Naturally, the textual descriptions of this data are typically far more complex than our simple schema, involving a wide variety of syntactic and semantic structures (some of which act as modifiers for tags that demarcate the main items). We use an XML-based representation to provide a set of markup tags that capture recognizable linguistic features of entities from our target representation and of additional entities to capture additional structure from the text. In Figure 2.7, we present two examples of text with accompanying XML markup to illustrate our methodology, the first relatively simple, the second more complex and more representative of our input data.

This illustrates how we use XML tags to demarcate phrases of interest (including names of brain structures, descriptions of labeling patterns, topographic terminology, *etc.*). Note that we have invented our new tags to provide additional processing structure for subsequent evaluation. For example, the `<injectionSpread>` tag denotes regions that may (or may not) be involved in the injection site. Constructing the tagset is an iterative ongoing process where we initially created a simple representation and then refined it as we mark up the text and run our NLP methods. The XML scheme serves two purposes: to capture the semantic detail sufficiently well to be able to populate the target representation and also to maximize performance of our system's ability to mark up the text. Consequently, there is not a one-to-one

A.
```
Injections of <tracerChemical abb="w"> wga-hrp </tracerChemical> were
confined to <injectionLocation region="XII"> xi1 </injectionLocation>
in 4 animals and extended beyond <injectionSpread> the boundaries of
xi1 </injectionSpread> in 6 animals.
```

B.
```
In this case , <labelingDescription density="6" type="f"> heavy
anterograde labeling </labelingDescription> was present in
<labelingLocation ipsiContra="b" region="MMm" topography="cv"> the
ventral portion of the posterior half of the medial mamillary nucleus
bilaterally </labelingLocation> ( fig . 4g , h ) ,
<labelingDescription density="4" type="f"> whereas moderate to light
anterograde labeling </labelingDescription> was present in
<labelingLocation ipsiContra="b" topography="rd" region="MM"> the
intermediate and dorsal parts of the anterior half of the medial
nucleus bilaterally </labelingLocation> ( fig . 4f , g ) .
```

Fig. 2.7. Text from tract-tracing experiments, marked up with XML tags under the current design of the text-mining process. Note the presence of a common 'OCR error' in the text extracted captured from the PDF file in (A): here 'xi1' is really 'XII', the hypoglossal nucleus in the rat.

correspondence between our markup tags and output representation shown in Figure 2.5. Traversing this step involves ongoing research that is currently at a preliminary stage. For the rest of this chapter, we describe our approach to automatically insert these tags into text across a corpus of papers describing tract-tracing experiments using modern NLP techniques.

2.7 Methodology

The overall challenge, from text to knowledge

The text-mining process when applied to our problem of tract-tracing experiments may be decomposed into subtasks: (a) identifying documents of interest, (b) delineating individual experiments in the text, (c) accurately tagging the appropriate text within the narrative, (d) annotating the marked-up text accurately, (e) composing the complete annotation into computable entities conforming to our target schema. Each one of these tasks requires the use of different sets of tools to accomplish the end goal of constructing database entries from the raw text input. Bringing all of these components together is an ongoing task within the project.

Existing computational approaches all contribute to address subtasks of this process. Fortunately, these separate subtasks are being addressed by research performed on several different topics within the community: Document Classification, Named Entity Recognition, Relation Extraction and Event Characterization (following the MUC competitions [87] and more recent competitions within the bio-NLP community [88]). Note that by our existing definitions, the overall task of extracting information pertaining to a specific complete experiment is synonymous with that of Event Detection and Characterization, a task that has been notoriously difficult to solve with high performance in the MUC and ACE evaluations (best performance tends to hover around 60% precision and recall, [89]). Even so, given the importance of biocuration and the high cost of maintaining biomedical databases, developing methods to improve efficency of constructing knowledge bases will still have a large impact.

The overall task has too many subcomponents to describe in detail here. Instead we will focus on the process of automatically inserting appropriate tags into the text and describe the methodology for this in detail.

Information extraction techniques: from Patterns to Conditional Random Fields

For the NLP community, IE has been a constantly active area since the 1970s. IE processes text corpora to populate a target representation, typically recorded in a database. Ideally, the specific information extracted should be concise and may contain several words or a phrase. Much of the current work in IE is pattern-based, that is, specific textual patterns are defined and associated with the data/knowledge types of interest. When the patterns match a fragment of text, they serve both to delimit the region of interest and to allocate it to a specific data type. For example, a pattern can be '<person> was born in <place> on <date>'. Whenever this pattern encounters a matching sentence, the person's name, the birth place and the birth date are extracted. This is the approach used within the Textpresso system [7].

Acquiring meaningful patterns is the key to this approach, and is the main restriction in terms of its usefulness. It is usually hard to create a complete pattern list with all variations that are naturally encountered in human language. Traditionally, these patterns were constructed either manually or programmatically, or they were acquired from human-annotated corpora, *e.g.*, [90–92]. In these cases, it is not generally guaranteed that all possible patterns can be included within such a manually compiled list. Therefore, these approaches tend to have unpredictable coverage. The cost of human annotation in these cases is non-trivial and must be repeated in each domain. It is also the case that required fields do not always follow fixed patterns and patterns cannot be derived with sparse data.

Depending on the extraction task, identifying the required information from the text may require additional knowledge beyond that expressible in a surface text pattern. This limited ability of expressivity arises since the only information represented is a sequence of words in a fixed order. Although some research reported to derive more complex patterns by mixing Part of Speech (POS) tags and surface words [63, 93], patterns cannot be integrated with other types of useful required knowledge, (such as the root form of a word).

A straightforward way to construct patterns is to annotate manually a large number of sentences with the required slots (a laborious task). It is possible to learn surface patterns by bootstrapping from a set of seed data [94, 95]. However, the power of this approach is somewhat limited and at most, only two slots are allowed in a single sentence. The ability to learn patterns with multiple slots has not been yet reported with reasonable performance.

In this bootstrapping procedure, a set of seed data pairs are prepared in advance. For example, we first manually create a list of person names and their birthdates for the relation 'birth date'. The system then scans a text corpus (or a corpus returned by querying search engines with these terms). Any sentence containing both search terms is automatically identified. Slots are renamed with two anchor names, for example, <person> and <birthdate> respectively in this case. A suffix tree traverse algorithm [96] then builds a suffix tree to strip off non-common portions of the sentences, leaving potential patterns. The learned patterns can be verified with a small validation set and used to extract relations in the future. Systems requiring averagely ten to twenty seed data pairs can obtain promising results while significantly reducing expensive human costs.

As mentioned above, pattern-based approaches learn useful patterns to pinpoint required fields values using seed data. Most approaches on binary relation extraction [94, 97] rely on the co-occurrence of two recognized terms as anchors in a single sentence. However, this approach cannot be generalized to more complex situations where the data corpus is not rich enough to learn variant surface patterns. Although surface pattern based techniques perform well when sentences are short and complete pattern lists are available, sentences within biomedical articles tend to be long and the prose structure tends to be complex, reducing the effectiveness of short contiguous patterns. What is required is the ability to recognize automatically, sequences of important indicator terms, regardless of intermediate material and then to assemble the pertinent parts as required.

A promising development within NLP research is the Conditional Random Field (CRF) model for sequential labeling [97, 98], which has been widely used for language processing, including improved model variants [99], web data extraction [100], scientific citation extraction [101], and word alignment [102]. The originators of the CRF model provide an open-source implementation in the form of the MALLET toolkit [103].

As given in [104], this model is simply a conditional probability $P(y|x)$ with an associated state-based graph structure. Within a labeling task, where the model traverses a set of tokens (words) and labels each one according to the current state of the model, the most likely transitions between states (to given the most likely label assigned to a given token) is given by summing a set of weighted feature functions. Here each feature, defined by the system builder, reflects some (potentially) pertinent aspect of the text: it may be a word, a part of speech, semantic or syntactic label, punctuation mark, formatting command, *etc*.

The structure of this graph is adaptable and when it takes the form of a linear chain, the CRF model has very similar properties to Hidden Markov Models (HMMs). CRF models have inherent characteristics that outperform the limitations of old pattern based approaches: they view all the required knowledge to extract useful information as features and given reasonable training data, they compile those features automatically to extract information. They can provide a compact way to integrate many different types of features (including explicit surface word patterns).

Therefore, CRF models have more powerful expressivity even when potential patterns have never been seen before by the system. In this situation, the CRF models utilize related information from heterogeneous sources. Additionally, they do not suffer from any limitation to the number of slots per sentence.

We use plain text as a token sequence for input and attempt to label each token with field labels. For each current state, we train the conditional probability of its output states given previously assigned values of input states. Formally, given a sentence of a separate input sequence of word tokens, $S = (w_1, w_2, ..., w_n)$, we attempt to obtain a corresponding labeling sequence of field names, $L = (l_1, l_2, ..., l_n)$, and each input token corresponds to only one label. The field names must include a default label, 'O', denoting that the token receives a null label.

The CRF model is trained to find the most probable labeling sequence L for an input sentence S by maximizing the probability of $P(L|S)$. The decision rule for this procedure is:

$$\hat{L} = \arg\max_{L} P(L|S) \quad (2.1)$$

As described above, this CRF model is characterized by a set of feature functions and their corresponding weights. The conditional probability can be computed using Equation 2.2 (as with Markov fields).

$$P(L|S) = \frac{1}{Z_S} \exp\left(\sum_{t=1}^{T} \sum_{k} \lambda_k * f_k(l_{t-1}, l_t, S, t)\right) \quad (2.2)$$

Where $f_k(l_{t-1}, l_t, S, t)$ is a feature function, including both the state transition feature $f_k(l_{t-1}, l_t, S)$ and the feature of output state given the input sequence $f_k(l_t, S)$. A detailed introduction to the mathematics of this formulation may be found in [98, 104] and will not be repeated here.

The individual feature functions are created by the system builder, often using standard computational linguistic tools such as parts of speech (POS) taggers, parsers, lexions *etc*. Since the CRF model automatically learns which features are relevant for which labels, the system builder is free to experiment with a variety of features.

The methodology we use is based on a supervised-learning approach. In order to learn which features predict which label(s), the CRF model requires a pre-labeled training set to learn and optimize system parameters. To avoid the over-fitting problem, a Gaussian prior over the parameters is typically applied to penalize the log-likelihood [105]. We calculate the first-derivative of this adjusted log-likelihood value, and use it to maximize this probability and estimate the values for λ_k. Once we have obtained these parameter values, the trained CRF model can be used to make predictions with previously unseen text.

The principal obstacle to the development of general-purpose information extraction systems based on supervised approaches is that obtaining enough suitably formatted training data upon which to train the system is either too expensive or too complex. Besides the bootstrapping approaches described previously, the procedure called 'active learning' strives to reduce the annotation cost by selecting the most informative training examples and presenting just them to the annotators, thereby obtaining from them the maximally useful feedback. Once these informative examples have been constructed they are added to the training set to improve system performance. Thus, one can start with a small annotation set, train a system, provide annotators with initial, largely inaccurate system results, and then use the corrections provided by the annotators to refine the learning process. Active learning approaches may be categorized on the basis of the selection criteria concerning data to be cycled through the annotation/correction process. 'Committee-based' approaches select data with the highest disagreement (in the classification task) to be reprocessed. 'Uncertainty/certainty score-based' approaches, require that all new data undergoing classification are assigned uncertainty/certainty scores based on predefined measurements. Those data with the highest uncertainty scores are then returned to be reprocessed by a human annotator and added to the training set.

These methods can significantly accelerate the process of annotating training data for machine learning systems. Although these methods were initially introduced into language processing for classification tasks [106, 107] many different NLP fields have adopted this idea to reduce the cost of training. These include information extraction and semantic parsing [108]; statistical parsing [109]; Named Entity Recognition [110]; and Word Sense Disambiguation [111].

Stage 1: Corpus Processing

The first stage of performing text mining work is to obtain and preprocess as large a body of textual information as possible. This involves downloading research articles from the web and extracting the text of these articles to remove the formatting used by individual journals. This is a vital but non-trivial step since the articles may only be available in formats that are difficult to manipulate (such as PDF). In addition to this, the publishing process places breaks, figure- and table-legends into the flow of the text so that an uninterrupted stream of the experimental narrative is not directly readable from the file without additional processing. Within our example application concerned with neuroanatomical connections, we used a geometric, rule-based approach built on top of a well-engineered, open-source document management system ('Multivalent' [112]) to parse the PDF files that make up our corpus.

We use the Journal of Comparative Neurology as the basis for our text corpus. This is an authoritative publication for neuroanatomists and for neuroscience in general [113]. We acted within the journal's copyright guidelines to download roughly 12,000 articles dating from 1970 to 2005. This coincides with the timeframe over which tract-tracing experiments have been performed. We used papers that had consistent formatting from volume 204 to 490 (1982-2005) providing a complete text corpus of 9,474 files and 99,094,318 words distributed into various article sections ('Abstract', 'Introduction', *etc.*). We restricted our attention to the results sections of these papers, which comprised roughly one quarter of the total text in the corpus.

As with many other researchers in the field of biomedical text mining, the preferred representation for text data is the Extensible Markup Language (XML). There are preexisting XML editors that support the process of adding annotations to text (see, for example, the Vex system [114]). This provides a convenient standardized user interface for the process of annotation (which is the most time-consuming and tedious component of this type of work). Vex also uses standard web-formatting (Cascading Style Sheets or 'CSS') to permit the user to define their own visual formatting for the text being annotated. For a review of tools to assist with managing corpora and their annotation, see [115].

Stage 2: The basic text processing and feature definition

In order to locate the text that pertains to the semantic structures specified in the schema, we use a set of morphological, lexical, grammatical or semantic functions to provide features that can train the CRF model to tag words appropriately. These feature functions implement NLP-based functions and may use downloadable tools within their implementation. The binary functions that we define for our target application are as follows:

- **Lexical features:** Entities defined within the schemas affiliated with each type of experiment are often identifiable through specific names. Note that in many domains that have not been centralized and regulated, the nomenclature of concepts is often quite messy, exceedingly complicated and contradictory (see [116, 117] for examples from neuroanatomy and [118, 119] for a discussions of this topic in the context of Named Entity Recognition for molecular biology). For our work with tract-tracing experiments, we use lexicons that are pre-chosen for different components of the schema. These include named neuroanatomical structures (taken from [120]), the neuroanatomical cardinal directions[1] (*e.g.*, 'caudal', 'rostral', *etc.*), names and abbreviations of tracer chemicals used (*e.g.*, 'PHAL'), and commonsense words that describe the density of labeling (*e.g.*, 'dense', 'weak', *etc.*). Given a different schema, we would select different features and would construct lexica from the expanding number of biomedical controlled vocabularies that are now avaiable (see [121] for review). Every word in a given lexicon forms a separate feature (*e.g.*, the feature **lexicon-region** only returns 1 if the word being labeled appears in the 'region' lexicon).
- **Surface and window words:** We employ the word itself and the immediately surrounding words as features for the labeling algorithm, (*e.g.*, the feature **surface-injection** only returns 1 if the word being labeled is 'injection'; the feature **previous-injection**, returns 1 only if the previous word is 'injection'; the **next-injection** feature function acts similarly for the following word).

---

[1] Six terms are typically used to denote directions along the three orthogonal axes within neuroanatomy: 'rostral' and 'caudal' denote the front-to-back direction; 'medial' and 'lateral' denotes towards or away from the midline; and 'dorsal' and 'ventral' denotes the top-to-bottom direction. These terms are often used in combination, so that 'dorsolateral' refers to a direction to the top and away from the midline.

- **Dependency relations:** We use a dependency parser ('MiniPar' [122]) to parse each sentence, and then derive four types of features from the parsing result. The first type is the root forms of words when this differs from the presented form (*e.g.*, the feature **root-inject**, only returns 1 if the being labeled is 'injected', 'injection' or some other derivation and 0 otherwise). The second and third types of dependency feature are based on the subject and object of the sentence. For example, the feature **syntax-subject**, only returns 1 if the word being labeled is the subject of the sentence. Similarly, the feature **syntax-object** only returns 1 if the word is the object of the phrase. The fourth type of feature is based on the governing verb for each word. We traverse dependency relations to the nearest verb within the parse and then base the definition of our feature on the root form of that verb (*e.g.*, the feature **govern-inject**, only returns 1 if the word being labeled is governed by the verb 'to inject' in the target sentence).

It should be remembered that the choice of features is not restricted for the set described above. These simply provide a working model for our tract-tracing example. Other types of features that can be used may be based on parts of speech, character n-grams, word-shapes, previously tagged words, short forms of abbreviations and other variants (see [123] as an example with a widespread choice of features). The choice of feature functions largely determines the performance of the system and is where the system designer can most greatly influence the outcome of the text-mining process. It is also possible to view the weight parameters for each individual feature for each state transition within the CRF model. This provides possible powerful insight into the reasoning learned within the labeling task.

Interestingly, studies of automated methods that evaluate the reliability of curated facts within the Geneways system also consider relationships and clustering between features themselves [124]. This illustrates the versatility and power of machine learning approaches in this context. Biomedical experts contribute to this process by providing training data for which computer scientists and NLP-experts may then devise suitable features.

Stage 3: Evaluating the results

As is usually the case within the field of NLP, quantitative evaluation is essential for the development of the techniques described here. The standard measurements that are most relevant to this question are measures of inter-annotator agreement (often based on the kappa statistic, [125]). This is calculated in the following formula where P(A) is equal to the proportion of times annotators agree, and P(E) is equal to the proportion of times annotators would be expected to agree according to chance alone.

$$Kappa = \frac{P(A) - P(E)}{1 - P(E)} \quad (2.3)$$

The recall (what proportion of target items have been correctly extracted?) and the precision (how many of these extracted items were themselves correct?) are routinely measured and reported for IE tasks. These two values may also be expressed as a single number by the use of the F-Score, see [126, 127].

$$Precision = \frac{\text{\# of correct extracted items}}{\text{\#of all extracted items}} \quad (2.4)$$

$$Recall = \frac{\text{\# of correct extracted items}}{\text{\#of target items from the 'gold standard' reference}} \quad (2.5)$$

$$F-score = \frac{2*Precision*Recall}{Precision+Recall} \quad (2.6)$$

Methods of evaluation within the field as a whole centers around shared evaluations where the task being addressed is standardized and presented to the community as a competition. Within biomedicine, recent evaluations include the KDD challenge cup task 1 (2002) [69], the TREC genomics track (2003-2006) [70, 71], BioCreAtIvE (2003-2004, 2006) [128].

Extrinsic measures of evaluation provide feedback from the perspective of domain experts and are based on subjective criteria such as 'is this useful?', and 'does this save time?'. Evaluating these type of criteria must depend on subject interviews and questionnaires. It is also possible to record behavioral statistics from the use of the system, which can provide valuable data to indicate how well the system performs at a specific task.

We focus on the development of systems that must be developed, implemented and tested. Whilst engaged in this pursuit, we use four extrinsic evaluation tasks. (1) requirements evaluation (are requirements fully specified, complete and attainable?); (2) system validation and verification (does the system fully represent the knowledge it is supposed to, and is the system built well technically?); (3) usability evaluation (is the system easy to learn and use?); (4) performance evaluation (how well does the system fulfill its requirements?). One important measure that we emphasize is the time taken to annotate documents by domain experts. Usage metrics (such as the number of system downloads over a given period) can also provide insight as to the impact of a given system on the community [129, 130].

2.8 Results

In a series of experiments, we marked up 21 documents by hand, providing 1047 sentences (at an approximate rate of 45 sentences per hour). We then randomly divided this data into training and testing sets (with 698 and 349 sentences respectively) to reconstruct our annotations. The system's performance based on different combinations of features is shown in Table 2.1. Performance of this task is acceptably high (F-Score = 0.79). This is especially encouraging because the number of training examples (14 documents) is relatively small. We then ran our labeling system on previously unseen text and corrected the machine driven annotations by hand. We found that this process had been accelerated to an approximate rate of 115 sentences per hour.

Table 2.1. NLP performance (Precision, Recall and F-Score) for text-mining from tract-tracing experiments. Features Key, L = Lexical, C = Current Word, P/F = Preceding or Following Word, W = Context Window, D = Dependency features.

Features	Precision	Recall	F-Score
Base	0.41	0.18	0.25
L	0.60	0.37	0.46
L + C	0.77	0.73	0.75
L + C + P/F	0.77	0.73	0.75
L + C + P/F + W	0.81	0.75	0.78
L + C + P/F + W + D	0.80	0.78	0.79

The confusion matrix describing the errors made by our system is shown in Figure 2.8. The leading diagonal holds the counts of our system's correct guesses for word-labels, and off-diagonal counts demonstrate errors. Note that the three labels for different types of neuroanatomical locations are frequently confused (`<injectionLocation>`, `<tracerChemical>`, and `<labelingLocation>`). Pooling these labels into a single category yields Recall = 0.81, Precision = 0.85, F-Score = 0.83. This emergent property of the textual descriptions may also have relevance to the design of the knowledge representations and ontological resources derived from text. Annotating the text of articles involves developing suitable labeling schemes and performing a large amount of annotation. This is particularly instructive concerning subtleties of representation that may be relevant to ontology engineers. We envisage that much of our future work will center on the actions of biocurators as knowledge engineers, enabled in their work by NLP approaches and KB systems.

Counts		O	Injection Location	Injection Spread	Injection Description	labeling Location	labeling	tracer Chemical	
machine labels	O	41087	141	97	338	1751		6	43420
	injectionLocation	545	744	48	6	820		1	2164
	injectionSpread	126	43	147	11	155		0	482
	labelingDescription	1121	5	0	3773	82		47	5028
	labelingLocation	1988	224	110	27	9251		0	11600
	tracerChemical	108	1	12	0	0		623	744
		44975	1158	414	4155	12059		677	

Fig. 2.8. A 'confusion matrix' for the tract-tracing experimental data.

2.9 Conclusions

This chapter is concerned with 'Intelligent Text Mining'; thus, the main component of our work described here is to describe an appropriate target for our text mining approaches. The central concept of this work is the view shown in Figure 2.2: we base our methodology primarily on experimental observations (that may be used to construct representations of 'facts' and 'models'). Each individual **experiment**, consists of a set of **independent variables** (that capture the constraints imposed on the experiment) and a set of **dependent variables** (that capture the measurements made within the experiment). Commonly used experimental designs provide templates for specific experiment-types that can be used to create effective data summaries of experimental observations.

Despite the astonishing scholarly abilities of top-level biologists, the number of individual experimental facts that typically pertain to any phenomenon of interest taxes the limits of human memory. The overall objective of this work is to provide large-scale knowledge-bases that serve as massive literature reviews. We observe that the process of constructing such systems mimics the process of performing a meta-analysis of the literature for specific experimental-types. Once such a knowledge-base has been compiled, new, previously unseen summaries of research data provide insight that is only possible from data-mining of such large-scale systems (see [3] for mathematical meta-analyses of neural connectivity based on these summary data).

The rate-determining step facing workers building such systems is knowledge acquisition, and many existing biomedical databases rely solely on the highly expensive process of human curation. This provides the underlying need for text-mining tools that fit can supply appropriately structured data. An interesting challenge of building these text-mining approaches lies in the possibility of providing tools that can be used by biocurators, which may then leverage their expertise and dedication into their functionality. It is crucial that advances in computer science translate effectively into application development for academic biomedical informatics systems. In our example of neuroanatomical tract-tracing experiments, we provide a system that may be used to support specific databases for this experiment-type [4, 5]. Given the performance of our system (F-Score = 0.79 for the text labeling task), we would not expect to provide a completely automated solution, but a significant increase in biocuration efficiency may permit these system-developers to provide a more comprehensive account of the literature with fewer curation resources.

It is currently an exciting time in the field of biomedical knowledge engineering. Advances in the performance and versatility of open-source machine-learning systems [98, 103], and in the maturity and infrastructure surrounding the use of ontologies in biomedicine [15] provide a rich, highly collaborative and productive environment for future work. We hope that this chapter encourages computer scientists to address these important questions through the development of new approaches and tools.

2.10 Acknowledgements

This work was funded under grant LM 07061 from the NIH and from seed funding generously provided by the Information Sciences Institute. We are grateful for the support and vision of the executive leadership of the Institute. The central role of independent and dependent variables within our strategy is attributed to discussion with Prof. Alan Watts at USC. The central theme of knowledge statements within our knowledge representations was arrived at in brainstorming sessions with Dr Arshad Khan. Many of the principles underlying this project emerged from lengthy discussions with the Watts and Swanson laboratories at USC. We are also grateful to Patrick Pantel for his good-natured brilliance and general support with this project.

References

[1] J. P. Jenuth (2000), Methods Mol Biol, 132: 301-12
[2] I. Sim, G. D. Sanders and K. M. McDonald (2002), J Gen Intern Med, 17(4): 302-8
[3] M. P. Young, J. W. Scannell and G. A. P. C. Burns (1995), The analysis of cortical connectivity. ed. ed. Vol., Austin, Texas: R. G. Landes.
[4] K. E. Stephan, L. Kamper, A. Bozkurt, G. A. Burns, M. P. Young and R. Kotter (2001), Philos Trans R Soc Lond B Biol Sci, 356(1412): 1159-86
[5] M. Bota, H. Dong and L. W. Swanson (2005), Neuroinformatics, 3(1): 15-48
[6] T. Reguly, A. Breitkreutz, L. Boucher, B. J. Breitkreutz, G. C. Hon, C. L. Myers, A. Parsons, H. Friesen, R. Oughtred, A. Tong, C. Stark, Y. Ho, D. Botstein, B. Andrews, C. Boone, O. G. Troyanskya, T. Ideker, K. Dolinski, N. N. Batada and M. Tyers (2006), J Biol, 5(4): 11
[7] H. M. Muller, E. E. Kenny and P. W. Sternberg (2004), PLoS Biol, 2(11): e309
[8] A. Rzhetsky, I. Iossifov, T. Koike, M. Krauthammer, P. Kra, M. Morris, H. Yu, P. A. Duboue, W. Weng, W. J. Wilbur, V. Hatzivassiloglou and C. Friedman (2004), J Biomed Inform, 37(1): 43-53
[9] R. Kotter (2004), Neuroinformatics, 2(2): 127-44
[10] R. Apweiler, A. Bairoch, C. H. Wu, W. C. Barker, B. Boeckmann, S. Ferro, E. Gasteiger, H. Huang, R. Lopez, M. Magrane, M. J. Martin, D. A. Natale, C. O'Donovan, N. Redaschi and L. S. Yeh (2004), Nucleic Acids Res, 32(Database issue): D115-9
[11] M. Kanehisa (2002), Novartis Found Symp, 247: 91-101; discussion 101-3, 119-28, 244-52
[12] H. Cooper and L. V. Hedges (1994), The Handbook of Research Synthesis. ed. ed. Vol., New York: Russell Sage Foundation.
[13] G. A. Burns, A. M. Khan, S. Ghandeharizadeh, M. A. O'Neill and Y. S. Chen (2003), Neuroinformatics, 1(1): 81-109
[14] G. A. Burns and W. C. Cheng (2006), J Biomed Discov Collab, 1(1): 10

[15] D. L. Rubin, S. E. Lewis, C. J. Mungall, S. Misra, M. Westerfield, M. Ashburner, I. Sim, C. G. Chute, H. Solbrig, M. A. Storey, B. Smith, J. Day-Richter, N. F. Noy and M. A. Musen (2006), Omics, 10(2): 185-98
[16] T. R. Gruber (1993), Towards principles for the design of ontologies used for knowledge sharing. in International Workshop on Formal Ontology. Padova, Italy.
[17] N. F. Noy, M. Crubezy, R. W. Fergerson, H. Knublauch, S. W. Tu, J. Vendetti and M. A. Musen (2003), AMIA Annu Symp Proc: 953
[18] D. Oberle, R. Volz, B. Motik and S. Staab (2004), An extensible ontology software environment, In, Handbook on Ontologies, Springer. 311-333.
[19] OBO-Edit - The OBO Ontology Editor [http://oboedit.org/]
[20] D. R. Swanson (1990), Bull Med Libr Assoc, 78(1): 29-37
[21] M. V. Blagosklonny and A. B. Pardee (2002), Nature, 416(6879): 373
[22] N. R. Smalheiser and D. R. Swanson (1998), Comput Methods Programs Biomed, 57(3): 149-53
[23] M. Ashburner, C. Ball, J. Blake, D. Botstein, H. Butler, J. Cherry, A. Davis, K. Dolinski, S. Dwight, J. Eppig, M. Harris, D. Hill, L. Issel-Tarver, A. Kasarskis, S. Lewis, J. Matese, J. Richardson, M. Ringwald, G. Rubin and G. Sherlock (2000), Nat Genet, 25(1): 25-9
[24] B. Latour and S. Woolgar (1979), Laboratory Life. 2 ed. ed. Vol., Princeton, New Jersey: Princeton University Press.
[25] G. D. Ruxton and N. Colegrave (2003), Experimental design for the life sciences. ed. ed. Vol., Oxford: Oxford University Press.
[26] S. S. Stevens (1946), Science, 103(2684): 677-680
[27] D. A. Sprott (2000), Statistical Inference in Science. ed. ed. Vol., New York: Springer Verlag.
[28] N. F. Noy, M. Crubezy, R. W. Fergerson, H. Knublauch, S. W. Tu, J. Vendetti and M. A. Musen (2003), AMIA Annu Symp Proc: 953
[29] P. D. Karp (2001), Science, 293(5537): 2040-4
[30] C. Brooksbank and J. Quackenbush (2006), Omics, 10(2): 94-9
[31] A. Brazma, P. Hingamp, J. Quackenbush, G. Sherlock, P. Spellman, C. Stoeckert, J. Aach, W. Ansorge, C. A. Ball, H. C. Causton, T. Gaasterland, P. Glenisson, F. C. Holstege, I. F. Kim, V. Markowitz, J. C. Matese, H. Parkinson, A. Robinson, U. Sarkans, S. Schulze-Kremer, J. Stewart, R. Taylor, J. Vilo and M. Vingron (2001), Nat Genet, 29(4): 365-71
[32] E. W. Deutsch, C. A. Ball, G. S. Bova, A. Brazma, R. E. Bumgarner, D. Campbell, H. C. Causton, J. Christiansen, D. Davidson, L. J. Eichner, Y. A. Goo, S. Grimmond, T. Henrich, M. H. Johnson, M. Korb, J. C. Mills, A. Oudes, H. E. Parkinson, L. E. Pascal, J. Quackenbush, M. Ramialison, M. Ringwald, S. A. Sansone, G. Sherlock, C. J. Stoeckert, Jr., J. Swedlow, R. C. Taylor, L. Walashek, Y. Zhou, A. Y. Liu and L. D. True (2006), Omics, 10(2): 205-8
[33] J. Leebens-Mack, T. Vision, E. Brenner, J. E. Bowers, S. Cannon, M. J. Clement, C. W. Cunningham, C. dePamphilis, R. deSalle, J. J. Doyle, J. A. Eisen, X. Gu, J. Harshman, R. K. Jansen, E. A. Kellogg, E. V. Koonin,

B. D. Mishler, H. Philippe, J. C. Pires, Y. L. Qiu, S. Y. Rhee, K. Sjolander, D. E. Soltis, P. S. Soltis, D. W. Stevenson, K. Wall, T. Warnow and C. Zmasek (2006), Omics, 10(2): 231-7

[34] G. A. Burns (2001), Philos Trans R Soc Lond B Biol Sci, 356(1412): 1187-208

[35] R. Homayouni, K. Heinrich, L. Wei and M. W. Berry (2005), Bioinformatics, 21(1): 104-15

[36] R. B. Norgren, Jr. and M. N. Lehman (1998), Neurosci Biobehav Rev, 22(6): 695-708

[37] M. Y. Galperin (2006), Nucleic Acids Res, 34(Database issue): D3-5

[38] The Neuroscience Database Gateway [http://ndg.sfn.org/]

[39] P. D. Karp, C. A. Ouzounis, C. Moore-Kochlacs, L. Goldovsky, P. Kaipa, D. Ahren, S. Tsoka, N. Darzentas, V. Kunin and N. Lopez-Bigas (2005), Nucleic Acids Res, 33(19): 6083-9

[40] R. Caspi, H. Foerster, C. A. Fulcher, R. Hopkinson, J. Ingraham, P. Kaipa, M. Krummenacker, S. Paley, J. Pick, S. Y. Rhee, C. Tissier, P. Zhang and P. D. Karp (2006), Nucleic Acids Res, 34(Database issue): D511-6

[41] I. M. Keseler, J. Collado-Vides, S. Gama-Castro, J. Ingraham, S. Paley, I. T. Paulsen, M. Peralta-Gil and P. D. Karp (2005), Nucleic Acids Res, 33(Database issue): D334-7

[42] C. Stark, B. J. Breitkreutz, T. Reguly, L. Boucher, A. Breitkreutz and M. Tyers (2006), Nucleic Acids Res, 34(Database issue): D535-9

[43] H. Ogata, S. Goto, K. Sato, W. Fujibuchi, H. Bono and M. Kanehisa (1999), Nucleic Acids Res, 27(1): 29-34

[44] L. Kreppel, P. Fey, P. Gaudet, E. Just, W. A. Kibbe, R. L. Chisholm and A. R. Kimmel (2004), Nucleic Acids Res, 32(Database issue): D332-3

[45] M. Ashburner and R. Drysdale (1994), Development, 120(7): 2077-9

[46] J. A. Blake, J. E. Richardson, M. T. Davisson and J. T. Eppig (1997), Nucleic Acids Res, 25(1): 85-91

[47] S. Twigger, J. Lu, M. Shimoyama, D. Chen, D. Pasko, H. Long, J. Ginster, C. F. Chen, R. Nigam, A. Kwitek, J. Eppig, L. Maltais, D. Maglott, G. Schuler, H. Jacob and P. J. Tonellato (2002), Nucleic Acids Res, 30(1): 125-8

[48] J. M. Cherry, C. Adler, C. Ball, S. A. Chervitz, S. S. Dwight, E. T. Hester, Y. Jia, G. Juvik, T. Roe, M. Schroeder, S. Weng and D. Botstein (1998), Nucleic Acids Res, 26(1): 73-9

[49] E. Huala, A. W. Dickerman, M. Garcia-Hernandez, D. Weems, L. Reiser, F. LaFond, D. Hanley, D. Kiphart, M. Zhuang, W. Huang, L. A. Mueller, D. Bhattacharyya, D. Bhaya, B. W. Sobral, W. Beavis, D. W. Meinke, C. D. Town, C. Somerville and S. Y. Rhee (2001), Nucleic Acids Res, 29(1): 102-5

[50] E. F. Kirkness and A. R. Kerlavage (1997), Methods Mol Biol, 69: 261-8

[51] T. W. Harris, R. Lee, E. Schwarz, K. Bradnam, D. Lawson, W. Chen, D. Blasier, E. Kenny, F. Cunningham, R. Kishore, J. Chan, H. M. Muller, A. Petcherski, G. Thorisson, A. Day, T. Bieri, A. Rogers, C. K. Chen, J. Spieth, P. Sternberg, R. Durbin and L. D. Stein (2003), Nucleic Acids Res, 31(1): 133-7

[52] M. Westerfield, E. Doerry, A. E. Kirkpatrick and S. A. Douglas (1999), Methods Cell Biol, 60: 339-55
[53] P. E. Bourne and J. McEntyre (2006), PLoS Comput Biol, 2(10): e142
[54] The Jackson Laboratory - Advancing Research in Human Health [http://www.jax.org/]
[55] J. D. Kim, T. Ohta, Y. Tateisi and J. Tsujii (2003), Bioinformatics, 19 Suppl 1: i180-2
[56] A. Yakushiji, Y. Tateisi, Y. Miyao and J. Tsujii (2001), Pac Symp Biocomput: 408-19
[57] P. D. Karp (2000), Bioinformatics, 16(3): 269-85
[58] The Signal Transduction Knowledge Environment (STKE) [http://stke.sciencemag.org/]
[59] A. Rzhetsky, T. Koike, S. Kalachikov, S. M. Gomez, M. Krauthammer, S. H. Kaplan, P. Kra, J. J. Russo and C. Friedman (2000), Bioinformatics, 16(12): 1120-8
[60] C. Friedman, P. Kra, H. Yu, M. Krauthammer and A. Rzhetsky (2001), Bioinformatics, 17 Suppl 1: S74-82
[61] D. L. Wheeler, T. Barrett, D. A. Benson, S. H. Bryant, K. Canese, V. Chetvernin, D. M. Church, M. DiCuccio, R. Edgar, S. Federhen, L. Y. Geer, W. Helmberg, Y. Kapustin, D. L. Kenton, O. Khovayko, D. J. Lipman, T. L. Madden, D. R. Maglott, D. Ostell, K. D. Pruitt, G. D. Schuler, L. M. Schriml, E. Sequeira, S. T. Sherry, K. Sirotkin, A. Souvorov, G. Starchenko, T. O. Suzek, R. Tatusov, T. A. Tatusova, L. Wagner and E. Yaschenko (2006), Nucleic Acids Res, 34(Database issue): D173-80
[62] A. Gass (2004), PLoS Biol, 2(10): e353
[63] P. Pantel, D. Ravichandran and E. H. Hovy (2004), Towards Terascale Knowledge Acquisition. in Proceedings of the COLING conference. Geneva, Switzerland.
[64] A. Khan, J. Hahn, W.-C. Cheng, A. Watts and G. Burns (2006), Neuroinformatics, 4(2): 139-160
[65] W.-C. Cheng and G. A. P. C. Burns (2006), NeuARt II Developers Manual, In, University of Southern California, Information Sciences Institute.: Los Angeles. 1-44.
[66] H. Cooper (1998), Synthesizing Research. A Guide for Literature Reviews. 3 ed. ed. Vol., Thousand Oaks: Sage Publications.
[67] G. Schrieber, H. Akkermans, A. Anjewierden, R. de Hoog, N. Shadbolt, W. Van de Velde and B. Wielinga (2000), Knowledge Engineering and Management. The CommonKADS Methodology. ed. ed. Vol., Cambridge, MA: MIT Press.
[68] D. Rebholz-Schuhmann, H. Kirsch, M. Arregui, S. Gaudan, M. Rynbeek and P. Stoehr (2006), Nat Biotechnol, 24(8): 902-3
[69] A. S. Yeh, L. Hirschman and A. A. Morgan (2003), Bioinformatics, 19 Suppl 1: i331-9
[70] A. M. Cohen and W. R. Hersh (2006), J Biomed Discov Collab, 1: 4

[71] W. Hersh, A. Cohen, J. Yang, R. T. Bhupatiraju, P. Roberts and M. Hearst (2005), TREC 2005 Genomics Track Overview. in Text REtrieval Conference (TREC) 2005. Gaithersburg, Maryland.
[72] S. J. Buckingham Shum, V. Uren, G. Li, J. Domingue and E. Motta (2003), Visualizing Internetworked Argumentation, In, Visualizing Argumentation, software tools for collaborative and educational sense making, Springer: London.
[73] T. Chklovski, Y. Gil, V. Ratnakar and J. Lee (2003), TRELLIS: Supporting Decision Making via Argumentation in the Semantic Web. in 2nd International Semantic Web Conference (ISWC 2003). Sanibel Island, Florida, USA. 20-23.
[74] I. Sim, G. D. Sanders and K. M. McDonald (2002), J Gen Intern Med, 17(4): 302-8
[75] P. Radivojac, N. V. Chawla, A. K. Dunker and Z. Obradovic (2004), J Biomed Inform, 37(4): 224-39
[76] W. P. Kuo, E. Y. Kim, J. Trimarchi, T. K. Jenssen, S. A. Vinterbo and L. Ohno-Machado (2004), J Biomed Inform, 37(4): 293-303
[77] R. Durbin, S. Eddy, A. Krogh and G. Mitchison (1998), Biological Sequence Analysis. ed. ed. Vol., Cambridge: University Press, Cambridge.
[78] M. P. Young (1992), Nature, 358(6382): 152-5
[79] G. A. Burns and M. P. Young (2001), Philos Trans R Soc Lond B Biol Sci, 355(1393): 55-70
[80] G. Hirst, C. DiMarco, E. H. Hovy and K. Parsons. (1997), Authoring and Generating Health-Education Documents that are Tailored to the Needs of the Individual Patient. in The Sixth International Conference on User Modeling (UM97). Sardinia, Italy.
[81] W. M. Cowan (1971), Brain Reserach, 37(1): 21-51
[82] C. Kobbert, R. Apps, I. Bechmann, J. L. Lanciego, J. Mey and S. Thanos (2000), Prog Neurobiol, 62(4): 327-51
[83] D. J. Felleman and D. C. Van Essen (1991), Cereb Cortex, 1(1): 1-47
[84] G. A. P. C. Burns (1997), Neural connectivity in the rat: theory, methods and applications, In, Department of Physiological Sciences, Oxford University: Oxford. 1-481.
[85] C. R. Gerfen and P. E. Sawchenko (1984), Brain Res, 290(2): 219-38
[86] L. C. Schmued (1989), Fluoro-Gold and 4-acetamindo-4'-isothiocyanostilbene-2-2'-disulpfonic acid: Use of substituted stilbenes in neuroanatomical studies., In, Methods in Neurosciences, Vol. 3. Quantitative and Qualitative Microscopy., Academic Press: New York.
[87] MUC (1988-95), Overview. in Message Understanding Conference (MUC). http://www.itl.nist.gov/iaui/894.02/related_projects/muc/.
[88] L. Hirschman and C. Blaschke (2006), Evaluation of Text Mining in Biology, In, Text Mining for Biology and Biomedicine, Artech House: Boston.
[89] D. Appelt and D. Israel (1999), Introduction to Information Extraction. in IJCAI-99. Stockholm, Sweden. http://www.ai.sri.com/appelt/ie-tutorial/.

[90] S. Soderland, D. Fisher, J. Aseltine and W. Lehnert (1995), CRYSTAL: Inducing a conceptual dictionary. in The Fourteenth International Joint Conference on Artificial Intelligence. Montreal, Canada.

[91] E. Riloff (1993), Automatically constructing a dictionary for information extraction tasks. in The 11th National Conference on Artificial Intelligence. Menlo Park, Calif. 811-816.

[92] J. Kim and D. Moldovan (1993), Acquisition of semantic patterns for information extraction from corpora. in The Ninth IEEE Conference on Artificial Intelligence for Applications.

[93] E. Riloff (1996), Automatically Generating Extraction Patterns from Untagged Text. in The Thirteenth National Conference on Artificial Intelligence (AAAI-96). 1044-1049.

[94] D. Ravichandran and E. Hovy (2002), Learning Surface Text Patterns for a Question Answering System. in Proceedings of the ACL conference. Philadelphia, PA.

[95] D. Feng, D. Ravichandran and E. H. Hovy (2006), Mining and Re-ranking for Answering Biographical Queries on the Web. in Proceedings of the Twenty-First National Conference on Artificial Intelligence.

[96] P. Weiner (1973), Linear Pattern Matching Algorithms. in 14th IEEE Annual Symp. on Switching and Automata Theory. 1-11.

[97] G. S. Mann and D. Yarowsky (2005), Multi-field information extraction and cross-document fusion. in The annual meeting for the Association for Computational Linguistics (ACL-2005). Ann Arbor, MI.

[98] J. Lafferty, A. McCallum and F. Pereira (2001), Conditional Random Fields: Probabilistic Models for Segmenting and Labeling Sequence Data. in Proceedings of the International Conference on Machine Learning.

[99] F. Jiao, S. Wang, C. Lee, R. Greiner and D. Schuurmans (2006), Semi-supervised conditional random fields for improved sequence segmentation and labeling. in The annual meeting for the Association for Computational Linguistics (ACL-2006).

[100] D. Pinto, A. McCallum, X. Wei and W. B. Croft (2003), Table Extraction Using Conditional Random Fields. in Proceedings of the ACM SIGIR.

[101] F. Peng and A. McCallum (2004), Accurate information extraction from research papers using conditional random fields. in Proceedings of HLT-NAACL. 329-336.

[102] P. Blunsom and T. Cohn (2006), Discriminative word alignment with conditional random fields. in The annual meeting for the Association for Computational Linguistics (ACL-2006).

[103] Mallet - Advanced Machine Learning for Language [http://mallet.cs.umass.edu/]

[104] C. Sutton and A. McCallum (2006), An Introduction to Conditional Random Fields for Relational Learning., In, In Introduction to Statistical Relational Learning., MIT Press.

[105] S. Chen and R. Rosenfeld (1999), A Gaussian prior for smoothing maximum entropy models, In, Technical Report CMUCS-99-108,, Carnegie Mellon University.
[106] D. D. Lewis and W. A. Gale (1994), A sequential algorithm for training text classifiers. in International Conference on Research and Development in Information Retrieval (SIGIR 1994). Dublin, Ireland.
[107] S. Tong and D. Koller (2000), Support vector machine active learning with applications to text classification. in Seventeenth International Conference on Machine Learning. Stanford University.
[108] C. A. Thompson, M. E. Califf and R. J. Mooney (1999), Active learning for natural language parsing and information extraction. in The Sixteenth International Conference on Machine Learning. Bled, Slovenia.
[109] M. Tang, X. Luo and S. Roukos (2002), Active learning for statistical natural language parsing. in Annual Meeting of the Association for Computational Linguistics (ACL-02). Pennsylvania, PA.
[110] D. Shen, J. Zhang, J. Su, G. Zhou and C. L. Tan (2004), Multi-criteria-based active learning for named entity recognition. in Annual Meeting of the Association for Computational Linguistics (ACL-04). Barcelona.
[111] J. Chen, A. Schein, L. Ungar and M. Palmer (2006), An empirical study of the behavior of active learning for word sense disambiguation. in Human Language Technology conference - North American chapter of the Association for Computational Linguistics annual meeting (HLT-NAACL) 2006. New York, NY.
[112] T. A. Phelps and R. Wilensky (2001), The Multivalent Browser: A Platform for New Ideas. in Document Engineering 2001. Atlanta, Georgia.
[113] C. B. Saper (1999), J Comp Neurol, 411(1): 1-2
[114] Vex - A Visual Editor for XML [http://vex.sourceforge.net/]
[115] J.-D. Kim and J. Tsujii (2006), Corpora and their annotation, In, Text Mining for Biology and Biomedicine, Artech House: Boston. 179-212.
[116] L. W. Swanson and G. D. Petrovich (1998), Trends Neurosci, 21(8): 323-31
[117] L. W. Swanson (2000), Trends Neurosci, 23(11): 519-27
[118] S. Ananiadou, C. Friedman and J. Tsujii. (2004), Journal of Biomedical Informatics, 37: 393-395
[119] M. Krauthammer and G. Nedadic (2005), Journal of Biomedical Informatics, 37: 512-526
[120] L. W. Swanson (2004), Brain Maps: Structure of the Rat Brain. 3 ed. ed. Vol., San Diego: Elsevier Academic Press.
[121] O. Bodenreider (2006), Lexical, Terminological and Ontological Resources for Biological Text Mining, In, Text Mining for Biology and Biomedicine, Artech House: London.
[122] MiniPar home page [http://www.cs.ualberta.ca/ lindek/minipar.htm]
[123] S. Dingare, J. Finkel, M. Nissim, C. Manning and C. Grover (2004), A System For Identifying Named Entities in Biomedical Text: How Results From Two Evaluations Reflect on Both the System and the Evaluations. in 2004

BioLink meeting: Linking Literature, Information and Knowledge for Biology at ISMB 2004. http://nlp.stanford.edu/manning/papers/ismb2004.pdf.
[124] R. Rodriguez-Esteban, I. Iossifov and A. Rzhetsky (2006), PLoS Comput Biol, 2(9):
[125] J. Fleiss (1971), Psychological Bulletin, 76: 378-81
[126] C. Manning and S. H (1999), Foundations of Statistical Natural Language Processing. ed. ed. Vol.: MIT Press.
[127] D. Jurafsky and J. H. Martin (2000), Speech and Language Processing. An introduction to Natural Language Processing, Computational Linguistics and Speech Recognition. ed. ed. Vol., Upper Saddle River, NJ: Prentice-Hall, Inc.
[128] L. Hirschman, A. Yeh, C. Blaschke and A. Valencia (2005), BMC Bioinformatics, 6 Suppl 1: S1
[129] L. Adelman and S. L. Riedel (1997), Handbook For Evaluating Knowledge-Based Systems. ed. ed. Vol., Boston: Kluwer Academic Publishers.
[130] The NeuroScholar SourceForge Project Page [http://www.sourceforge.net/projects/neuroscholar]

3

Intuitionistic Fuzzy Set: Application to Medical Image Segmentation

Tamalika Chaira[1] and Tridib Chaira[2]

[1] India, tchaira@yahoo.com
[2] Ranbaxy Reseach Laboratory, Gurgaon, India
   tridib.chaira@ranbaxy.com

"When everything seems a murky mess
And you are forced to second guess
The way you are headed when you're going straight
And whether you're there on time 'cause early may be late!
When your eyes start playing tricks - it's neither night nor day
But the magic hour; when you just can't fat sure say
The white from the black as mostly all is grey
Take a moment to close your eyes and thank Zedah!
For inventing a way to tell black is black or how tall is tall!
'Cause when chance becomes a possibility, you know you sure can bet
That you're in one group or the other, 'cause you're in a fuzzy set!"
- Sukanto Bhattarcharya

Summary: From year to year the number of investigations on intelligent systems grow rapidly and it reflects the worldwide tendencies for the leading role of the research on intelligent systems theoretically and practically. Object description in medical image often has the property of fuzziness, and with the development of computing, fuzzy logic theory are progressively used in medical image processing. In this chapter, computational intelligence and their applications in medical informatics are the essential topics being covered. From recent publications, it seems that as the area of intuitionistic fuzzy image processing is just beginning to develop, there are hardly few methods in the literature. Intuitionistic fuzzy set theory has been used to extract information by reflecting and modeling the hesitancy present in real-life situations.

Also, a new image segmentation technique using intuitionistic fuzzy set has been proposed and may be applied to many potential real applications such as medical informatics and bioinformatics, where information is imprecise or uncertain. The method has the advantages of high accuracy and flexibility to many situations. Experiments on brain image and blood cell for edge detection; tissue and blood cell for thresholding have proved to be fast and effective method. The method works well even on poor quality image. Lastly, the comparison with proposed intuitionistic fuzzy method and existing fuzzy methods has been shown. It is concluded that the fuzzy approach to the development of artificial intelligence in application systems is beneficial in these contexts because of the need to focus on uncertainty as a main issue.

Key words: Intuitionistic fuzzy set, hesitation degree, edge detection, thresholding

3.1 Introduction

Uncertainty effects all decision making and appears in a number of different forms. The concept of information is fully connected with the concept of uncertainty. The most fundamental aspect of this connection is that uncertainty involved in any problem-solving situation is a result of some information deficiency, which may be incomplete, imprecise, vague or deficient in some other ways and this uncertainty can be solved by using fuzzy set theory. Computerized decision-support tools or computational intelligence can now be used to generate patient specific instructions for therapy that can be carried out with very little interclinician variability. Computational intelligence in medicine systems or precisely medical informatics is created to support healthcare workers in the normal daily duties. Medical informatics is defined as a science developing methods for medical data processing and providing methodologies in the diagnosis and treatment of patients. It covers a variety of disciplines: medical classification and coding, medical image processing, medical decision support and department systems, biostatistics and biosignal analysis, health information systems, medical computer-based education and training, clinical support systems, medical telecommunication and networking. They are best at assisting with tasks that rely on manipulation of data and knowledge and can contribute in many ways to healthcare and patient care. Moreover, computer-based tools can help to discover ways of reducing costs, optimize clinical outcomes, and improve care. Scientific research, quality assessment, and in many instances the day-to-day practice of medicine are almost no longer possible without computers. The end objective of (bio)medical informatics is the coalescing of data, knowledge, and the tools necessary to apply that data and knowledge in the decision-making process, at the time and place that a decision needs to be made. The focus on the structures and algorithms necessary to manipulate the information, separates biomedical informatics from other medical disciplines where information content is the focus. It is the comprehensive application of mathematics (e.g.probability and statistics), science (e.g. biochemistry), and a core set of problem-solving methods (e.g. computer algorithms).

With the advent of digital imaging technology and digital computers, digital image processing has emerged as a practical and useful tool with diverse applications such as biomedical informatics, medical imaging, remote sensing, document imaging, forensic science, and the movie industry. Image processing is the science of manipulating and using images to fulfill some purpose or benefit, such as extracting data automatically or assisting in the human interpretation. The role of image processing is becoming increasingly important in medical imaging as many new digital modalities reach the clinical environment. On the other hand, many difficulties in medical image processing arise because the data/tasks/results are uncertain. This uncertainty, however, is not always due to the randomness but also to the ambiguity and vagueness. Beside randomness, which can be managed by probability theory, the other three kinds of imperfection in the image processing are i) grayness ambiguity, ii) geometrical fuzziness and iii) vague (complex/ill-defined) knowledge.

Since Zadeh [1] in 1965 introduced the concept of fuzzy sets, various notions of higher-order fuzzy sets have been proposed. Among the fuzzy sets and higher order fuzzy sets, intuitionistic fuzzy set has drawn the attention of many researches in the last decades. Thus Atanassov in 1983 [2, 3] introduced the concept of intuitionistic fuzzy set(IFS) theory, which is a generalization of ordinary fuzzy set theory that takes into account the membership degree (degree of belongingness) $\mu_A(x)$ and non-membership degree $\nu_A(x)$. As with ordinary fuzzy set, intuitionistic fuzzy set does not always assign the degree of non-membership equal to 1 minus degree of membership, but there may be some hesitation degree present in defining the membership degree. Hesitation degree is nothing but the lack of knowledge in defining the membership degree. With the insertion of hesitation degree, the membership degree lies in the interval range, i.e., $[\mu_A(x), 1 - \nu_A(x)]$. In this way, a whole spectrum of knowledge not accessible to fuzzy sets can be expressed. Unsurprisingly, their applicability in such various domains as medical informatics, approximate reasoning, expert systems, medical imaging etc. continues to inspire researchers to consider and incorporate them fruitfully into their work.

In this chapter an attempt has been made to overview the computational intelligence in biomedical informatics. Intuitionistic fuzzy set theory and its application on medical images for thresholding and edge detection have also been discussed. Also, a new method on medical image thresholding has been proposed and compared with other intuitionistic fuzzy methods.

The rest of this chapter is organized as follows. Section 3.2 provides a brief overview of related work, with a strong focus on epilepsy detection in electroencephalogram, angiogenesis, and calcification detection in mammogram. Section 3.3 is based on the concept of intuitionistic fuzzy set. Section 3.4 desribes the intuitionistic fuzzy set in segmentation specially in indexedge detection and thresholding. Also some related work on these two types of segmentation is described. Section 3.5 discusses a proposed intuitionistic fuzzy set method on thresholding of medical images using Gamma membership function is described along with the method of computation and it is followed by results and discussion in Section 3.6. Finally, conclusion is drawn in Section 3.7.

3.2 Related work in medical informatics

Computational intelligence in medical practice is undoubtedly a remarkably fast growing fields of research and real-world applications. Computer processing and analysis of medical images covers a broad number of potential topic areas including image acquisition, storage, analysis, and image visualization. To encourage the development of formal computing methods and their application in biomedical research, computer processing has been used in analysing the medical images.

In this section, few applications to medical informatics are overviewed. Kannathal et al. [4] detected the epilepsy in electroencephalogram (EEG). EEG is a signal, mainly the shape of the wave, contains the information in the brain. Since biosignals are highly subjective and appear at random at time scales, computer analysis is very useful in diagnosis. They worked on different entropy estimators to detect the epilepsy. They used spectral entropy which is a normalized form of Shannon's entropy [5], Renyi's entropy [6], Kolmogorov- Sinai entropy [7], and approximate entropy [8]. Shannon's entropy is the spectral complexity of the time series. Using Fourier transformation, power spectral density is obtained and hence the total power at different frequencies is calculated. Data with broad, flat probability distribution will have higher entropy. In higher frequency bands (20-50 Hz), Renyi and Shannon's entropy are similar. KS entropy use time series directly to estimate entropy. It is determined in time series data by finding the points that are closer together in phase space but occurred at different times. These two points help to observe how rapidly they move apart from one another. They used neuro-fuzzy classifier to classify the epilepsy using the entropy measures. The adaptive neuro-fuzzy inference system (ANFIS) uses 81 fuzzy rules. The results show that the entropies of epileptic activity are less than that of non-epileptic activity.

Rodriguez [9] segmented the blood vessels to study the detection angiogenesis which is an important process in a hispathological research. It is a normal process that occurs in all tissues but in pathology the increase in blood vessels is abnormal. For example, in mammary, prostrate, bladder, and brain cancer, the increase in blood vessels leads to the increase severity of the disease. In the study of angiogenesis, pathologists normally analyze through microscope which is very tedious and time-consuming. The easiest way is to use digital image processing to segment the blood vessels. In this, the image is initially filtered using Gaussian filter $g_\sigma(x)$ at different scales i.e. at $\sigma = 0.5, 2, 7$, and 11 and then divided into several windows. The Gaussian filter kernel is expressed in (3.1).

$$g_\sigma(x) = \frac{1}{(2\pi\sigma^2)^{\frac{d}{2}}} e^{\frac{-x^2}{\sigma^2}} \qquad (3.1)$$

where d is the dimension of the domain and σ is the standard deviation of the Gaussian. The threshold is selected by subtracting the standard deviation at each window area from the threshold obtained by Otsu's [10]. Otsu's method is based on discriminant analysis. It separates the pixels into two classes, as object and background, by a threshold level. An optimum threshold is obtained by maximizing the ratio of the between class variance and the within-class variance. A sample result is shown in Fig.

3.1, where the segmentation is carried out with σ = 0.5 and window size 40 × 80 for the image size 160 × 160. Window sizes less than 40 × 80 will pick fine particles and therefore not considered.

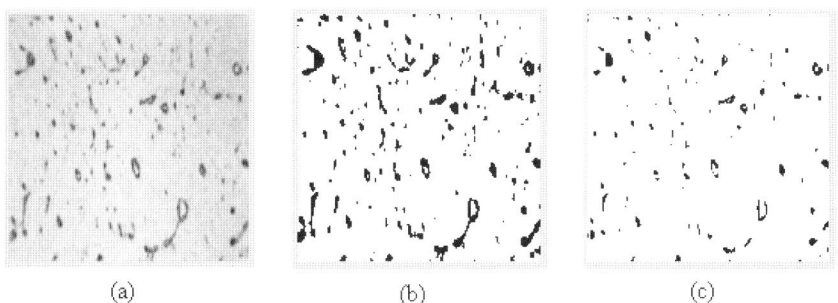

(a)　　　　　　　　　(b)　　　　　　　　　(c)

Fig. 3.1. Blood vessel segmentation, i) original image, ii) Otsu's method, and iii) Rodriguez's method

Arodz et al. [11] detected clustered microcalcification in digital mammography. Initially they filtered the image with 3 × 3 median filter to de-noise the image. Thereafter, they developed a filter to accentuate the standard appearance of this type of lesion. The filter belongs to a family of finite impulse response filter. Such filter produces a sharp responses in places where microcalcification is located by suppressing the lower responses elsewhere. The poor contrast of the mammogram image is enhanced using 2D discrete wavelet transform. Discrete wavelet transform decomposes the image into approximation coefficients and detailed coefficients i.e., horizontal, vertical, and diagonal. The mammograph is then subjected to five level discrete wavelet transform using Daubechis wavelet of order 4. After decomposition, the algorithm performs inverse wavelet transform using these five sets of detailed coefficients. As the microcalcification appear in the image as small, bright spot-like protrusions, wavelet decomposition of the image will contain the microcalcification in the detailed coefficients. The resulting image $I_r(i,j)$ is used to create a mask $M_e(i,j)$ using (3.2).

$$M_e(i,j) = e^{tI_r(i,j)} \quad (3.2)$$

$t > 0$ is used to control the strength of enhancement of the image. Before it is presented to radiologists, the original image is multiplied by the normalized mask to obtain an enhanced image $I_e(i,j)$ as in (3.3).

$$I_e(i,j) = M_e(i,j)I(i,j) \quad (3.3)$$

A sample result is shown in Fig. 3.2.

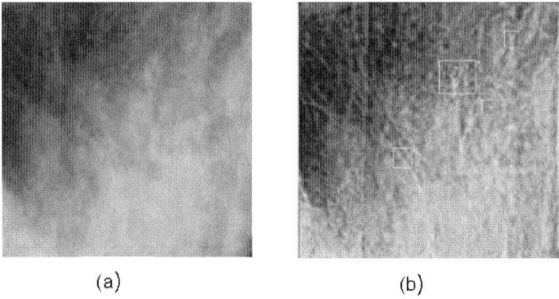

(a)   (b)

Fig. 3.2. Detection of microcalcification (Arodz) i) original image and ii) detection regions in square

3.3 Prelimineries on intuitionistic fuzzy set

In this section, we will briefly describe on intuitionistic fuzzy set. A fuzzy subset A in a finite set X, $[x_1, x_2, x_3 \cdots, x_n]$, may be represented mathematically by:

$$A = \{(x, \mu_A(x)) | x \in X\}$$

where $\mu_A(x)$ is the membership value of an element x in the finite set A. According to Atanassov, an intuitionistic fuzzy subset A in a finite set X may also be represented mathematically by:

$$A = \{(x, \mu_A(x), \nu_A(x)) | x \in X\}$$

where $\mu_A(x), \nu_A(x): X \to [0,1]$ are respectively the membership and non-membership function of an element x in a finite set X with the necessary condition

$$0 \leq \mu_A(x) + \nu_A(x) \leq 1$$

Again, every fuzzy set corresponds to an intuitionistic fuzzy subset:

$$A = \{(x, \mu_A(x), 1 - \nu_A(x)) | x \in X\}$$

Furthermore, in 2000, Szmidt stressed that it is necessary to take into account a third parameter $\pi_A(x)$, known as intuitionistic fuzzy index or hesitation degree (c.f. Atanassov [2], [3], [12]) for calculating the distances between intuitionistic fuzzy sets. So with the introduction of hesitation degree, $\pi_A(x)$, an intuitionistic fuzzy subset A in X may be represented as:

$$A = \{(x, \mu_A(x), \nu_A(x), \pi_A(x)) | x \in X\}$$

with the condition as

$$\mu_A(x) + \nu_A(x) + \pi_A(x) = 1 \qquad (3.4)$$

It is obvious that

$$0 \leq \pi_A(x) \leq 1$$

for each $x \in X$.

3.4 Use of intuitionistic fuzzy set theory in medical informatics - segmentation

Computers and information technology have become major forces in transforming medicine. Segmentation is an important step for any kind of medical image processing. Only after splitting an image into primitives (segmenting), it is possible to address and use the primitives, such as organs or tissues, separately. Pathologists often make diagnostic decisions by observing the specimen cells, particularly, the geometrical properties of cells such as radius, diameter, circumferance etc. Radiologists also diagnose the defects in the CT scanned image of the patient. In an automated system, it is very useful to accurately measure the geometrical properties. Many methods of segmentation are in the literature e.g. edge detection, contour detection, thresholding, and clustering algorithms. Below which are described two segmentation methods of medical images- edge detection and thresholding using intuitionistic fuzzy set theory.

3.4.1 Edge detection

Classification based on gray-scale value can often be useful in medical images e.g. in computed tomography (CT) and magnetic resonance imaging (MRI). Edge detection methods are fundamental to computer vision, because edge detection is often the first stage of a lengthy image interpretation process. Edges characterize boundaries and are therefore a problem of fundamental importance in image processing. Edges in images are areas with strong intensity contrasts, a jump in intensity from one pixel to the next pixel. Edge based segmentation represents a set of methods based on information about edges, found in an image by edge detecting operators. This is usually done with a first and/or second derivative measurement following by a test which marks the pixel as either belonging to an edge or not. The result is a binary image which contains only the detected edge pixels. These operators find out the edges in an image, which are manifested by the discontinuities in gray level, color, textures, etc. There are varieties of edge detection algorithms and edge operators such as Roberts, Sobel, Prewitt etc. [13].

Edge detection is commonly used in medical imaging and mapping applications. It is sometimes used to highlight small and low contrast vascular structures. It is used to increase the contrast between adjacent structures in an image, allowing the viewer to discriminate greater detail and thus helps in detecting many diseases such as prostrate carcinoma etc. The algorithms detect well-localized, unfragmented thin edges in medical images.

There are many fuzzy and crisp edge detection methods in literature [14, 15, 17]. As the area of intuitionistic fuzzy in image processing is just beginning to develop, there are a few work in image processing literature. Chaira et al. [17] suggested an intuitionistic method for edge detection on medical images. They proposed a new distance measure using Attanassov's intuitionistic fuzzy set and used the measure for detecting the edges of an image. In their approach, using intuitionistic fuzzy set theory, a new distance measure is proposed called intuitionistic fuzzy divergence.

Let $A = \{x, \mu_A(x), \nu_A(x) | x \in X\}$ and $B = \{x, \mu_B(x), \nu_B(x) | x \in X\}$ be the two intuitionistic fuzzy sets where $\mu_A(x), \mu_B(x)$ are the membership values and $\nu_A(x), \nu_B(x)$ are the non-membership values. As explained earlier, for intuitionistic fuzzy sets, there may be some hesitation degree present while defining the membership function. If the hesitation degrees are $\pi_A(x)$ and $\pi_B(x)$ such that $\pi_A(x) = 1 - \mu_A(x) - \nu_A(x)$ and $\pi_B(x) = 1 - \mu_B(x) - \nu_B(x)$, the membership values lie in the interval $[\mu_A(x), \mu_A(x) + \pi_A(x)]$ and $[\mu_B(x), \mu_B(x) + \pi_B(x)]$.

For two images A and B at $(i, j)^{th}$ pixels i.e. a_{ij} and b_{ij} of the image, the information of discrimination of images A and B is given as follows:

i) due to $\mu_A(a_{ij})$ and $\mu_B(b_{ij})$ of the $(i, j)^{th}$ of the image:

$$e^{\mu_A(a_{ij})}/e^{\mu_B(b_{ij})} = e^{\mu_A(a_{ij}) - \mu_B(b_{ij})}$$

ii) due to $\mu_A(a_{ij}) + \pi_A(a_{ij})$ and $\mu_B(b_{ij}) + \pi_B(b_{ij})$ of the $(i, j)^{th}$ of the image:

$$e^{\mu_A(a_{ij}) + \pi_A(a_{ij})}/e^{\mu_B(b_{ij}) + \pi_B(b_{ij})}$$

Corresponding to the fuzzy entropy, the discrimination between images A and B due to $\mu_A(a_{ij})$ and $\mu_B(b_{ij})$ may be expressed as:

$$D_1(A, B) = \sum_{i=0}^{M-1} \sum_{j=0}^{M-1} \left[1 - (1 - \mu_A(a_{ij}))e^{(\mu_A(a_{ij}) - \mu_B(b_{ij}))} \right.$$
$$\left. - \mu_A(a_{ij})e^{\mu_B(b_{ij}) - \mu_A(a_{ij})} \right] \quad (3.5)$$

Similarly, the discrimination of B against A may be given as:

$$D_1(B, A) = \sum_{i=0}^{M-1} \sum_{j=0}^{M-1} \left[1 - (1 - \mu_B(b_{ij}))e^{\mu_B(b_{ij}) - \mu_A(a_{ij})} \right.$$
$$\left. - \mu_B(b_{ij})e^{\mu_A(a_{ij}) - \mu_B(b_{ij})} \right] \quad (3.6)$$

Combining (3.5) and (3.6), total divergence or the divergence between the pixels a_{ij} and b_{ij} of the images A and B due to $\mu_A(a_{ij})$ and $\mu_B(b_{ij})$ may be written as:

$$Div - 1(A, B) = D_1(A, B) + D_1(B, A) =$$
$$\sum_{i=0}^{M-1} \sum_{j=0}^{M-1} \left[2 - (1 - \mu_A(a_{ij}) + \mu_B(b_{ij}))e^{\mu_A(a_{ij}) - \mu_B(b_{ij})} \right.$$
$$\left. - (1 - \mu_B(b_{ij}) + \mu_A(a_{ij}))e^{\mu_B(b_{ij}) - \mu_A(a_{ij})} \right] \quad (3.7)$$

In a likewise manner, the divergence between a_{ij} and b_{ij} of the images A and B due to membership values $[\mu_A(a_{ij}) + \pi_A(a_{ij})]$ and $[\mu_B(b_{ij}) + \pi_B(b_{ij})]$ may be given as:

$$Div-2(A,B) = \sum_{i=0}^{M-1}\sum_{j=0}^{M-1}\left[2-(1-(\mu_A(a_{ij})-\mu_B(b_{ij}))+\pi_B(b_{ij})-\pi_A(a_{ij}))\right.$$
$$e^{\mu_A(a_{ij})-\mu_B(b_{ij})-(\pi_B(b_{ij})-\pi_A(a_{ij}))}$$
$$-(1-(\pi_B(b_{ij})-\pi_A(a_{ij}))+\mu_A(a_{ij})-\mu_B(b_{ij}))$$
$$\left.e^{\pi_B(b_{ij})-\pi_A(a_{ij})-(\mu_A(a_{ij})-\mu_B(b_{ij}))}\right] \tag{3.8}$$

Using Hausdorff distance in any two intervals, the intuitionistic fuzzy divergence between two images due to the membership interval range using (3.7) and (3.8) may be written as:

$$D_H(A,B) = \sum_{i=0}^{M-1}\sum_{j=0}^{M-1}\max\left\{2-(1-\mu_A(a_{ij})+\mu_B(b_{ij}))e^{\mu_A(a_{ij})-\mu_B(b_{ij})}\right.$$
$$-(1-\mu_B(b_{ij})+\mu_A(a_{ij}))e^{\mu_B(b_{ij})-\mu_A(a_{ij})},$$
$$2-(1-(\mu_A(a_{ij})-\mu_B(b_{ij}))+\pi_B(b_{ij})-\pi_A(a_{ij}))$$
$$e^{\mu_A(a_{ij})-\mu_B(b_{ij})-(\pi_B(b_{ij})-\pi_A(a_{ij}))}$$
$$-(1-(\pi_B(b_{ij})-\pi_A(a_{ij}))+\mu_A(a_{ij})-\mu_B(b_{ij}))$$
$$\left.e^{\pi_B(b_{ij})-\pi_A(a_{ij})+\mu_B(b_{ij})-\mu_A(a_{ij})}\right\} \tag{3.9}$$

Next, edge detection is performed using (3.9). A set of sixteen fuzzy templates, each of size 3×3, representing the edge profiles of different types are used as in Fig. 3.4.1. The choice of templates is crucial which reflects the type and direction of edges that

0 b a	a a a	a a b	b b b	b a a	b a 0	a 0 b	0 0 0
0 b a	0 0 0	a b 0	0 0 0	0 b a	b a 0	a 0 b	b b b
0 b a	b b b	b 0 0	a a a	0 0 b	b a 0	a 0 b	a a a

a a a	a b 0	0 0 0	0 a b	b b b	b 0 a	b 0 0	0 0 b
b b b	a b 0	a a a	0 a b	a a a	b 0 a	a b 0	0 b a
0 0 0	a b 0	b b b	0 a b	0 0 0	b 0 a	a a b	b a a

Fig. 3.3. A set of sixteen templates

occur. The templates are the examples of the edges, which are also the images. 'a', 'b', and 0 represent the pixels of the edge templates. The values of $a = 0.3$ and $b = 0.8$ are chosen by trial and error method. These values remain same for all the images. It is further observed that on increasing the number of templates beyond 16, there is no remarkable change in the edge results and on decreasing the number of templates, many edges were found missing. With 16 templates all the edges are almost satisfactorily detected. The center of each template is placed at each pixel position (i, j) over a normalized image. The intuitionistic fuzzy divergence measure IFD – measure(i, j) at each pixel position (i, j) in the image, where the template was centered, is calculated between the image window (same size as that of the template) and the template using max-min relationship as follows:

$$\text{IFD} - \text{measure}(i, j) = \max_N [\min_r (\text{IFD}(A, B))]$$

The IFD between A and B, IFD(A,B), is calculated by finding the IFD between each of the elements a_{ij} and b_{ij} of image A and of template B. IFD(a_{ij}, b_{ij}) is the intuitionistic fuzzy divergence measure between each element in the template b_{ij} and those in image window a_{ij}. N is the number of templates and r is the number of elements in the square template, i.e., $3^2 = 9$.

3.4.2 Calculation of membership, non-membership degree and intuitionistic fuzzy index

Here the image represents the chosen window in the test image of same size as template and the image B is the template. Normalized values of the pixel of image A are the membership values, $\mu_A(a_{ij})$, while the values of the template are the membership value of the template $\mu_B(b_{ij})$.

From (3.4), $\mu_A(a_{ij}) + \nu_A(a_{ij}) + \pi_A(a_{ij}) = 1$
     or $\nu_A(a_{ij}) = 1 - \mu_A(a_{ij}) - \pi_A(a_{ij})$
i.e.   non-membership value = 1 – membership – hesitation degree.

The intuitionistic fuzzy index is calculated as:

$$\text{intuitionistic fuzzy index} = c \times (1 - \text{membership}) \quad (3.10)$$

where 'c' is a intuitionistic fuzzy constant. The value of 'c' should be such that (3.4) should hold.

    Hesitation constant 'c' is introduced to edge templates and also to images. For edge template, the hesitation constant is marked as 'c'_t'. But for images, though the images are considered as fuzzy images, the hesitation or the lack of knowledge in the membership values is less. For the edge templates, the hesitation constants are varied to obtain the good edge-detected image. Change in hesitation constants, different edges are detected. The values of hesitation constant 'c' for the images are chosen '0.05'. In each of the images, the values of 'c'_t' and 'th' denote respectively the edge template hesitation constant and the threshold values. Threshold values are obtained by trial and error method only to binarize the image where only the edges will be present. Results with different values of hesitation degree are presented in Figs. 3.4-3.5 and also Canny's [16] edge detected results are shown along with Chaira et al. results. It is observed from the figures, that with intuitionitic fuzzy set, better edge detected images are obtained.

(a) The CT scanned *brain image* of size 316×316 containing the gray and white matter is shown in Fig. 3.4(a). The new matrix as mentioned above has been thresholded, depending on the value of c in the hesitation degree in (3.10), and then thinned. Figure 3.4 shows the edge results on different hesitation constants. It is seen that changing the hesitation degree, desired and better edges are detected. Result with '$c_t = 0.3$' produces better edge detected image as shown in Fig. 3.4(d), where all the edges of the inner part of the brain are clearly detected with the outer edges slightly broken. Results of Chaira et al. is compared with Canny's edge detector. Canny's method shows good outer edges but the edge details of the inner part of the brain are not properly detected.

(b) The *blood image* of size 120×120 is shown in Fig. 3.5(a). Figure 3.5 shows the edge results on different hesitation constants. As above, it is seen that changing the hesitation degree desired and better edges are detected. Better edge detected results are obtained when '$c_t = 0.35$ and more' as shown in Fig. 3.5(d) and Fig. 3.5(e), where all the boundaries are prominent. In Canny's edge detector, the boundaries are not uniformly detected.

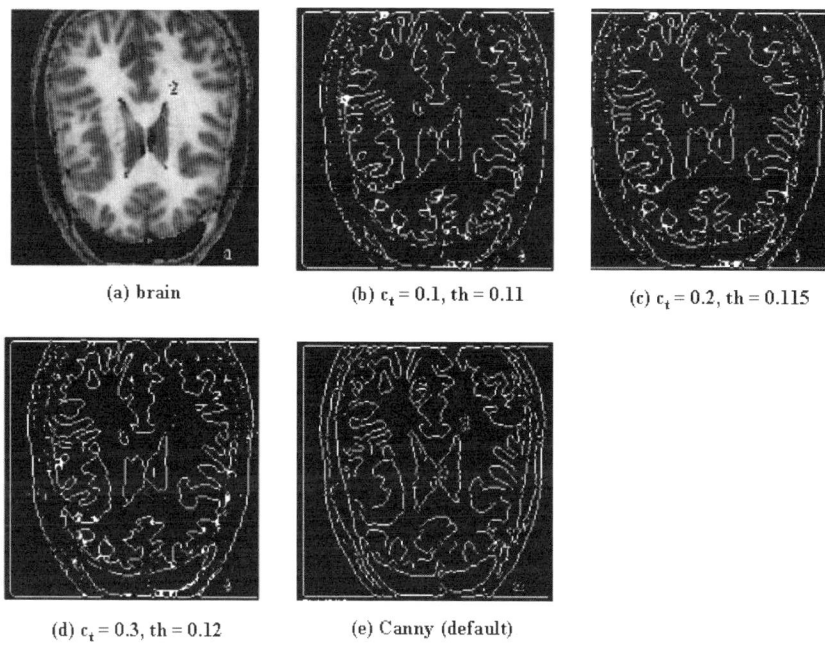

(a) brain (b) $c_t = 0.1$, th = 0.11 (c) $c_t = 0.2$, th = 0.115

(d) $c_t = 0.3$, th = 0.12 (e) Canny (default)

Fig. 3.4. Brain image

3.4.3 Application of intuitionistic fuzzy set theory in image thresholding

Thresholding is a popular tool in image segmentation. This section deals with a segmentation technique that classifies the pixels based on their gray levels. It is a

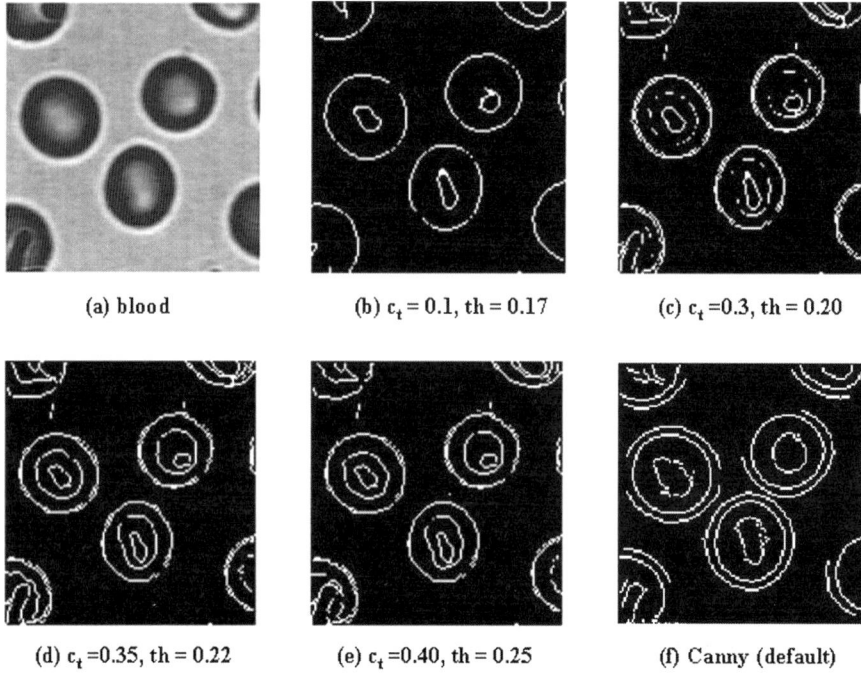

(a) blood (b) $c_t = 0.1$, th = 0.17 (c) $c_t = 0.3$, th = 0.20
(d) $c_t = 0.35$, th = 0.22 (e) $c_t = 0.40$, th = 0.25 (f) Canny (default)

Fig. 3.5. Blood image

simple and oldest segmentation technique and computationally inexpensive but fast. The gray level histogram of the picture should display peaks correspondingly to the two gray levels such as the objects and the background. Choosing a threshold that separates these peaks can thus segment the picture: one for the object and other for the background.

Thresholding is one way to try and separate useful information out of raw data. In medical imaging, this might mean finding a bone in a CT scan of the leg. It works by taking the range of grey shades in an image and redrawing it with only two colours. All shades darker than the threshold value become black, whilst those lighter become white. It is simple yet often effective means for obtaining segmentation in images where different structures have contrast intensities. Surgeons can look at these on computerised displays and interpret them. We want computers to be able to automate, or semi-automate, this expert task.

In pathological side, for many disease detection such as counting the blood cells or blood vessels (for angiogenesis detection), pathologists have to go through a tedious job by counting the cells and blood vessels. In that case, computers are very useful in giving the information which is very fast. We want the computer to be able to pick out the blood cells and blood vessels in the picture by itself. If a voxel has a 'high' intensity, we colour it white, otherwise we colour it black.

Thresholding is a transformation of an input image A into a segmented output image B which is given as follows:

$$bij = \begin{cases} 1 & \text{if } a_{ij} \geq T \\ 0 & \text{if } a_{ij} < T \end{cases}$$

where T is the threshold.
$b_{ij} = 1$, for the image elements which are contributed to the object and $b_{ij} = 0$, for the image elements which are contributed to the background region. If objects are disjoint and their gray levels are clearly distinct from the background, then the thresholding is a suitable segmentation method.

There are many fuzzy and crisp methods in literature [18–20]. As the area of intuitionistic fuzzy in image processing is just beginning to develop, there are a few work in literature. Some of the work in image thresholding are described here. Bustince et el. [21] proposed a technique using intuitionistic fuzzy set theory and restricted equivalence function. They constructed a membership function from restricted equivalence function as:

$$\mu_t(q) = \begin{cases} (1 - 0.5|q - m_b(t)|) & \text{if } a_{ij} \leq t, \text{ for background} \\ (1 - 0.5|q - m_o(t)|) & \text{if } a_{ij} > t, \text{ for object} \end{cases}$$

where $m_b(t)$ and $m_o(t)$ are the means of the background and object regions that are explained in the following section. With this membership function, non-membership function is calculated and an intuitionistic fuzzy set is constructed as:

$$\tilde{A} = \{(x, \mu_A^\alpha(x), 1 - \mu_A^{\frac{1}{\beta}}(x) | x \in X)\}$$

The threshold is selected using intuitionistic fuzzy entropy, $IFE(A_{t\alpha\beta})$, using (3.11).

$$IFE(A_{t\alpha\beta}) = \frac{1}{n} \sum_{k=0}^{L-1} h(q)(\mu_{At}^{\frac{1}{\beta}}(q) - \mu_{At}^\alpha(q)) \qquad (3.11)$$

where L is the total number of gray levels, t is the threshold gray level, q is the gray level, and $\alpha, \beta > 0$.

3.5 The proposed method

In this section, using intuitionistic fuzzy set, a new method that uses Gamma membership function and Hausdorff metric distance measure is proposed for medical image segmentaion.

Let A be an image of size $M \times M$ having L gray levels where $\mu_A(a_{ij})$, $0 \leq \mu_A(a_{ij}) \leq 1$, is the membership value of the $(i, j)^{th}$ pixel in A. Mathematically, the intuitionistic fuzzy image may be represented as

$$A = \{a_{ij}, \mu_A(a_{ij}), \nu_A(a_{ij})\}, \forall a_{ij} \in A$$

Let $'count\, f'$ denotes the number of occurrences of the gray level in the image. Given a certain threshold value t, which separates the object and the background, the average gray level of the background (m_0) and object region (m_1) are respectively given as:

$$m_0 = \frac{\sum_{f=0}^{t} f\, count(f)}{\sum_{f=0}^{t} f\, count(f)}$$

and

$$m_1 = \frac{\sum_{f=t+1}^{L-1} f\, count(f)}{\sum_{f=t+1}^{L-1} f\, count(f)}$$

The membership function of each pixel in the image depends on its affinity to the region to which it belongs. The membership values of the pixels are determined by the proposed Gamma membership function [19] which is another way of representing the membership function as is described below.

The Gamma Membership function

The probability density function of the Gamma distribution is given as

$$f(x) = \frac{(\frac{x-m}{\beta})^{(\gamma-1)} e^{-\frac{x-m}{\beta}}}{\Gamma(\gamma)}, \quad x \geq m; \gamma, \beta > 0 \tag{3.12}$$

where γ is the shape parameter, m is the location parameter β is the scale parameter and Γ is the Gamma function, which is defined as:

$$\Gamma(a) = \int_0^\infty t^{a-1} e^{-t} dt$$

The case where $m = 0$ and $\beta = 1$ is called the standard Gamma distribution. The equation for the standard Gamma distribution reduces to:

$$f(x) = \frac{x^{(\gamma-1)} e^{-x}}{\Gamma(\gamma)}, \quad x \geq 0, \gamma > 0$$

The case when $\beta = 1, \gamma = 1$ and $m \neq 0$, then the Gamma distribution in (3.12) becomes

$$f(x) = \frac{e^{-(x-m)}}{\Gamma(1)} \tag{3.13}$$

Now as the membership values denote the belongingness to a region, or, said in another way that the membership values are more when the pixels belong to the region, the membership function for the background and object is given as:

$$\mu(a_{ij}) = \begin{cases} \frac{e^{-c|a_{ij}-m_0|}}{\Gamma(1)} & \text{if } a_{ij} \leq t, \text{ for background region} \\ \frac{e^{-c|a_{ij}-m_1|}}{\Gamma(1)} & \text{if } a_{ij} > t \text{ for object region} \end{cases}$$

where t is the any chosen threshold and a_{ij} is the $(i,j)^{th}$ pixel in the image A. The constant $c = \frac{1}{max-min}$, where $'max'$ and $'min'$ are the maximum and minimum gray levels of an image and m_0, m_1 are the means of background and object regions as defined above.

Method of computation

Threshold region is chosen from the searching strategy discussed in the next section. For each threshold, membership values and non-membership values of all the pixels in the experimental thresholded image are calculated, and compared with an ideally segmented image [22] using intuitionistic fuzzy divergence. The IFD used in this experiment is (3.9).

For an ideally thresholded image, the membership values $\mu_B(b_{ij})$ are 1, the non-membership values $\nu_B(b_{ij})$ are 0, and the hesitation degrees $\pi_B(b_{ij})$ are 0. Therefore (3.9) may be rewritten as:

$$D_H(A,B) = \sum_{i=0}^{M-1}\sum_{j=0}^{M-1} \max\left\{2 - (1-\mu_A(a_{ij})+1)e^{\mu_A(a_{ij})-1}\right.$$
$$-(1-1+\mu_A(a_{ij}))e^{1-\mu_A(a_{ij})},$$
$$2-(1-(\mu_A(a_{ij})-1)+0-\pi_A(a_{ij}))e^{\mu_A(a_{ij})-1-0+\pi_A(a_{ij}))}$$
$$\left.-(1-(0-\pi_A(a_{ij}))+\mu_A(a_{ij})-1)e^{0-\pi_A(a_{ij})+1-\mu_A(a_{ij})}\right\}$$

$\Longleftrightarrow$

$$D_H(A,B) = \sum_{i=0}^{M-1}\sum_{j=0}^{M-1} \max\left\{2 - (2-\mu_A(a_{ij}))e^{\mu_A(a_{ij})-1}\right.$$
$$-\mu_A(a_{ij})e^{1-\mu_A(a_{ij})},$$
$$2-(2-\mu_A(a_{ij})-\pi_A(a_{ij}))e^{\mu_A(a_{ij})-1+\pi_A(a_{ij}))}$$
$$\left.-(\pi_A(a_{ij})+\mu_A(a_{ij}))e^{1-\pi_A(a_{ij})-\mu_A(a_{ij})}\right\} \quad (3.14)$$

Calculation of the membership value, non-membership value, and hesitation degree are discussed earlier. The hesitation constant 'c' is chosen as 0.2. The threshold value, corresponding to the minimum intuitionistic fuzzy divergence is chosen as the optimum threshold.

3.6 Results and Discussion

Experiments are performed on several images. Two sets of the thresholded images on tissue and blood cells using intuitionistic fuzzy divergence are presented here. In a multimodal histograms, a selection strategy searches threshold values in the region between the two consecutive peaks of the histogram, while in unimodal thresholding linear search is used from minimum to maximum value of the gray level. We have restricted the searching length, so the time required is less. Also, along with the proposed result, the intuitionistic fuzzy method of Bustince et al. is shown for comparison.

a) Figure 3.6(a) is a *hestain* image which is an image of tissue stained with hemotoxylin and eosin. Figure 3.6(b) shows the result using Bustince method where the tissues are not clearly segmented specially at the upper left part of the image i.e. the figure is less segmented. In the proposed intuitionistic fuzzy method in Fig. 3.6(c), all the tissues are clearly segmented and very little noise is present.
b) Figure 3.7(a) shows the image of *blood cell*. Figure 3.7(b) shows the result using Bustince method with noise present mainly at the lower left portion of the image whereas in the proposed intuitionistic fuzzy method in Fig. 3.7(c), all the cells specially in the left lower portion of the image are clearly segmented. So the result with the proposed method is giving better result.

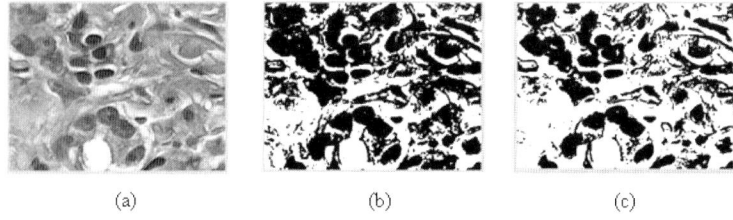

Fig. 3.6. a) hestain image, b) Bustince method, and c) proposed method

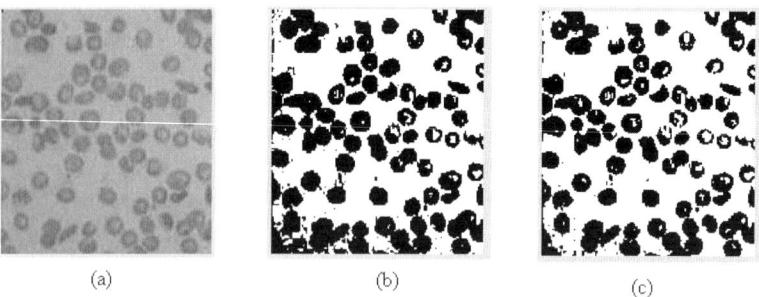

Fig. 3.7. a) blood cell image, b) Bustince method, and c) proposed method

3.7 Conclusions

This chapter overviews the computational intelligence in medical informatics. As intuitionistic fuzzy set theory in image processing is just beginning to develop, so there are hardly few methods in literature. Among them some thresholding and edge detection techniques on medical images are discussed. Also, a new method is proposed using intuitionistic fuzzy set theory to threshold medical images and the results are found better. In our opinion, the use of Atanassov's intuitionistic fuzzy set deals with the uncertainty in the form of hesitation degree when we choose wrong membership degree, and so the results improve when the membership values are adequate and we obtain the results that are similar or better than the fuzzy method.

References

[1] Zadeh LA (1985) Concept of a linguistic variable and its application to approximate reasoning I, II, III, Information Sciences 8: 199-249, 301-357, 43-80.
[2] Atanassov KT (1999) Intuitionistic fuzzy sets, theory and applications. (Series in Fuzziness and Soft Computing), Phisica-Verlag, 1999.
[3] Atanassov KT, Stoeva S (1993) Intuitionistic fuzzy set. in Polish Symposium on Interval and Fuzzy Mathematics, Poznan 23-26.
[4] Kannathal N, Choo ML, Acharya UR, Sadasivan PK (2005) Entropy for detection of epilepsy in EEG. Computer Methods and Programs in Biomedicine 80: 187-194.
[5] Shannon CE (1948) A mathematical theory of communication. Bell System Technical Journal 27: 379-423, 623-656.
[6] Renyi A (1970) Probabilty theory. Americal Elsevier Publishing Co, New York.
[7] Kolmogorov AN (1958) New metric invariant of transitive dynamical systems and endomorphisms of lebesgue spaces. Doklady of Russian Academy of Sciences 119: N5, 861-864.
[8] Pincus SM (1991) Approximate entropy as a measure of system complexity. Proc National Academy of Sciences, USA 88:2297-2301.
[9] Rodriguez R (2006) A stategy for blood vessel segmentation based on threshold which combines statistical and scale space filter: Application to study of angiogenesis. Computer Methods and Programs in Biomedicine 80: 1-1.
[10] Otsu N (1979) A threshold selection method from gray level histograms. IEEE Transactions on Systems, Man, and Cybernetics SMC-9:62-66.
[11] Arodz T, Kurdziel M, Popiela TJ, Sevre EOD, Yuen DA (2006) Detection of clustered microcalcification in small field digital mammography. Computer Methods and Programs in Biomedicine 80: 56-65.
[12] Atanassov KT (1986) Intuitionistic fuzzy set. Fuzzy Sets and Systems: 87-97.
[13] Gonzalez RC and Woods RE (1992) Digital image processing. Addison-Wesley, Reading, M.A.

[14] Ho KHL, Ohnishi N (1995) FEDGE - Fuzzy edge detection by fuzzy categorization and classification of edges. Fuzzy Logic in Artificial Intelligence, 182-196.
[15] Kim TY, Joon JH (1998) Edge representation with fuzzy sets in blurred images. Fuzzy Sets and Systems, 77-87.
[16] Canny J (1986) A Computational approach to edge detection. IEEE Transaction on Pattern Analysis and Machine Intelligence 8(6): 679-698.
[17] Chaira T, De S, Salvetti O (2007) A new measure on intuitionistic fuzzy set using Hausdorff metric and its application to edge detection. The Journal of Fuzzy Mathematics (accepted).
[18] Huang LK, Wang MJJ (1995) Image thresholding by minimizing the measure of fuzziness. Pattern Recognition 28: 41-51.
[19] Chaira T, Ray AK (2004) Threshold selection using fuzzy set theory. Elsevier Pattern Recognition Letters 25(8): 865-874.
[20] Chaira T, Ray AK (2003) Segmentation using fuzzy divergence. Pattern Recognition Letters 24(12): 1837-1844.
[21] Bustince H, Mohedano V, Barrenechea E, Pagola M (2006) An algorithm for calculating the threshold of an image representing the uncertainty through A-IFS. in Proc. of the 11th IPMU International Conference, France.
[22] Chaira T (2004) Image segmentation and color retrieval - a fuzzy and intuitionistic fuzzy set theoretic approach. PhD Thesis, Indian Institute of Technology, Kharagpur, India.

4

Decomposable Aggregability in Population Genetics and Evolutionary Computations: Algorithms and Computational Complexity

Vladik Kreinovich and Max Shpak

University of Texas at El Paso, El Paso, TX 79968, USA vladik@utep.edu, mshpak@utep.edu

Summary Many dynamical systems are *decomposably aggregable* in the sense that one can divide their (micro) variables $x_1, \ldots, x_n$ into several (k) non-overlapping blocks and find combinations $y_1, \ldots, y_k$ of variables from these blocks (*macrovariables*) whose dynamics depend only on the initial values of the macrovariables. For example, the state of a biological population can be described by listing the frequencies x_i of different genotypes i; in this example, the corresponding functions $f_i(x_1, \ldots, x_n)$ describe the effects of mutation, recombination, and natural selection in each generation.

Another example of a system where detecting aggregability is important is a one that describes the dynamics of an evolutionary algorithm – which is formally equivalent to models from population genetics.

For very large systems, finding such an aggregation is often the only way to perform a meaningful analysis of such systems. Since aggregation is important, researchers have been trying to find a general efficient algorithm for detecting aggregability.

In this chapter, we show that in general, detecting aggregability is NP-hard even for linear systems, and thus (unless P=NP), we can only hope to find efficient detection algorithms for specific classes of systems. Moreover, even detecting *approximate* aggregability is NP-hard.

We also show that in the linear case, once the blocks are known, it is possible to efficiently find appropriate linear combinations y_a.

4.1 What is Aggregability

Many systems in nature can be described as *dynamical systems*, in which the state of a system at each moment of time is characterized by the values of (finitely many) variables $x_1, \ldots, x_n$, and the change of the state over time is described by an equation $x'_i = f_i(x_1, \ldots, x_n)$, where

- for continuous-time systems, in which the time t can take any real value, x'_i is the first time derivative of x_i:

$$\frac{dx_i}{dt} = f_i(x_1, \ldots, x_n); \qquad (4.1)$$

- for discrete-time systems, in which the time t can only take integer values, x'_i is the value of x_i at the next moment of time:

$$x_i(t+1) = f_i(x_1(t), \ldots, x_n(t)). \qquad (4.2)$$

For example, the state of a biological population can be described by listing the frequencies x_i of different genotypes i; in this example, the corresponding functions $f_i(x_1, \ldots, x_n)$ describe the effects of mutation, recombination, and natural selection.

For natural systems, the number of variables is often very large. For example, for a system with g loci on a chromosome in which each of these genes can have two possible allelic states, there are $n = 2^g$ possible genotypes. For large g, dues to the large number of state variables, the corresponding dynamics is extremely difficult to analyze.

Many biological systems (and in many systems from other fields such as economics [22] and queuing theory [1] etc.) are *aggregable* in the sense that for appropriate functions $y_a = c_a(x_1, \ldots, x_n)$, $a = 1, \ldots, k$ ($k \ll n$, equations (4.1) or (4.2) lead to simpler equations

$$\frac{dy_a}{dt} = h_a(y_1, \ldots, y_k) \qquad (4.3)$$

or, correspondingly,

$$y_a(t+1) = h_i(y_1(t), \ldots, y_k(t)) \qquad (4.4)$$

for appropriate functions $h_1, \ldots, h_k$.

In other words, if the dynamics of x_i is described by the equation (4.1) or (4.2), then for the resulting dynamics of $y_a = c_a(x_1, \ldots, x_n)$, we have, correspondingly, the equations (4.3) or (4.4).

The corresponding combinations $y_a = c_a(x_1, \ldots, x_n)$ (where c_a are functions from real numbers to real numbers) are called *macrovariables*. If a system is aggregable, then the original variables $x_1, \ldots, x_n$ are also called *microvariables*.

Aggregability property has been actively studied; see, e.g., [1, 9, 10, 12, 17, 18, 20–22]. In most practical cases, the aggregation is *decomposable* in the sense that variables $x_1, \ldots, x_n$ can be divided into non-overlapping blocks $I_1 = \{i(1,1), \ldots, i(1,n_1)\}, \ldots, I_k = \{i(k,1), \ldots, i(k,n_k)\}$ ($\cup I_a = \{1, \ldots, n\}$ and $I_a \cap I_b = \emptyset$ for $a \neq b$) with $n_1, \ldots, n_k$ elements $\left(\sum_{a=1}^{k} n_a = n\right)$ so that each macrovariable y_a depends only on the variables x_i from the a-th block: $y_1 = c_1(x_{i(1,1)}, \ldots, x_{i(1,n_1)}), \ldots, y_k = c_k(x_{i(k,1)}, \ldots, x_{i(k,n_k)})$; see, e.g., [20].

In this case, macrovariables take the form $y_a = c_a(x_{i(a,1)}, \ldots, x_{i(a,n_a)})$, where $I_a = \{i(a,1), \ldots, i(a,n_a)\}$; if the dynamics of x_i is described by the equation (4.1) or (4.2), then for the resulting dynamics of $y_a = c_a(x_{i(a,1)}, \ldots, x_{i(a,n_a)})$, we have, correspondingly, the equations (4.3) or (4.4).

Since most practical aggregable systems are decomposable, in this chapter, we will concentrate on decomposable aggregations. For readability, we will simply refer to decomposable and aggregable systems as *aggregable*.

Comment. In analyzing aggregability, we should take into consideration that perfect aggregability usually occurs only in idealized mathematical models. In many practical situations, we only have *approximate* aggregability, so that the aggregate dynamics (4.3) or (4.4) differs only marginally from the actual microdynamics of the macrovariables variables $y_a = c_a(x_{i(a,1)}, \ldots, x_{i(a,n_a)})$.

Note that many dynamical systems are only approximately aggregable during certain time intervals in their evolution, or over certain subspaces of their state space [10, 22].

4.2 Exact Aggregability: A Simple Example

If there are g genetic loci such that allelic substitutions at each locus have identical effects, then instead of $n = 2^g$ original variables $x_{0\ldots0}, x_{0\ldots1}, \ldots, x_{1\ldots1}$, we can consider $k = g + 1$ ($\ll 2^g$) macrovariables $y_1 = x_{0\ldots0}$ (the frequency of the original state), $y_2 = x_{0\ldots01} + x_{0\ldots010} + \ldots + x_{0\ldots010\ldots0} + \ldots + x_{10\ldots0}$ (the frequency of states with a single mutation), y_3 – overall frequency of states with 2 mutations, ..., $y_{g+1} = x_{1\ldots1}$. This example is described in detail in [19, 20, 23]; let us give a brief description of the simplest case.

In this scenario, we assume that reproduction is asexual, without crossing-over (recombination). We assume the simplest model of non-overlapping generations. In this case, we can select the discrete time variable t in such a way that at moment t, only members of t-th generation are present.

Since there is no crossing-over, the only possible changes in a genotype are caused by mutations. Since individual mutations are rare events, the probability of multiple mutations is negligible. Therefore, in the corresponding first order approximation, we do not consider multiple mutations. In this approximation, each genotype can mutate into g possible *mutational neighbors*, corresponding to the change in each of g cites. For example, a genotype $00\ldots0$ can evolve into one of g mutational neighbors $10\ldots0$, $010\ldots0$, ..., $00\ldots01$. In precise terms, a genotype g' is a mutational neighbor of g if they differ only in one locus, i.e., if the Hamming distance between them is equal to 1.

The per-locus mutation rate, i.e., the probability that a mutation occurs at a given locus, is assumed to be constant; we will denote this constant by μ.

We also make a similar assumption about the *fitness* w_i of the genotype i, i.e., its rate of replication (expected number of offspring of an individual). Specifically, we assume that this fitness w_i depends only on the number of 0s and 1s in the description of i. In evolutionary computation, such a fitness function is called a *function of unitation*; see, e.g., [16] and Chapter 6 of [15]. In population genetics, this fitness function is often called the *Eigen model* after Manfred Eigen's work on error thresholds and quasispecies (see, e.g., [5]).

For this fitness function, we will denote the number of ones in a genotype i by o_i; then, the number of 0s in this genotype is equal to $g - o_i$, and the fitness w_i is equal to $w_i = w(o_i)$.

Let us describe the discrete-time genotype frequency dynamics under these assumptions. It is assumed that at moment t, the (relative) frequency of i-th genotype is equal to $x_i(t)$. Let N be the total number of individuals; this means that out of N individuals, we have $N \cdot x_i(t)$ individuals of genotype i.

The replication rate w_i means that $N \cdot x_i(t)$ individuals of genotype i result, in the next generation, in $w_i \cdot (N \cdot x_i(t))$ individuals. Thus, the total number of individuals in the next generation $t + 1$ is equal to $N(t+1) = \sum_i w_i \cdot (N \cdot x_i(t)) = N(t) \cdot \overline{w}$, where $\overline{w} = \sum_i w_i \cdot x_i(t)$. The ratio $\overline{w} = \dfrac{N(t+1)}{N(t)}$ is called the *mean fitness*.

An individual of the next generation has a genotype i if either its parent had the same genotype and did not mutate, or if its parent had a genotype j which differed from i in a single locus, and it mutated at this locus at which it mutated. The mutation rate at each locus is equal to μ, and we ignore multiple mutations. Thus, the probability that one of g loci mutates is $g \cdot \mu$, and the probability of no mutation is $1 - g \cdot \mu$. As a result, the total number of individuals N_i with genotype i in the next generation can be determined as

$$N_i(t+1) = (1 - g \cdot \mu) \cdot w_i \cdot x_i(t) + \sum_{j \sim i} \mu \cdot x_j(t), \tag{4.5}$$

where $j \sim i$ means that j and i are mutational neighbors (i.e., that their Hamming distance is 1). Dividing the above formula for the number of individuals $N_i(t+1)$ with genotype i by the expression for the total number of individuals $N(t+1)$, and canceling the common factor N in both numerator and denominator, we get the desired formula for the frequencies $x_i(t+1)$ at the next moment of time:

$$x_i(t+1) = \dfrac{1}{\overline{w}} \cdot \left[(1 - g \cdot \mu) \cdot w_i \cdot x_i + \sum_{j \sim i} \mu \cdot w_j \cdot x_j \right], \tag{4.6}$$

where $\overline{w} = \sum_i w_i \cdot x_i$ is the mean fitness.

In this example, it is natural to subdivide all the variables x_i into $g + 1$ blocks $I_1, \ldots, I_{g+1}$, where I_a consists of all genotypes i with $o_i = a - 1$, i.e., with $a - 1$ zeros, and, correspondingly, $g - (a - 1)$ ones. Each genotype i has g neighbors corresponding to a change at one locus. Thus, each genotype i from the class I_a has $a - 1$ mutational neighbors from the class I_{a+1} (with an additional "1") and $g - (a - 1)$ mutational neighbors from the class I_{a-1} (with one fewer "1").

As macrovariables, we can take $y_a = \sum_{i \in I_a} x_i$. Let us find the dynamic equations for these macrovariables. Each genotype i from the class I_a, by definition, has $a - 1$ zeros and $g - (a - 1)$ ones. Since we are only allowing single mutations, there are only three possibility to get this genotype in the next generation:

- One possibility is that we had exactly this genotype in the previous generation, and no mutation occurred. As we have mentioned, the probability that no mutations occurred is equal to $1 - g \cdot \mu$. Thus, the corresponding term in x'_i is $(1 - g \cdot \mu) \cdot x_i$. By adding these terms, we conclude that the corresponding term in $y'_a = \sum_{i \in I_a} x'_i$ is equal to $(1 - g \cdot \mu) \cdot y_a$.

- Another possibility is that we had one more zero, i.e., the original genotype x_j belonged to the class I_{a+1}, and there was a mutation that changed an additional zero to a one. The probability of such a mutation is μ, so the corresponding term in $y'_a = \sum_{i \in I_a} x'_i$ is thus proportional to $\mu \cdot \sum_{j \in I_{a+1}} x_j$. Each genotype $j \in I_{a+1}$, with a zeros, has a possible mutations that lead to a genotype from I_a. Thus, in the formula for $y'_a = \sum_{i \in I_a} x'_i$, we have a occurrences of each term x_j for $j \in I_{a+1}$. So, the corresponding term in y'_a takes the form $a \cdot \mu \cdot y_{a+1}$.

- Finally, it is possible that original genotype x_j belonged to the class I_{a-1}, with one more "1" than in x'_j, and there was a mutation that changed one of its 1s to a zero. The probability of such a mutation is μ, so the corresponding term in $y'_a = \sum_{i \in I_a} x'_i$ is thus proportional to $\mu \cdot \sum_{j \in I_{a-1}} x_j$. Each genotype $j \in I_{a-1}$, with $g - a$ ones, has $g - a$ possible mutations that lead to a genotype from I_a. Thus, in the formula for $y'_a = \sum_{i \in I_a} x'_i$, we have $g - a$ occurrences of each term x_j for $j \in I_{a-1}$. So, the corresponding term in y'_a takes the form $(g - a) \cdot \mu \cdot y_{a-1}$.

We assumed that the fitness w_i of a genotype $i \in I_a$ depends only on the number $a - 1$ of zeros in this genotype, i.e., $w_i = w(a)$ for all $i \in i_a$. Thus, $\overline{w} = \sum_i w_i \cdot x_i = \sum_{a=1}^{g+1} w(a) \cdot y_a$, and the dynamics of the macrovariables y_a takes the form:

$$y_a(t+1) = \frac{1}{\overline{w}} \cdot [(1 - g \cdot \mu) \cdot y_a + a \cdot \mu \cdot y_{a+1} + (g - a) \cdot \mu \cdot y_{a-1}], \quad (4.7)$$

where

$$\overline{w} \stackrel{\text{def}}{=} \sum_{a=1}^{g+1} w(a) \cdot y_a. \quad (4.8)$$

4.3 Detecting Aggregability is Important

In many actual problems, the variables can be subdivided into blocks based on identity or symmetry properties. In the previous example from population genetics (or genetic algorithms), if we know the fitness effects of all the genes, it is natural to group together all the genotypes with similar effects.

Another example of a system where detecting aggregability is important is a one that describes the dynamics of an evolutionary algorithm – which is formally equivalent to models from population genetics. In genetic algorithms, the resulting group of "genes" is called a *schema* [8].

Genetic algorithms are used in bioinformatics for multiple sequence alignment and for a number of other standard bioinformatics applications; see, e.g., [13, 14]. Genetic algorithms are also used in predicting RNA and protein secondary structure.

Other examples of multivariable biological systems where aggregation of variables may prove useful include gene regulatory networks [3], metabolic control theory [6], and community ecology [9]. In all of these systems, there are always blocks of microvariables that behave in a similar or concerted fashion.

In many other situations, however, we only know the equations (4.1) or (4.2) (we may know these equation from the the analysis of the empirical data), but we do not yet know how to properly divide and combine the variables. For example, one may not know the functional role or epistatic interactions of genes on a chromosome a priori, only the phenotypes or Darwinian fitnesses of different genotypes. In such situations, it is important to be able to detect whether an aggregation is possible – and, if possible, to find such an aggregation. The aggregation itself may be instructive as to the function and interaction of genes, and may inform one as to which system components are relevant. For a detailed discussion see, e.g., [1, 9, 10, 12, 17, 18, 20–22]. (The reader should be aware that some of these papers deal with the general notion of aggregability, when blocks may overlap.)

Usually, we have some *partial* information about the variables – e.g., we may know that a certain variable x_i should affect one of the combinations y_a. In such situations, it is desirable to restrict the search to blocks which are consistent with this partial information.

4.4 What We Do in This Chapter

For some special systems with known symmetry properties, there exist efficient techniques that detect decomposable aggregability and find the corresponding aggregations. Since it is important to detect aggregability, researchers have been trying to find a *general* efficient method for its detection.

In this chapter, we show that even in the simplest case when the system is *linear* (i.e., all the dependencies f_i in (4.1), (4.2) are linear), the number of classes is $k = 2$, and the additional information consists of a single variable that has to be involved in one of the combinations y_a, the problem of detecting decomposable aggregability is NP-hard. This means that even for linear systems (unless P=NP), there is no hope of finding a *general* method for detecting decomposable aggregability; we should therefore concentrate our efforts on detecting decomposable aggregability for *specific* classes of dynamic systems.

Comment. For readers who are not very familiar with the notion of NP-hardness, here is a brief and informal explanation.

The complexity of a computational problem is usually described by the computation time that is needed to solve this problem. This time grows with the number of variables (and with the number of bits which are needed to represent each of these variables).

For some computational problems, this time grows as a polynomial of the size n of the input. For example, the standard algorithms for multiplying two $n \times n$ matrices or solving a system of linear equations with n unknowns grows as $\text{const} \cdot n^3$. For large n, this is still feasible. These problems are called *polynomial time* (or P, for short), and the class of such problem is denoted by P.

For some other computational problems, however, the computation time grows exponentially with n, as 2^n or even faster. For example, this growth occurs when we need to search for a subset of the set of n variables, and we need to do an exhaustive search over all 2^n subsets in order to find the desired set. For such algorithms, for reasonable $n \approx 300 - 400$, the number of computational steps exceeds the number of particles in the Universe; thus, such exhaustive-search algorithms are not practically feasible.

In most of these problems, once we have guessed a solution, we can check, in feasible (polynomial) time, whether this guess is indeed a correct solution. Such problems can be "solved" in polynomial time on a hypothetical "non-deterministic" machine, i.e., on a Turing machine that allows non-deterministic (= guess) steps. Because of this possibility, these problems are usually called *non-deterministic polynomial* (NP, for short), and the class of such problems is denoted by NP.

Most computer scientists believe that there are problems in the class NP which cannot be solved in polynomial time, i.e., that NP$\neq$P; however, this has not been proven yet.

Not all the problems from the class of NP are of the same complexity. Some problems from the class NP – e.g., the problem of solving systems of linear equations – are relatively easy in the sense that they can be solved by polynomial time algorithms. Some problem are more difficult than others – because we can reduce every particular case of the first problem to special cases of the second problem. For example, we can reduce solution of a system of linear equations to solving quadratic equations (with 0 coefficients at x_i^2); this means that the general problem of solving systems of quadratic equations is more difficult (or at least not less difficult) than the general problem of solving systems of linear equations.

Some general problems from the class NP are known to be the most difficult ones, in the sense that every other problem from the class NP can be reduced (in the above sense) to this particular problem. Such problems are called *NP-complete*. A similar notion of complexity can be extended to problems outside the class NP, for which we may not know how to check the correctness of the proposed solution in polynomial time. If any problem from the class NP can be reduced to such a problem, then this problem is called *NP-hard*. In these terms, a problem is NP-complete if it is NP-hard and belongs to the class NP.

It is worth mentioning that even if a general problem is NP-hard, its particular instance may be easy to solve. There may be efficient algorithms which solve particular instances from an important subclass of an NP-hard problem, there may be efficient heuristics which, in many cases, solve these problems.

Let us now formulate our results in precise terms. Some of these results were previously presented in [11].

4.5 First Theoretical Result: Detecting Decomposable Aggregability Is NP-Hard

Let us start by presenting the (known) formal definitions of a linear dynamical system.

Definition 1. *Let n be an integer. This integer will be called the* number of microvariables *(or* variables, *for short). These variables will be denoted by $x_1,\ldots,x_n$.*

Definition 2. *Let the number of microvariables n be given. By a* microstate *(or* state*), we mean an n-dimensional vector $x = (x_1,\ldots,x_n)$. By a* trajectory, *we means a function which maps integers t into states $x(t)$. The state $x(t)$ is called* a state at moment t.

Definition 3. *For a given n, by a* linear dynamical system, *we mean an $n \times n$ rational-valued matrix c with entries $c_{i,j}$, $1 \le i \le n$, $1 \le j \le n$. We say that a trajectory $x(t)$ is* consistent *with the linear dynamical system $c_{i,j}$ if for every t, we have*

$$x_i(t+1) = \sum_{j=1}^{n} c_{i,j} \cdot x_j(t). \tag{4.9}$$

Comment. In reality, the coefficients $c_{i,j}$ can be real numbers (not necessarily rational). However, our main objective is to analyze the corresponding algorithms. So, instead of the actual (unknown) value of each coefficient, we can only consider the (approximate) value represented in the computer, and in the computer, usually, only rational numbers are represented.

Now that we have reminded the reader about the formal definition of a dynamical system, let us formally describe what it means for a system to be decomposably aggregable. The main objective of this section is to prove that detecting decomposable aggregability is NP-hard even in the simplest case when we only have two blocks. In view of this objective, to simplify our notations, let us present the definitions of decomposable aggregability only for this case (when we only have 2 blocks I_1 and I_2).

To simplify the situation even more, let us fix a microvariable x_{i_0} (i.e., an index from 1 to n). In a partition, this microvariable can belong either to the first block or to the second block. Without losing generality, let us assume that it belongs to the first block I_1 (if it belong to the second block, we can simply rename the blocks).

Since i_0 belongs to the first block and the blocks do not overlap, only the first macrovariable y_1 can depend on this microvariable. We would also like to avoid a degenerate case in which the macrovariables do not depend on this microvariable x_{i_0} at all, so we require that y_1 actually depend on x_{i_0}. Let us describe this requirement in precise terms.

Definition 4. *Let us fix an index $i_0 \le n$.*

- *By a* 2-partition, *we mean a pair (I_1, I_2) of non-empty sets $I_1 \subseteq \{1,\ldots,n\}$ and $I_2 \subseteq \{1,2,\ldots,n\}$ such that $i_0 \in I_1$, $I_1 \cup I_2 = \{1,\ldots,n\}$, and $I_1 \cap I_2 = \emptyset$.*

- By decomposable aggregation, *we mean a triple* (I_1, I_2, α), *where* (I_1, I_2) *is a 2-partition, and* $\alpha = (\alpha_1, \ldots, \alpha_n)$ *is a tuple for for which* $\alpha_{i_0} \neq 0$.
- *For every microstate* $x = (x_1, \ldots, x_n)$, *by the corresponding* macrostate *we mean a pair* $y = (y_1, y_2)$, *where* $y_a = \sum_{i \in I_a} \alpha_i \cdot x_i$.

Definition 5. *We say that a decomposable aggregation* (I_1, I_2, α) *is consistent with the linear dynamical system* $c_{i,j}$ *if for every moment of time t, when two microstates* $x(t)$ *and* $\tilde{x}(t)$ *correspond to the same macrostate* $y(t) = \tilde{y}(t)$, *then in the next moment of time, the resulting microstates* $x_i(t+1) = \sum_{j=1}^{n} c_{i,j} \cdot x_j(t)$ *and* $\tilde{x}_i(t+1) = \sum_{j=1}^{n} c_{i,j} \cdot \tilde{x}_j(t)$ *also lead to the same macrostate:* $y(t+1) = \tilde{y}(t+1)$.

Comment. In other words, we require that the next macrostate $y(t+1)$ is uniquely determined by the previous macrostate $y(t)$ (and does not depend on a specific microstate $x(t) = (x_1(t), \ldots, x_n(t))$. Since we only consider linear systems, this definition is equivalent to the following:

Definition 6. *We say that a decomposable aggregation* (I_1, I_2, α) *is consistent with the linear dynamical system* $c_{i,j}$ *if there exist values* $h_{a,b}$ ($a = 1, 2$, $b = 1, 2$) *such that for every* $x_1, \ldots, x_n$, $x'_i = \sum_{j=1}^{n} c_{i,j} \cdot x_j$ *implies that*

$$y'_a = \sum_{b=1}^{2} h_{a,b} \cdot y_b, \tag{4.10}$$

where $y_a \stackrel{\text{def}}{=} \sum_{i \in I_a} \alpha_i \cdot x_i$ *and* $y'_a \stackrel{\text{def}}{=} \sum_{i \in I_a} \alpha_i \cdot x'_i$.

Definition 7. *Let* $c_{i,j}$ *be a linear dynamical system and let* i_0 *be a selected index. We say that the pair* (c, i_0) *is* (decomposably) 2-aggregable *if there exists a decomposable aggregation which is consistent with this linear dynamical system.*

Theorem 1. *Detecting decomposable 2-aggregability is NP-hard.*

Comments.

- The computational complexity of the problem comes from the fact that we are looking for decomposable aggregability, when the blocks I_a should be non-overlapping. For general aggregability (not necessarily decomposable), we allow overlapping blocks. In this case, we can easily find the corresponding combinations y_a, e.g., as the coordinates $y_a = \sum x_i \cdot e_i^{(a)}$ of the vector $x = (x_1, \ldots, x_n)$ in the basis formed by the eigenvectors $e^{(a)}$ of the matrix $c_{i,j}$.
- For the readers' convenience, the proofs of all our results are presented in the special (last) section.
- For readers who are more accustomed to matrix notations, a linear combination $\sum \alpha_i \cdot x_i$ can be represented as a matrix product $\alpha^T x$, where α^T denotes a transposition of the vector α.

- In the following text, we prove that for linear systems, once we have found the partition $I_1, \ldots, I_k$, we can then find the corresponding weights α_i in polynomial time. Thus, the problem of detecting decomposable aggregability belongs to the class NP; hence, our theorem actually implies that detecting decomposable 2-aggregability is NP-complete.

4.6 Approximate Aggregability: Possible Definitions

We have mentioned that in mathematical terms, the (exact) aggregability means that the dynamics of the macrovariables y_a is uniquely determined by the macrovariables themselves. For linear systems, this means that for each a, the value y'_a (that describes the dynamics of y_a) is equal to the expression $\sum_{b=1}^{k} h_{a,b} \cdot y_b$ determined only by the values of the macrovariables themselves.

In many practical cases, we do not have *exact* aggregability, we only have an *approximate* one. In other words, the difference Δy_a between the aggregation y'_a of x'_i and $\sum_{b=1}^{k} h_{a,b} \cdot y_b$ should be small.

The macrovariables are defined modulo multiplying by arbitrary scaling constants; so, in principle, for every real number $\delta > 0$, we consider the new macrovariables $Y_a \stackrel{\text{def}}{=} \delta \cdot y_a$. For these new macrovariables, the difference ΔY_a between Y'_a and $\sum_{b=1}^{k} h_{a,b} \cdot Y_b$ is equal to $\delta \cdot \Delta y_a$. Thus, no matter how large the original difference Δy_a is, the new difference ΔY_a can be arbitrarily small if we select an appropriate small value $\delta > 0$. Therefore, to come up with a meaningful definition of approximate aggregability, we must either provide a scale-independent criterion for approximate aggregability or, alternatively, assume that the macrovariables are appropriately scaled.

For linear systems, it is easy to scale the macrovariables in this manner. For example, once we fixed an index i_0, we can take the group that contains i_0 as I_1 (as we did before). Then, we can require that $\alpha_{i_0} = 1$ and that for every $a > 1$, we have $\alpha_i = 1$ for one of the values $i \in I_a$. Clearly, an arbitrary set of macrovariables Y_a can be thus rescaled if we replace Y_1 with $y_1 = Y_1/\alpha_{i_0}$ and Y_a ($a > 1$) with $y_a = Y_a/\alpha_i$ for some $i \in I_a$.

In the following text, we assume that we are looking for thus rescaled macrovariables.

Since both y'_a and $\sum_{b=1}^{2} h_{a,b} \cdot y_b$ depend on the initial state x_i, the difference Δy_a is a function of the variables $x_1, \ldots, x_n$. In particular, for linear systems, Δy_a is a linear function of x_i, i.e., $\Delta y_a = \sum_{i=1}^{n} c_{ai} \cdot x_i$ for some coefficients c_{ai}.

A natural way to describe the smallness of the difference Δy_a is explained in [10] and [20]. Namely, we assume that we know the probability of different possible initial states. It is reasonable to assume that this probability distribution is non-degenerate, i.e., that it is not concentrated on a single surface within the n-dimensional space with probability 1.

In this case, it is natural to say that Δy_a is small if the mean value of its norm is small: $\int \|\Delta y\|^2 \cdot \rho(x)\,dx \le \varepsilon^2$, where $\varepsilon > 0$ is a given small number,

$$\|\Delta y\| = \|(\Delta y_1,\ldots,\Delta y_k)\| = \sqrt{\Delta y_1^2 + \ldots + \Delta y_k^2} \tag{4.11}$$

is the standard Euclidean (l^2-) norm of a vector $\Delta y = (\Delta y_1,\ldots,\Delta y_k)$, and $\rho(x)$ is the probability density corresponding to the actual distribution of the initial states.

In terms of the vector $c = \{c_{ai}\}$ of the coefficients c_{ai}, this definition of smallness can be described as $\|c\| \le \varepsilon$, where

$$\|c\| \stackrel{\text{def}}{=} \sqrt{\int \sum_{a=1}^{k}\left(\sum_{i=1}^{n} c_{ai}\cdot x_i\right)^2 \cdot \rho(x)\,dx}. \tag{4.12}$$

In some practical situations, we do not know the probabilities of different initial states. In such situations, we can define Δy_a to be small if, e.g., $|\Delta y_a| \le \varepsilon \cdot \max_i |x_i|$ for all a. In terms of the vector c, this is equivalent to requiring that $\|c\| \le \varepsilon$, where

$$\|c\| \stackrel{\text{def}}{=} \max_{a,x} \frac{\left|\sum_{i=1}^{n} c_{ai}\cdot x_i\right|}{\max_i |x_i|}. \tag{4.13}$$

These two examples can be naturally generalized. Indeed, in both cases (4.12) and (4.13), we can check that the corresponding "smallness measure" $\|c\|$ is a *norm* on a linear space $\mathbb{R}^{k\cdot n}$ of all $(k\cdot n)$-dimensional vectors $c = \{c_{ai}\}$, in the sense that it satisfies the usual properties of the norm on a vector space (see, e.g., [4]):

- $\|c\| = 0$ if and only if $c_{ai} = 0$ for all a and i;
- for every real number λ and for every vector c, we have $\|\lambda \cdot c\| = |\lambda| \cdot \|c\|$;
- for every two vectors c and c', we have $\|c + c'\| \le \|c\| + \|c'\|$.

Thus, we can give a more general definition of smallness by requiring that $\|c\| \le \varepsilon$ for some norm $\|c\|$.

In some reasonable sense, the resulting definition of approximate aggregability does not depend on the choice of the norm. Indeed, it is known (see, e.g., [4]) that all the norms on a finite-dimensional linear space are equivalent, i.e., that for every two norms $\|\cdot\|_1$ and $\|\cdot\|_2$, there exist real numbers r_{12} and R_{12} such that for every vector c, we have

$$r_{12} \cdot \|c\|_1 \le \|c\|_2 \le R_{12} \cdot \|c\|_1. \tag{4.14}$$

Thus, if we use a norm $\|\cdot\|_1$ to define smallness, i.e., if we require that this norm does not exceed a threshold value ε ($\|c\|_1 \le \varepsilon$), then we can conclude that for this same vector c, the value $\|c\|_2$ of the second norm is also small: it does not exceed the value $\varepsilon' \stackrel{\text{def}}{=} R_{12} \cdot \varepsilon$. When the original threshold ε tends to 0, the new threshold $\varepsilon' = R_{12} \cdot \varepsilon$ tends to 0 as well.

Conversely, if we use a norm $\|\cdot\|_2$ to define smallness, i.e., if we require that this norm does not exceed a threshold value ε ($\|c\|_2 \leq \varepsilon$), then we can conclude that for the same vector c, the value $\|c\|_1$ of the first norm is also small: it does not exceed the value $\varepsilon'' \stackrel{\text{def}}{=} R_{21} \cdot \varepsilon$. When the original threshold ε tends to 0, the new threshold $\varepsilon'' = R_{21} \cdot \varepsilon$ tends to 0 as well.

In view of this equivalence, in the following text, we will provide the detailed proof for only one norm. Proofs for other norms are similar.

Comment. Approximate aggregability means, crudely speaking, that for the same initial state $x_i(0)$, the values of the macrovariables $y_a(1)$ after a one-step iteration of the actual system are close to the result $y_a^{\text{aggr}}(1)$ of the one-step iteration of the corresponding aggregable system. From this, we can conclude that the values of the macrovariables $y_a(2)$ after a two-step iteration of the actual system are close to $y_a^{\text{aggr}}(2)$, and that the same is true for an arbitrary (fixed) number of steps t.

It should be mentioned, however, that in many important cases, the difference between the values $y_a(t)$ and $y^{\text{aggr}}(t)$ grows with time t. So, if we fix the initial state $x_i(0)$ and a threshold ε, then the values $y_a(t)$ and $y^{\text{aggr}}(t)$ are ε-close only until some critical time t_{critical}; after this critical time, the difference exceeds the desired threshold.

4.7 Second Theoretical Result: Detecting Approximate Decomposable Aggregability Is Also NP-Hard

Let us show that detecting *approximate* decomposable aggregability is also NP-hard, even in the simplest case of 2-aggregability ($k = 2$). As we have mentioned, in the linear case, macrovariables are defined modulo multiplying by arbitrary scaling constants; so, by applying appropriate "normalizing" re-scaling, we can safely assume, e.g., that $\alpha_{i_0} = 1$ for $i_0 \in I_1$ and that $\alpha_i = 1$ for some $i \in I_2$. Instead of requiring that the dynamics of the macrovariables y_a is uniquely determined by the macrovariables themselves, we can now require that the difference between y'_a and $\sum_{b=1}^{2} h_{a,b} \cdot y_b$ should be small, i.e., that the absolute value of this difference does not exceed $\varepsilon \cdot \max |x_i|$ for some small ε. We thus arrive at the following definition.

Definition 8. *We say that a decomposable aggregation (I_1, I_2, α) is normalized if $\alpha_{i_0} = 1$ and $\alpha_i = 1$ for some $i \in I_2$.*

Definition 9. *Let $\varepsilon > 0$ be a real number. We say that a normalized decomposable aggregation (I_1, I_2, α) is ε-consistent with the linear dynamical system $c_{i,j}$ if there exist values $h_{a,b}$ ($a = 1, 2$, $b = 1, 2$) such that for every $x_1, \ldots, x_n$, $x'_i = \sum_{j=1}^{n} c_{i,j} \cdot x_j$ implies that $\left| y'_a - \sum_{b=1}^{2} h_{a,b} \cdot y_b \right| \leq \varepsilon \cdot \max_i |x_i|$, where*

$$y_a \stackrel{\text{def}}{=} \sum_{i \in I_a} \alpha_i \cdot x_i, \quad y'_a \stackrel{\text{def}}{=} \sum_{i \in I_a} \alpha_i \cdot x'_i. \tag{4.15}$$

Definition 10. *Let $c_{i,j}$ be a linear dynamical system, let i_0 be a selected index, and let $\varepsilon > 0$ be a real number. We say that the pair (c, i_0) is ε-approximately (decomposably) 2-aggregable if there exists a decomposable aggregation which is ε-consistent with this linear dynamical system.*

Theorem 2. *Detecting approximate decomposable 2-aggregability is NP-hard.*

Comment. We have already mentioned that all norms on $\mathbb{R}^n$ are equivalent. Thus, the proof of our result can be easily modified into a proof that we if we use other norm-based definitions of approximate decomposable aggregability, e.g., for the definition from [10], then detecting approximate decomposable aggregability is also NP-hard.

4.8 Once We Find the Partition, Finding the Combinations is Feasible

4.8.1 Algorithm

We have shown that finding the partition is NP-hard. Our original problem was not only to find a partition, but also to find the appropriate combinations y_a. Let us show that, in the linear case, once the partition is found, finding the weights of the corresponding combinations y_a is easy.

Indeed, in matrix terms, the original dynamic equation has the form $x' = cx$. Once the partition $I_1, \ldots, I_k$ is fixed, we can represent each n-dimensional state vector x as a combination of vectors $x^{(a)}$ formed by the components x_i, $i \in I_a$. In these terms, the equation $x' = cx$ can be represented as $x'^{(a)} = \sum_b c^{(a),(b)} x^{(b)}$, where $c^{(a),(b)}$ denotes the corresponding block of the matrix c (formed by elements $c_{i,j}$ with $i \in I_a$ and $j \in I_b$). For the corresponding linear combinations $y_a = \alpha^{(a)T} x^{(a)}$, the dynamics takes the form $y'_a = \sum_b \alpha^{(a)T} c^{(a),(b)} x^{(b)}$. The only possibility for this expression to only depend on the combinations $y_b = \alpha^{(b)T} x^{(b)}$ is when for each b, the coefficients of the dependence of y'_a on x_i, $i \in I_b$, are proportional to the corresponding weights α_i, i.e., when for every a and b, we have $\alpha^{(a)T} c^{(a),(b)} = \lambda_{a,b} \alpha^{(b)T}$ for some number $\lambda_{a,b}$. By transposing this relation, we conclude that

$$c^{(a),(b)T} \alpha^{(a)} = \lambda_{a,b} \alpha^{(b)}. \tag{4.16}$$

In particular, for $a = b$, we conclude that $\alpha^{(a)}$ is an eigenvector of the matrix $c^{(a),(a)T}$. Since the weight vectors $\alpha^{(a)}$ are defined modulo a scalar factor, we can thus select one of the (easy-to-compute) eigenvectors of $c^{(a),(a)T}$ as $\alpha^{(a)}$.

Once we know $\alpha^{(a)}$ for one a, we can determine all other weight vectors $\alpha^{(b)}$ from the condition (4.16), i.e., as $\alpha^{(b)} = c^{(a),(b)T} \alpha^{(a)}$.

Comment. A similar – but more complex – algorithms can be used in the nonlinear case as well. We will describe this nonlinear generalization in detail in a forthcoming paper.

4.8.2 Calculating aggregate dynamics

Once we know the partitions I_a and the corresponding weights $y_a = \sum_{i \in I_a} \alpha_i \cdot x_i$, we can use the results from [20] to calculate the coefficients $h_{a,b}$ that describe the aggregate dynamics $y'_a = \sum_b h_{a,b} \cdot y_b$. Namely, if we describe a $k \times n$ matrix α as $\alpha_{a,i} = \alpha_i^{(a)}$ if $i \in I_a$ and 0 otherwise, then $h = \alpha c \alpha^T (\alpha \alpha^T)^{-1}$.

4.8.3 Example

We now illustrate this algorithm on the above simple example, i.e., selection-mutation system where the fitness of each genotype depends only on the number of 0s and 1s.

It is assumed that we already know the partition of microvariables into clusters $I_1 = \{0\ldots0\}, I_2 = \{10\ldots0, 010\ldots0, \ldots, 0\ldots01\}$, etc. For each of these clusters, we consider the linear space whose dimension is equal to the number of microvariables in each cluster: the linear space corresponding to I_1 has dimension 1, the linear space corresponding to cluster I_2 has dimension g, the linear space corresponding to cluster I_3 has dimension $\dfrac{g \cdot (g-1)}{2}$, etc. The simplest, thus, easiest-to-analyze space is the space corresponding to I_1. For this space, the corresponding 1×1 matrix $c_{ij}^{(1),(1)}$ consists of the single element $1 - g \cdot \mu$, and so, its eigenvector is the 1-element vector $\alpha_i = \alpha_{0\ldots0} = 1$.

According to our algorithm, we can now find the weights α_i for $i \in I_2$ by considering equation (4.16) for the matrix $c_{ij}^{(2),(1)}$. For each genotype $i \in I_2$ with one "1" and for the genotype $i \in I_1$ with all 0s, the term $c_{ij} \cdot x_j$ in the expression for $x'_i = x_i(t+1)$ is the same, i.e., $c_{ij}^{(2),(1)} =$ const. Thus, because of the formula (4.16), all the elements i for $i \in I_2$ have the same weight: $\alpha_i =$ const. So, the combination $y_2 = \sum_{i \in I_2} \alpha_i \cdot x_i$ is proportional to the sum $\sum_{i \in I_2} x_i$.

Similarly, by applying the formula (4.16) to the matrix $c_{ij}^{(3),(2)}$, we conclude that the weights α_i of all the genotypes $i \in I_3$ are also equal to each other, i.e., that the combination $y_3 = \sum_{i \in I_3} \alpha_i \cdot x_i$ is also proportional to the sum $\sum_{i \in I_3} x_i$, etc. Eventually, we will conclude that for each a, the macrovariable y_a is proportional to $\sum_{i \in I_a} x_i$ – i.e., we get exactly the aggregation which is, as we have shown, consistent with the system's dynamics.

In this example, In this example, the matrix formula for h in terms of α and c [20] discussed in the previous subsection leads to the desired aggregate dynamics from Section 2.

4.8.4 What to Do in the Case of Approximate Aggregation

In the previous sections, we assumed that we know the partition for which an exact aggregation is possible, and we described n algorithm for finding the weights (i.e., macrovariables) corresponding to the exact aggregation. In practice, the aggregation is rarely exact. So, a more realistic setting is as follows: we know the partition, we must find the macrovariables that provide the approximate aggregation.

A natural way to proceed is to assume that the aggregation is exact and use the above algorithm to find the weights corresponding to this assumption.

It is reasonable to apply this heuristic algorithm for all the approximate aggregation situations. Moreover, it has been shown that for many reasonable continuous-time [9, 10] and discrete-time systems ([20], pp. 40–41), this approach leads to the best possible approximation.

4.9 Proofs

4.9.1 Proof of Theorem 1

As we have mentioned earlier, NP-hardness of a general problem means that any problem from the class NP can be reduced to this problem. Some problems are already known to be NP-hard. An example of such a problem is a *subset problem* (see, e.g., [7]). The subset problem is as follows: given n positive integers $s_1, \ldots, s_m$ and a positive integer s_0, whether there exists a subset $I \subseteq \{1, \ldots, m\}$ such that $\sum_{i \in I} s_i = s_0$.

In order to prove that our problem is NP-hard, it is therefore sufficient to show that the subset problem can be reduced to our problem. Since we already know that every problem from the class NP can be reduced to the subset problem, and the subset problem can be reduced to our problem, then we will be able to conclude that an arbitrary problem from the class NP can be reduced to our problem – i.e., that our problem is indeed NP-hard.

Therefore, to prove our theorem, it is sufficient to prove that the subset problem can be reduced to the problem of checking 2-aggregability, i.e., that for every instance of the subset problem, we can find an equivalent instance of the 2-aggregation problem. Let us show how this can be done.

The subset problem does not have a solution if $s_0 > \sum_{i=1}^{m} s_i$, so it is sufficient to consider only instances of the subset problem for which $s_0 \leq \sum_{i=1}^{m} s_i$. When $s_0 = \sum_{i=1}^{m} s_i$, then $I = \{1, \ldots, m\}$ is an obvious solution. Thus, it is sufficient to only consider instances of this problem for which $s_0 < \sum_{i=1}^{m} s_i$, i.e. (since s_0 and s_i are integers), for which $s_0 \leq \sum_{i=1}^{m} s_i - 1$.

For every instance of the subset problem that satisfies this condition, we take $s_{m+1} \stackrel{\text{def}}{=} -s_0$, $n = m+2$, $i_0 = m+2$, and we form the following linear system:

- for $1 \leq i \leq m+1$, we take $c_{i,i} = 1$, $c_{i,n+1} = s_i$, and $c_{i,j} = 0$ for all other j;

- for $i = m+2$, we take $c_{m+2,m+2} = 1 + \beta$, where $\beta \stackrel{\text{def}}{=} 1 + s_0 - \sum_{i=1}^{m} s_i$, and $c_{m+2,i} = 1$ for all other i.

Since $s_0 \leq \sum_{i=1}^{m} s_i - 1$, we have $\beta \leq 0$.

Let us prove that this system is consistent if and only if the original instance of the subset problem has a solution.

"If" part.

If the original instance has a solution I, with $CI \stackrel{\text{def}}{=} \{1,\ldots,m\} - I$, then we take $I_1 = CI \cup \{m+2\}$, $I_2 = I \cup \{m+1\}$, $\alpha_i = 1$ for all i, $h_{1,1} = 2$, $h_{1,2} = h_{2,2} = 1$, and $h_{2,1} = 0$. Then, we should have $y_1' = 2y_1 + y_2$ and $y_2' = y_2$.

Indeed, the fact that I is a solution means that $\sum_{i \in I} s_i = s_0$. For our choice of weights α_i, we get $y_1 = \sum_{i \in CI} x_i + x_{m+2}$ and $y_2 = \sum_{i \in I} x_i + x_{m+1}$. For y_2', we get

$$y_2' = \sum_{i \in I} x_i' + x_{m+1}' = \sum_{i \in CI} x_i + x_{m+1} + \left(\sum_{i \in I} -s_0\right) \cdot x_{m+2}. \quad (4.17)$$

Since $\sum_{i \in I} s_i = s_0$, we conclude that $y_2' = y_2$.

Similarly,

$$y_1' = \sum_{i \in CI} x_i' + x_{m+2}'. \quad (4.18)$$

Describing the sum $\sum_{i=1}^{m+2} x_i$ in the expression for x_{m+2}' as the sum of the values from I, CI, $m+1$, and $m+2$, we conclude that

$$y_1' = \sum_{i \in CI} x_i + \left(\sum_{i \in CI} s_i\right) \cdot x_{m+2} + \sum_{i \in CI} x_i + \sum_{i \in I} x_i + x_{m+1} + x_{m+2} + \beta \cdot x_{m+2} =$$

$$\left(\sum_{i \in I} x_i + x_{m+1}\right) + 2 \cdot \sum_{i \in CI} x_i + \left(\sum_{i \in CI} s_i + 1 + \beta\right) \cdot x_{m+2}. \quad (4.19)$$

Since $\sum_{i \in I} s_i = s_0$, we have $\sum_{i \in CI} s_i = \sum_{i=1}^{m} s_i - \sum_{i \in I} s_i = \sum_{i=1}^{m} s_i - s_0$. Due to our choice of β, we thus have $\sum_{i \in CI} s_i + 1 + \beta = 2$, hence $y_1' = 2y_1 + y_2$.

"Only if" part.

Conversely, let us assume that the system is 2-aggregable, i.e., that there exist sets $I_1 \ni m+2$, and the values α_i and $h_{a,b}$ for which all the above conditions are satisfied. In other words, $\alpha_{m+2} \neq 0$, and from the equations

$$x_i' = x_i + s_i \cdot x_{m+2}, \quad 1 \leq i \leq m+1, \quad (4.20)$$

4 Aggregability: Algorithms and Computational Complexity

$$x'_{m+2} = \sum_{i=1}^{m+2} x_i + \beta \cdot x_{m+2}, \qquad (4.21)$$

we should be able to conclude that for

$$y_1 = \sum_{i \in I_1} \alpha_i \cdot x_i, \quad y_2 = \sum_{i \in I_2} \alpha_i \cdot x_i, \qquad (4.22)$$

$$y'_1 = \sum_{i \in I_1} \alpha_i \cdot x'_i, \quad y'_2 = \sum_{i \in I_2} \alpha_i \cdot x'_i, \qquad (4.23)$$

we have

$$y'_1 = h_{1,1} \cdot y_1 + h_{1,2} \cdot y_2 \qquad (4.24)$$

and

$$y'_2 = h_{2,1} \cdot y_1 + h_{2,2} \cdot y_2. \qquad (4.25)$$

Let us denote $I'_1 \stackrel{\text{def}}{=} I_1 - \{m+2\}$. From (4.20), (4.21), and (4.23), we conclude that

$$y'_1 = \sum_{i \in I'_1} \alpha_i \cdot x_i + \left(\sum_{i \in I'_1} \alpha_i \cdot s_i \right) \cdot x_{m+2} + \alpha_{m+2} \cdot \sum_{i=1}^{m+2} x_i + \alpha_{m+2} \cdot \beta \cdot x_{m+2}. \qquad (4.26)$$

Thus, the equation (4.24) takes the form

$$\sum_{i \in I'_1} \alpha_i \cdot x_i + \left(\sum_{i \in I'_1} \alpha_i \cdot s_i \right) \cdot x_{m+2} + \alpha_{m+2} \cdot \sum_{i=1}^{m+2} x_i + \alpha_{m+2} \cdot \beta \cdot x_{m+2} = $$

$$h_{1,1} \cdot \left(\sum_{i \in I'_1} \alpha_i \cdot x_i + \alpha_{m+2} \cdot x_{m+2} \right) + h_{1,2} \cdot \sum_{i \in I_2} \alpha_i \cdot x_i. \qquad (4.27)$$

Since this equality must hold for all possible values of x_i, for each i, the coefficient at x_i in the left-hand side of (4.27) must be equal to the coefficient at x_i in the right-hand side of (4.27).

In particular, for $i \in I'_1$, we conclude that $\alpha_i + \alpha_{m+2} = h_{1,1} \cdot \alpha_i$, i.e., that $(h_{1,1} - 1) \cdot \alpha_i = \alpha_{m+2}$. Since $\alpha_{m+2} \neq 0$, we conclude that $\alpha_i \neq 0$ and $h_{1,1} - 1 \neq 0$, hence $\alpha_i = \alpha_{m+2}/(h_{1,1} - 1)$ for all such i – i.e., all the values α_i, $i \in I'_1$ are equal to each other. Let us denote the common value of these α_i by $\alpha^{(1)} \neq 0$.

For $i \in I_2$, we similarly conclude that $\alpha_{m+2} = h_{1,2} \cdot \alpha_i$. Since $\alpha_{m+2} \neq 0$, we similarly conclude that $\alpha_i \neq 0$, and that $\alpha_i = \alpha_{m+2}/h_{1,2}$ is the same for all $i \in I_2$. Let us denote the common value of these α_i by $\alpha^{(2)} \neq 0$. Thus, the formulas (4.22)–(4.23) take the following form:

$$y_1 = \alpha^{(1)} \cdot \sum_{i \in I'_1} x_i + \alpha_{m+2} \cdot x_{m+2}, \quad y_2 = \alpha^{(2)} \cdot \sum_{i \in I_2} x_i, \qquad (4.28)$$

$$y'_1 = \alpha^{(1)} \cdot \sum_{i \in I'_1} x'_i + \alpha_{m+2} \cdot x'_{m+2}, \quad y'_2 = \alpha^{(2)} \cdot \sum_{i \in I_2} x'_i. \tag{4.29}$$

By using the expressions (4.20)–(4.22) and (9a), we conclude that y'_2 takes the form

$$y'_2 = \alpha^{(2)} \cdot \sum_{i \in I_2} x_i + \alpha^{(2)} \cdot \left(\sum_{i \in I_2} s_i \right) \cdot x_{m+2}. \tag{4.30}$$

Thus, the equation (4.25) takes the form

$$\alpha^{(2)} \cdot \sum_{i \in I_2} x_i + \alpha^{(2)} \cdot \left(\sum_{i \in I_2} s_i \right) \cdot x_{m+2} =$$

$$h_{2,1} \cdot \left(\alpha^{(1)} \cdot \sum_{i \in I'_1} x_i + \alpha_{m+2} \cdot x_{m+2} \right) + h_{2,2} \cdot \alpha^{(2)} \cdot \sum_{i \in I_2} x_i. \tag{4.31}$$

For $i \in I'_1$, by equating coefficients at x_i in both sides of (4.31), we conclude that $h_{2,1} \cdot \alpha^{(1)} = 0$. Since $\alpha^{(1)} \neq 0$, we thus conclude that $h_{2,1} = 0$. By comparing coefficients at x_{m+2}, we now conclude that $\alpha^{(2)} \cdot \sum_{i \in I_2} s_i = 0$. Since $\alpha^{(2)} \neq 0$, we thus conclude that $\sum_{i \in I_2} s_i = 0$. Since all the values s_i are positive except for $s_{m+1} = -s_0$, the only possibility to have $\sum_{i \in I_2} = 0$ is when $m+1 \in I_2$. In this case, for $I \stackrel{\text{def}}{=} I_2 - \{m+1\}$, we get $\sum_{i \in I} s_i + (-s_0) = 0$, i.e., $\sum_{i \in I} s_i = s_0$. So, the original instance of the subset problem has a solution.

This completes the proof of the theorem.

4.9.2 Proof of Theorem 2

To prove NP-hardness of approximate 2-aggregability, we use the same reduction to subset problem that we used in Theorem 1. Namely, for every instance of the subset problem, we define the same linear system: as in the previous proof; we will show that this system is approximately 2-aggregable if and only if the original instance of the subset problem has a solution.

We have already shown that if the original instance has a solution I, then the corresponding system is 2-aggregable and therefore, approximately 2-aggregable.

Conversely, let us assume that the system is approximately 2-aggregable, i.e., that there exist sets $I_1 \ni m+2$ and I_2, and the values α_i and $h_{a,b}$ for which all the above conditions are satisfied. In other words, $\alpha_{m+2} = 1$, and from the equations (4.20) and (4.21), we should be able to conclude that for the values y_a and y'_a we have

$$|y'_1 - h_{1,1} \cdot y_1 - h_{1,2} \cdot y_2| \leq \varepsilon \cdot \max_i |x_i| \tag{4.32}$$

and

4 Aggregability: Algorithms and Computational Complexity

$$|y'_2 - h_{2,1} \cdot y_1 - h_{2,2} \cdot y_2| \leq \varepsilon \cdot \max_i |x_i|. \quad (4.33)$$

By using the expression for y'_1 from the previous proof, and taking into account that $\alpha_{m+2} = 1$, we conclude that the condition (4.32) takes the form

$$\left| \sum_{i \in I'_1} \alpha_i \cdot x_i + \left(\sum_{i \in I'_1} \alpha_i \cdot s_i \right) \cdot x_{m+2} + \sum_{i=1}^{m+2} x_i + \beta \cdot x_{m+2} - h_{1,1} \cdot \left(\sum_{i \in I'_1} \alpha_i \cdot x_i + x_{m+2} \right) - h_{1,2} \cdot \sum_{i \in I_2} \alpha_i \cdot x_i \right| \leq \varepsilon \cdot \max_i |x_i|. \quad (4.34)$$

This inequality must hold for all possible values of x_i. In particular, for each i, we can take $x_i = 1$ and $x_j = 0$ for all $j \neq i$, and conclude that the coefficient at x_i at the left-hand side of (4.34) should not exceed ε.

In particular, for $i \in I'_1$, we conclude that

$$|\alpha_i \cdot (1 - h_{1,1}) + 1| \leq \varepsilon. \quad (4.35)$$

For $i \in I_2$, we conclude that

$$|1 - h_{1,2} \cdot \alpha_i| \leq \varepsilon, \quad (4.36)$$

and for $i = m+2$, we conclude that

$$\left| \sum_{i \in I'_1} \alpha_i \cdot s_i + 1 + \beta - h_{1,1} \right| \leq \varepsilon. \quad (4.37)$$

Let us first use (4.35) to prove, by reduction to a contradiction, that $|h_{1,1}| \leq \sum_{i=1}^{m} s_i + 1$. In this proof, we will use the known fact that for every two numbers b and c, we have $||b| - |c|| \leq |b+c| \leq |b| + |c|$.

Indeed, suppose that $|h_{1,1}| > \sum_{i=1}^{m} s_i + 1$; then $|1 - h_{1,1}| \geq ||h_{1,1}| - 1| = \sum_{i=1}^{m} s_i$. From (4.35), we conclude that $|\alpha_i| \cdot |1 - h_{1,1}| \leq 1 + \varepsilon$, hence $|\alpha_i| \leq \dfrac{1+\varepsilon}{\sum_{i=1}^{m} s_i}$. Thus,

$$\left| \sum_{i=1}^{m} \alpha_i \cdot s_i \right| \leq \sum_{i=1}^{m} |\alpha_i| \cdot s_i \leq \sum_{i=1}^{m} s_i \cdot \frac{1+\varepsilon}{\sum_{i=1}^{m} s_i} = 1 + \varepsilon. \quad (4.38)$$

Since we assumed that $|h_{1,1}| > \sum_{i=1}^{m} s_i + 1$ and we know that $\beta \leq 0$, we conclude that

$$\left| h_{1,1} - 1 - \beta - \sum_{i=1}^{m} \alpha_i \cdot s_i \right| > \left(\sum_{i=1}^{m} s_i + 1 \right) - 1 - (-\beta) - (1+\varepsilon). \quad (4.39)$$

Substituting $\beta = 1 + s_0 - \sum_{i=1}^{m}$ into this expression, we conclude that

$$\left| h_{1,1} - \beta - \sum_{i=1}^{m} \alpha_i \cdot s_i \right| > s_0 - \varepsilon. \tag{4.40}$$

Since s_0 is a positive integer, we have $s_0 - \varepsilon > 1 - \varepsilon$; so for $\varepsilon < \dfrac{1}{2}$, we get $s_0 - \varepsilon > \dfrac{1}{2} > \varepsilon$ and thus, $\left| h_{1,1} - 1 - \beta - \sum_{i=1}^{m} \alpha_i \cdot s_i \right| > \varepsilon$, which contradicts to the inequality (4.37).

This contradiction shows that $|h_{1,1}|$ cannot be larger than $\sum_{i=1}^{m} s_i + 1$, so $|h_{1,1}| \le \sum_{i=1}^{m} s_i + 1$. In this case,

$$|1 - h_{1,1}| \le \sum_{i=1}^{n} s_i + 2. \tag{4.41}$$

From the equation (4.35), we conclude that $|\alpha_i \cdot (1 - h_{1,1})| \ge 1 - \varepsilon$, and therefore, due to (4.41), that

$$|\alpha_i| \ge \frac{1 - \varepsilon}{\sum_{i=1}^{n} s_i + 2}. \tag{4.42}$$

Let us now analyze the consequences of the condition (4.36). We have requested that for some $i \in I_2$, we have $\alpha_i = 1$. For this i, the condition (4.36) takes the form $|1 - h_{1,2}| \le \varepsilon$, i.e.,

$$1 - \varepsilon \le h_{1,2} \le 1 + \varepsilon. \tag{4.43}$$

For all other i, we get

$$1 - \varepsilon \le h_{1,2} \cdot \alpha_i \le 1 + \varepsilon. \tag{4.44}$$

Dividing (4.44) by (4.43), we conclude that for all $i \in I_2$, we have

$$\frac{1-\varepsilon}{1+\varepsilon} \le \alpha_i \le \frac{1+\varepsilon}{1-\varepsilon}, \tag{4.45}$$

hence

$$-\frac{2\varepsilon}{1+\varepsilon} \le \alpha_i - 1 \le \frac{2\varepsilon}{1-\varepsilon}, \tag{4.46}$$

and

$$|\alpha_i - 1| \le \frac{2\varepsilon}{1-\varepsilon}. \tag{4.47}$$

For y_2', we have

$$y_2' = \sum_{i \in I_2} \alpha_i \cdot x_i + \left(\sum_{i \in I_2} \alpha_i \cdot s_i \right) \cdot x_{m+2}, \tag{4.48}$$

and therefore, taking into account that $\alpha_{m+2} = 1$, we can describe the condition (4.33) in the form

$$\left| \sum_{i \in I_2} \alpha_i \cdot x_i + \left(\sum_{i \in I_2} \alpha_i \cdot s_i \right) \cdot x_{m+2} - \right.$$
$$\left. h_{2,1} \cdot \left(\sum_{i \in I_1'} \alpha_i \cdot x_i + x_{m+2} \right) - h_{2,2} \cdot \sum_{i \in I_2} \alpha_i \cdot x_i \right| \le \varepsilon \cdot \max_i |x_i|. \quad (4.49)$$

Similarly to the previous case, we conclude that the coefficient at x_i at the left-hand side of (4.49) should not exceed ε. So, for $i \in I_1'$, we conclude that

$$|h_{2,1} \cdot \alpha_i| \le \varepsilon. \quad (4.50)$$

For $i \in I_2$, we conclude that

$$|\alpha_i - h_{2,2} \cdot \alpha_i| \le \varepsilon, \quad (4.51)$$

and for $i = m + 2$, we conclude that

$$\left| \sum_{i \in I_2} \alpha_i \cdot s_i - h_{2,1} \right| \le \varepsilon. \quad (4.52)$$

From (4.50) and (4.42), we conclude that

$$|h_{2,1}| = \frac{|h_{2,1} \cdot \alpha_i|}{|\alpha_i|} \le \frac{\varepsilon}{1 - \varepsilon} \cdot \left(\sum_{i=1}^{m} s_i + 2 \right). \quad (4.53)$$

The condition (4.52) can be rewritten as

$$\left| \sum_{i \in I_2} s_i + \sum_{i \in I_2} (\alpha_i - 1) \cdot s_i - h_{2,1} \right| \le \varepsilon, \quad (4.54)$$

hence

$$\left| \sum_{i \in I_2} s_i \right| \le \sum_{i \in I_2} |\alpha_i - 1| \cdot s_i + |h_{2,1}| + \varepsilon. \quad (4.55)$$

Using (4.47) and (4.53), we conclude that

$$\left| \sum_{i \in I_2} s_i \right| \le \frac{2\varepsilon}{1 - \varepsilon} \cdot \sum_{i \in I_2} s_i + \frac{\varepsilon}{1 - \varepsilon} \cdot \left(\sum_{i=1}^{m} s_i + 2 \right) + \varepsilon. \quad (4.56)$$

Replacing the sum $\sum_{i \in I_2} s_i$ in the right-hand side with a larger sum $\sum_{i=1}^{m} s_i$, we get

$$\left| \sum_{i \in I_2} s_i \right| \le \frac{2\varepsilon}{1 - \varepsilon} \cdot \sum_{i=1}^{m} s_i + \frac{\varepsilon}{1 - \varepsilon} \cdot \left(\sum_{i=1}^{m} s_i + 2 \right) + \varepsilon. \quad (4.57)$$

If $\varepsilon < \dfrac{1}{8 \cdot \sum_{i=1}^{m} s_i}$, then $\varepsilon < \dfrac{1}{8}$, hence $1 - \varepsilon > \dfrac{7}{8}$ and $\dfrac{1}{1 - \varepsilon} < \dfrac{8}{7}$. Hence, the condition (4.57) implies that

$$\left|\sum_{i\in I_2} s_i\right| \leq 2\varepsilon \cdot \frac{8}{7} \cdot \sum_{i=1}^{m} s_i + \varepsilon \cdot \frac{8}{7} \cdot \sum_{i=1}^{m} s_i + \frac{8}{7} \cdot (2\varepsilon) + \varepsilon. \qquad (4.58)$$

Because of our choice of ε, the first two terms in the right-hand side of (4.58) can be bounded as follows:

$$3 \cdot \frac{8}{7} \cdot \left(\varepsilon \cdot \sum_{i=1}^{m} s_i\right) \leq 3 \cdot \frac{8}{7} \cdot \frac{1}{8} = \frac{3}{7} < \frac{1}{2}. \qquad (4.59)$$

Similarly, since $\varepsilon < \frac{1}{8}$, we conclude that

$$\frac{8}{7} \cdot (2\varepsilon) + \varepsilon < \frac{8}{7} \cdot \left(2 \cdot \frac{1}{8}\right) + \frac{1}{8} = \frac{2}{7} + \frac{1}{8} = \frac{23}{56} < \frac{1}{2}. \qquad (4.60)$$

Therefore, (4.58) implies that

$$\left|\sum_{i\in I_2} s_i\right| < \frac{1}{2} + \frac{1}{2} = 1. \qquad (4.61)$$

Since all the values s_i are integers, the sum $\sum_{i\in I_2} s_i$ is also an integer, and the fact that the absolute value of this sum is smaller than 1 means that this sum must be equal to 0.

We have already shown, in the proof of Theorem 1, that this equality implies that the original instance of the subset problem has a solution. This completes the proof of the theorem.

4.10 Conclusions

In most biological system, we deal with a large number of microvariables. To simplify the analysis of such systems, it is desirable to reduce the dimensionality of the system's description by introducing *macrovariables* – combinations of microvariables from different classes. From the practical viewpoint, it is therefore very important to identify possible aggregations of microvariables into macrovariables which are consistent with the system's dynamics.

In addition to the practical importance of reducing the complexity of the dynamical system, aggregation of the variables allows us to identify components of the system (subsets of variables) that are quasi-independent modules or otherwise have significant equivalence or symmetry properties. This aspects has been explored formally from the group-symmetry prospective in [17, 18].

Our main result shows, crudely speaking, that no general efficient algorithm is possible for identifying such aggregation. This means that, in general, for a system with n microvariables, we need $\approx 2^n$ computational steps (i.e., in effect, an exhaustive search) to find an appropriate aggregation. For biological systems, with a large number n of microvariables, such an exhaustive search is not possible. For example, for a genetic system with g possible loci with two allels, there are 2^g possible genotypes and thus, 2^{2^g} possible subsets of microvariables. Even for a relatively small number of loci $g = 10$, we need $2^{2^{10}} = 2^{1024} \approx 10^{300}$ computational steps – much more than the number of particles in the universe.

Thus, to efficiently aggregate a system, we must, in general, specify some additional information about the grouping of the variables. When we do have such information, then it is possible to efficiently generate the desired aggregations. In this chapter, we describe the corresponding algorithm for the case of linear systems. These results can be readily extended to nonlinear systems with differentiable state equations by local linearization at all states; we will explore this approach in a forthcoming paper.

Acknowledgments

This work was supported in part by NASA under cooperative agreement NCC5-209, NSF grants EAR-0225670 and DMS-0532645, and by Texas Department of Transportation grant No. 0-5453.

The authors are thankful to Pierre-Jacques Courtois and Michael Vose for useful ideas, references, and suggestions, and to the anonymous referees for valuable suggestions.

References

[1] Courtois PJ (1977) Decomposability: queueing and computer system applications. Academic Press, New York
[2] Crow J, Kimura M (1970) An introduction to population genetics theory. Harper and Row, New York
[3] Davidson EH (2006) The regulatory genome: gene regulatory networks in development and evolution. Academic Press, New York
[4] Edwards RE (1995) Functional analysis: theory and applications. Dover, New York
[5] Eigen M, McCaskill J, Schuster P (1989) The molecular quasispecies. Advances in Chemistry and Physics 75:149–263
[6] Fell D (1996) Understanding the control of metabolism (Frontiers in metabolism). Ashgate Publ., London
[7] Garey MR, Johnson DS (1979) Computers and intractability, a guide to the theory of np-completeness. WH Freeman and Company, San Francisco, California
[8] Holland JH (1975) Adaptation in natural and artificial systems. The University of Michigan Press, Ann Arbor, Michigan
[9] Iwasa Y, Andreasen V, Levin SA (1987) Aggregation in model ecosystems. I. Perfect aggregation. Ecological Modelling 37:287–302

[10] Iwasa Y, Levin SA, Andreasen V (1989) Aggregation in model ecosystems. II. Approximate aggregation. IMA Journal of Mathematics Applied in Medicine and Biology 6:1–23
[11] Kreinovich V, Shpak M (2006) Aggregability is NP-hard. ACM SIGACT, 37(3):97–104
[12] Moey CCJ, Rowe JE (2004). Population aggregation based on fitness. Natural Computing 3(1):5–19.
[13] Notredame C, Higgins DG (1996) SAGA: sequence alignment by genetic algorithm. Nucleic Acids Research 24:1515–24.
[14] Notredame C, O'Brien EA, Higgins DG (1997) RAGA: RNA sequence alignment by genetic algorithm. Nucleic Acids Res. 25:4570–4580.
[15] Reeves CR, Rowe JE (2002) Genetic algorithms: principles and perspectives. Kluwer Academic Publishers, Dordrecht
[16] Rowe J (1998) Population fixed-points for functions of unitation. In: Reeves C, Banzhaf W (Eds), Foundations of Genetic Algorithms, Morgan Kaufmann Publishers, Vol. 5
[17] Rowe JE, Vose MD, Wright AH (2005). Coarse graining selection and mutation. In: Proceedings of the 8th International Workshop on Foundations of Genetic Algorithms FOGA'2005, Aizu-Wakamatsu City, Japan, January 5–9, 2005, Springer Lecture Notes in Computer Science, Vol. 3469, pp. 176–191
[18] Rowe JE, Vose MD, Wright AH (2005) State aggregation and population dynamics in linear systems. Artificial Life 11(4):473–492
[19] Schuster P, Swetina J (1988) Stationary mutant distributions and evolutionary optimization. Bulletin of Mathematical Biology 50:635–650
[20] Shpak M, Stadler PF, Wagner GP, Hermisson J (2004) Aggregation of variables and system decomposition: application to fitness landscape analysis. Theory in Biosciences 123:33–68
[21] Shpak M, Stadler PF, Wagner GP, Altenberg L (2004). Simon-Ando decomposability and mutation-selection dynamics. Theory in Biosciences 123:139–180
[22] Simon H, Ando F (1961) Aggregation of variables in dynamical systems. Econometrica 29:111–138
[23] Stadler PF, Tinhofer G (2000). Equitable partitions, coherent algenras, and random walks: applications to the correlation structure of landscapes. MATCH 40:215–261

5

Evolutionary Learning of Neural Structures for Visuo-Motor Control

Nils T Siebel[1], Gerald Sommer[1], and Yohannes Kassahun[2]

[1] Cognitive Systems Group, Institute of Computer Science, Christian-Albrechts-University of Kiel, Germany
nils@siebel-research.de, gs@ks.informatik.uni-kiel.de
[2] Group for Robotics, DFKI Lab Bremen, University of Bremen, Germany
kassahun@informatik.uni-bremen.de

Summary: Evolutionary Learning of Neural Structures for Visuo-Motor Control Artificial neural networks are computing tools, modeled after the human brain in order to make its vast learning and data processing potential available to computers. These networks are known to be powerful tools with natural learning capabilities. However, learning the structure and synaptic weights of an artificial neural network to solve a complex problem can be a very difficult task. With a growing size of the required network the dimension of the search space can make it next to impossible to find a globally optimal solution. We apply a relatively new method called EANT to develop a network that moves a robot arm in a visuo-motor control scenario with the goal to align its hand with an object. EANT starts from a simple initial network and gradually develops it further using an evolutionary method. On a larger scale new neural structures are added to a current generation of networks. On a smaller scale the current individuals (structures) are optimised by changing their parameters. Using a simulation to evaluate the individuals a reinforcement learning procedure for neural topologies has been realised. We present results from experiments with two types of optimisation strategies for the parameter optimisation. It is shown that while the original evolutionary method has the advantage of realising cascaded learning at a smaller scale, a new CMA-ES based method achieves better convergence in the parameter space.

5.1 Introduction

Artificial neural networks are computer constructs inspired by the neural structure of the brain. The aim is to approximate the vast learning and signal processing power of the human brain by mimicking its structure and mechanisms. In an artificial neural network (often simply called "neural network"), interconnected neural nodes allow the flow of signals from special input nodes to designated output nodes. With this very general concept neural networks are capable of modelling complex mappings between the inputs and outputs of a system up to an arbitrary precision [13, 21]. This allows neural networks to be applied to problems in the sciences, engineering and even economics [4, 15, 25, 26, 30]. A further advantage of neural networks is the fact that learning strategies exist that enable them to adapt to a problem.

Neural networks are characterised by their *structure (topology)* and their *parameters* (which includes the weights of connections) [27]. When a neural network is to be developed for a given problem, two aspects need therefore be considered:

1. What should be the *structure* (or, *topology*) of the network? More precisely, how many neural nodes does the network need in order to fulfil the demands of the given task, and what connections should be made between these nodes?
2. Given the structure of the neural network, what are the optimal values for its *parameters*? This includes the weights of the connections and possibly other parameters.

5.1.1 Current Practice

Traditionally the solution to aspect 1, the network's *structure*, is found by trial and error, or somehow determined beforehand using "intuition". Finding the solution to aspect 2, its *parameters*, is therefore the only aspect that is usually considered in the literature. It requires optimisation in a parameter space that can have a very high dimensionality – for difficult tasks it can be up to several hundred. This so-called "curse of dimensionality" is a significant obstacle in machine learning problems [3, 22].[3] Most approaches for determining the parameters use the backpropagation algorithm [27, chap. 7] or similar methods that are, in effect, simple stochastic gradient descent optimisation algorithms [28, chap. 5].

5.1.2 Problems and Biology-inspired Solutions

The traditional methods described above have the following deficiencies:

1. The common approach to pre-design the network structure is difficult or even infeasible for complicated tasks. It can also result in overly complex networks if the designer cannot find a small structure that solves the task.
2. Determining the network parameters by local optimisation algorithms like gradient descent-type methods is impracticable for large problems. It is known from mathematical optimisation theory that these algorithms tend to get stuck in local minima [24]. They only work well with very simple (e.g., convex) target functions or if an approximate solution is known beforehand *(ibid.)*.

---

[3] When training a network's parameters by examples (e.g. supervised learning) it means that the number of training examples needed increases exponentially with the dimension of the parameter space. When using other methods of determining the parameters (e.g. reinforcement learning, as it is done here) the effects are different but equally detrimental.

In short, these methods lack generality and can therefore only be used to design neural networks for a small class of tasks. They are engineering-type approaches; there is nothing wrong with that if one needs to solve only a single, more or less constant problem[4] but it makes them unsatisfactory from a scientific point of view.

In order to overcome these deficiencies the standard approaches can be replaced by more general ones that are inspired by biology. Evolutionary theory tells us that the *structure* of the brain has been developed over a long period of time, starting from simple structures and getting more complex over time. In contrast to that, the *connections* between biological neurons are modified by experience, i.e. learned and refined over a much shorter time span.

In this chapter we will introduce such a method, called *EANT*, *Evolutionary Acquisition of Neural Topologies*, that works in very much the same way to create a neural network as a solution to a given task. It is a very general learning algorithm that does not use any pre-defined knowledge of the task or the required solution. Instead, EANT uses evolutionary search methods on two levels:

1. In an outer optimisation loop called *structural exploration* new neural *structures* are developed by gradually adding new structure to an initially minimal network that is used as a starting point.
2. In an inner optimisation loop called *structural exploitation* the *parameters* of all currently considered structures are adjusted to maximise the performance of the networks on the given task.

To further develop and test this method, we have created a simulation of a *visuo-motor control* problem, also known in robotics as *visual servoing*. A robot arm with an attached hand is to be controlled by the neural network to move to a position where an object can be picked up. The only sensory data available to the network is visual data from a camera that overlooks the scene. EANT was used with a complete simulation of this visuo-motor control scenario to learn networks by reinforcement learning.

The remainder of this chapter is organised as follows. In Section 5.2 we briefly describe the visuo-motor control scenario and review related work. Section 5.3 presents the main EANT approaches: genetic encoding of neural networks and evolutionary methods for structural exploration and exploitation. In Section 5.4 we analyse a deficiency of EANT and introduce an improved version of EANT to overcome this problem. Section 5.5 details the results from experiments where a visuo-motor control has been learnt by both the original and our new, improved version of EANT. Section 5.6 concludes the chapter.

---

[4]The No Free Lunch Theorem states that solutions that are specifically designed for a particular task always perform better at this task than more general methods. However, they perform worse on most or all other tasks, or if the task changes.

5.2 Problem Formulation and Related Work

5.2.1 Visuo-Motor Control

Visuo-motor control (or visual servoing, as it is called in the robotics community) is the task of controlling the actuators of a manipulator (e.g. a human or robot arm) by using visual feedback in order to achieve and maintain a certain goal configuration. The purpose of visuo-motor control is usually to approach and manipulate an object, e.g. to pick it up.

In our setup a robot arm is equipped with a camera at the end-effector and has to be steered towards an object of unknown pose[5] (see Figure 5.1). This is realised in the visual feedback loop depicted in Figure 5.2. In our case a neural network shall be used as the controller, determining where to move the robot on the basis of the object's appearance in the image. Using the standard robotics terminology defined by Weiss et al. [32] our visuo-motor controller is of the type "Static Image-based Look-and-Move".

The object has 4 circular, identifiable markings. Its appearance in the image is described by the *image feature vector* $y_n \in \mathbf{R}^8$ that contains the 4 pairs of image coordinates of these markings. The desired pose relative to the object is defined by the object's appearance in that pose by measuring the corresponding *desired image features* $y^\star \in \mathbf{R}^8$ ("teaching by showing"). Object and robot are then moved so that no Euclidean position of the object or robot is known to the controller. The system has the task of moving the arm such that the current image features resemble the desired image features. This is an iterative process. In some of our experiments the orientation of the robot hand was fixed, allowing the robot to move in 3 degrees of freedom, DOFs. In others the orientation of the hand was also controllable, which means the robot could move in 6 DOFs.

The *input* to the controller is the *image error* $\Delta y_n := y^\star - y_n$ and additionally image measurements which enable the neural network to make its output dependent on the context. In some of the experiments this was simply y_n, resulting in a 16-dimensional input to the network. In other experiments the additional inputs were the 2 distances in the image of the diagonally opposing markings, resulting in a 10-dimensional input vector. The *output* of the controller/neural network is a relative movement u_n of the robot in the camera coordinate system: $u_n = (\Delta x, \Delta y, \Delta z)$ when moving the robot in 3 DOFs, $u_n = (\Delta x, \Delta y, \Delta z, \Delta yaw, \Delta pitch, \Delta roll)$ when moving in 6 DOFs. This output is given as an input to the robot's internal controller which executes the movement. The new state x_{n+1} of the environment (i.e. the robot and scene) is perceived by the system with the camera. This is again used to calculate the next input to the controller, which closes the feedback loop shown in Figure 5.2.

In order to be able to learn and train the neural network by reinforcement learning a simulation of the visuo-motor control scenario was implemented. For the assessment of the fitness (performance) of a network N it is tested by evaluating it in the simulated visual servoing setup. For this purpose s different robot start poses and 29 teach poses (desired poses) have been generated. In case of the 3 DOF scenario

---

[5]The *pose* of an object is defined as its position and orientation.

5 Evolutionary Learning of Neural Structures for Visuo-Motor Control

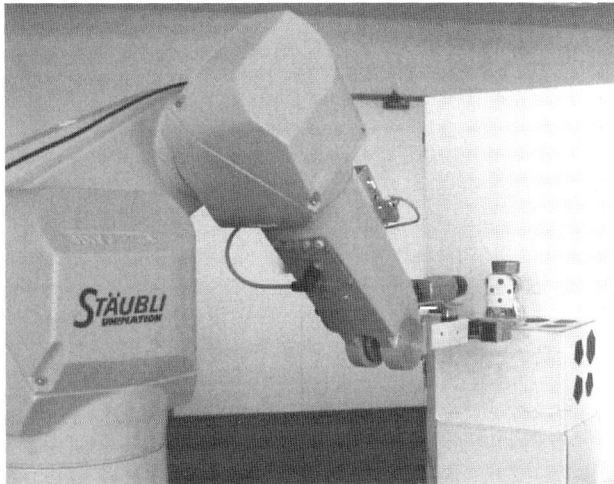

Fig. 5.1. Robot Arm with Camera and Object

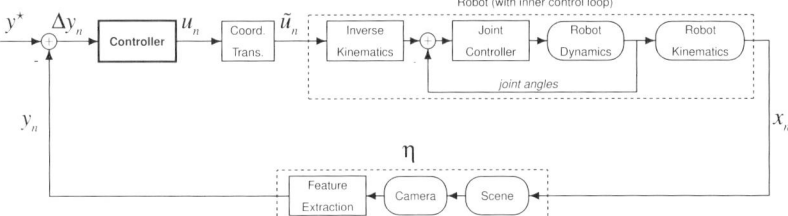

Fig. 5.2. Visual Feedback Control Loop

we used $s = 1023$ start poses, in the 6 DOF scenario $s = 58,677$ start poses. Each start pose is paired with a teach pose to form a task. These tasks contain all ranges and directions of movements. For each task, N is given the visual input data corresponding to the start and teach poses, and its output is executed by a simulated robot. The *fitness function* $F(N)$ measures the negative RMS (root mean square) of the remaining image errors after the robot movements, over all tasks. This means that our fitness function $F(N)$ always takes on negative values with $F(N) = 0$ being the optimal solution. Let y_i denote the new image features after executing one robot movement starting at start pose i. Then $F(N)$ is calculated as follows:

$$F(N) := -\sqrt{\frac{1}{s}\sum_{i=1}^{s}\left(\frac{1}{4}\sum_{j=1}^{4}d_j(y_i)^2 + b(y_i)\right)} \qquad (5.1)$$

where

$$d_j(y_i) := \left\| (y^\star)_{2j-1,2j} - (y_i)_{2j-1,2j} \right\|_2 \qquad (5.2)$$

is the distance of the jth marker position from its desired position in the image, and $(y)_{2j-1,2j}$ shall denote the vector comprising of the $2j-1$th and $2j$th component of a vector y. The inner sum of (5.1) thus sums up the squared deviations of the 4 marker positions in the image. $b(y)$ is a "badness" function that adds to the visual deviation an additional positive measure to punish potentially dangerous situations. If the robot moves such that features are not visible in the image or the object is touched by the robot, $b(y) > 0$, otherwise $b(y) = 0$. All image coordinates are in the camera image on the sensor and have therefore the unit 1 mm. The sensor (CCD chip) in this simulation measures $\frac{8}{3}$ mm $\times$ 2 mm.

For the 3 DOF data set the average (RMS) image error is -0.85 mm at the start poses, which means that a network N that avoids all robot movements (e.g. a network with all weights $= 0$) has $F(N) = -0.85$. $F(N)$ can easily reach values below -0.85 for networks that tend to move the robot away rather than towards the target object.

An analysis of the data set used for training the network in the 3 DOF case was carried out to determine its intrinsic dimensionality. The dimensionality is (approximately) 4, the Eigenvalues being 1.70, 0.71, 0.13, 0.04 and the other 6 Eigenvalues below 1e-15. It is not surprising that the dimensionality is less than 10 (the length of the input vector). This redundancy makes it more difficult to train the neural networks, however, we see this challenge as an advantage for our research, and the problem encoding is a standard one for visual servoing.

5.2.2 Related Work: Visuo-Motor Control

Visuo-motor control is one of the most important robot vision tasks [14, 32]. Traditionally it uses a simple P-type controller—an approach known from engineering [5]. In these controllers the output is determined as the minimal vector that solves the locally linearised equations describing the image error as a function of the robot movement. This output is often multiplied by a constant scale factor α, $0 < \alpha < 1$ (dampening). Sometimes, more elaborate techniques like trust-region methods are also used to control the step size of the controller depending on its current performance [16]. From a mathematical point of view, visuo-motor control is the iterative minimisation of an error functional that describes differences of objects' appearances in the image, by moving in the search space of robot poses. The traditional approach to a solution then becomes an iterative Gauss-Newton method [9] to minimise the image error, using a linear model ("Image Jacobian") of the objective function.

There have also been approaches to visuo-motor control using neural networks, or combined Neuro-Fuzzy approaches like the one by Suh and Kim [11]. Urban et al. use a Kohonen self-organising map (SOM) to estimate the Image Jacobian for a semi-traditional visuo-motor control [31]. Zeller et al. also train a model that uses a Kohonen SOM, using a simulation, to learn to control the position of a pneumatic robot arm based on 2 exteroceptive and 3 proprioceptive sensor inputs [35].

Many of these methods reduce the complexity of the problem (e.g. they control the robot in as few as 2 degrees of freedom, DOFs) to avoid the problems of learning a complex neural network. Others use a partitioning of the workspace to learn a network of "local experts" that are easier to train [6, 12]. A neural network that controls a robot to move around obstacles is presented in [23]. The network is optimised by a genetic algorithm, however, its structure (topology) is pre-defined and does not evolve.

There are a few methods that develop both the structure and the topology of a neural network by evolutionary means. These methods will be discussed in section 5.3.5 below. However, we have not seen these methods applied to visuo-motor control problems similar to ours.

To our mind it is a shortcoming of most (if not, all) existing visuo-motor control methods that the solution to the control task is modelled by the designer of the software. Whether it be using again an Image Jacobian, or whether it be selecting the size and structure of the neural network "by hand"—that is, by intuition and/or trial and error—*these methods learn only part of the solution by themselves*. Training the neural network then becomes "only" a parameter estimation, even though the curse of dimensionality still makes this very difficult.

We wish to avoid this pre-designing of the solution. Instead, *our method learns both the structure (topology) and the parameters of the neural network* without being given any information about the nature of the problem. To achieve this, we have used our own, recently developed method, *EANT, Evolutionary Acquisition of Neural Topologies* [19] and improved its convergence with an optimisation technique called CMA-ES [10] to *develop a neural network from scratch by evolutionary means* to solve the visuo-motor control problem.

5.3 Developing Neural Networks with EANT

EANT, Evolutionary Acquisition of Neural Topologies [18, 19], is an evolutionary reinforcement learning system that is suitable for learning and adapting to the environment through interaction. It combines the principles of neural networks, reinforcement learning and evolutionary methods.

5.3.1 EANT's Encoding of Neural Networks: The Linear Genome

EANT uses a unique genetic encoding that uses a linear genome of genes that can take different forms. A gene can be a neuron, an input to the neural network or a connection between two neurons. We call "irregular" connections between neural genes "jumper connections". Jumper genes are introduced by structural mutation along the evolution path. They can encode either forward or recurrent connections.

Figures 3(a) through 3(c) show an example encoding of a neural network using a linear genome. The figures show (a) the neural network to be encoded. It has one forward and one recurrent jumper connection; (b) the neural network interpreted as a tree structure; and (c) the linear genome encoding the neural network. In the linear genome, N stands for a neuron, I for an input to the neural network, JF for a forward

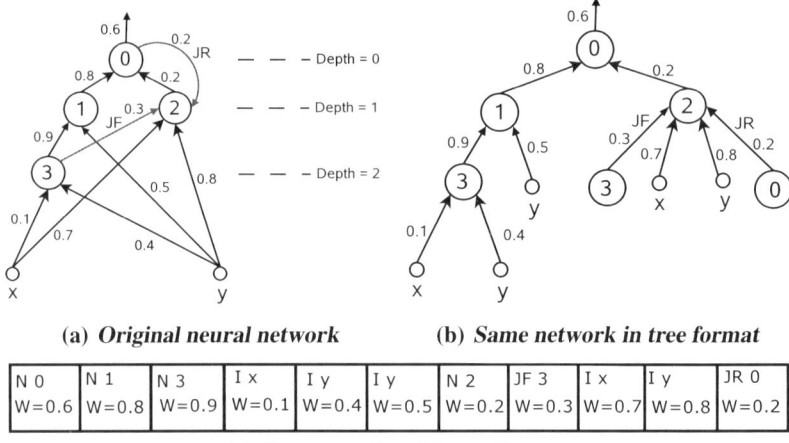

Fig. 5.3. An example of encoding a neural network using a linear genome

jumper connection, and JR for a recurrent jumper connection. The numbers beside N represent the global identification numbers of the neurons, and x or y represent the inputs coded by the input gene. As can be seen in the figure, a linear genome can be interpreted as a tree based program if one considers all the inputs to the network and all jumper connections as terminals.

The linear genome encodes the topology of the neural network implicitly in the ordering of the elements of the linear genome. This enables one to evaluate the represented neural controller without decoding it. The evaluation of a linear genome is closely related to executing a linear program using a postfix notation. In the genetic encoding the operands (inputs and jumper connections) come before the operator (a neuron) if one goes from right to left along the linear genome. The linear genome is *complete* in that it can represent any type of neural network. It is also a *compact* encoding of neural networks since the length of the linear genome is the same as the number of synaptic weights in the neural network. It is *closed* under structural mutation and under a specially designed crossover operator (see below). An encoding scheme is said to be closed if all genotypes produced are mapped into a valid set of phenotype networks [17].

If one assigns integer values to the genes of a linear genome such that the integer values show the difference between the number of outputs and number of inputs to the genes, one obtains the following rules useful in the evolution of the neural controllers:

1. The sum of integer values is the same as the number of outputs of the neural controller encoded by the linear genome.
2. A sub-network (sub-linear genome) is a collection of genes starting from a neuron gene and ending at a gene where the sum of integer values assigned to the genes between and including the start neuron gene and the end gene is 1.

Figure 5.4 illustrates this concept. Please note that only the number of inputs to neural genes is variable, so in order to achieve a compact representation only this number is stored within the linear genome.

5.3.2 Initialisation of the EANT Population of Networks

EANT starts with initial structures that are generated using either the full or the grow method as known from genetic programming [2]. Given a maximum initial depth of a tree (or in our case, a neural network), the full method generates trees where each branch has exactly the maximum depth. The grow method, on the other hand, adds more stochastic variation such that the depth of some (or all) branches may be smaller. Initial structures can also be chosen to be minimal, which is done in our experiments. This means that an initial network has no hidden layers or jumper connections, only 1 neuron per output with each of these connected to all inputs. Starting from simple initial structures is the way it is done by nature and most of the other evolutionary methods [33].

Using this simple initial network structure as a starting point, EANT incrementally develops it further using evolutionary methods. On a larger scale new neural structures are added to a current generation of networks. We call this process the "exploration" of new structures. On a smaller scale the current individuals (neural networks) are optimised by changing their parameters, resulting in an "exploitation" of these existing structures. Both of these optimisation loops are implemented as evolutionary processes. The main search operators in EANT are structural mutation, parametric mutation and crossover. The search stops when a neural controller is obtained that can solve the given task.

5.3.3 Structural Exploration: Search for Optimal Structures

Starting from a simple initial network structure, EANT gradually develops it further using structural mutation and crossover.

The *structural mutation* adds or removes a forward or a recurrent jumper connection between neurons, or adds a new sub-network to the linear genome. It does not remove sub-networks since removing sub-networks causes a tremendous loss of performance of the neural controller. The structural mutation operates only on neuron genes. The weights of a newly acquired topology are initialised to zero so as not to disturb the performance of the network. Figure 5.5 shows an example of structural mutation where a neuron gene lost connection to an input and received a self-recurrent connection.

As a recently added new feature to EANT, new hidden neurons that are added by structural mutation are only connected to a subset of inputs. These inputs are randomly chosen. This makes the search for new structures "more stochastic".

The *crossover* operator exploits the fact that structures originating from the same initial structure have some parts in common. By aligning the common parts of two randomly selected structures, it is possible to generate a third structure which contains the common and disjoint parts of the two parent structures. This type of

N 0	N 1	N 3	I x	I y	I y	N 2	JF 3	I x	I y	JR 0
W=0.6	W=0.8	W=0.9	W=0.1	W=0.4	W=0.5	W=0.2	W=0.3	W=0.7	W=0.8	W=0.2
[-1]	[-1]	[-1]	[1]	[1]	[1]	[-3]	[1]	[1]	[1]	[1]

Fig. 5.4. An example of the use of assigning integer values to the genes of the linear genome. The linear genome encodes the neural network shown in Figure 3(a). The numbers in the square brackets below the linear genome show the integer values assigned to the genes of the linear genome. Note that the sum of the integer values is 1 showing that the neural network encoded by the linear genome has only 1 output. The shaded genes form a sub-network. The sum of these values assigned to a sub-network is always 1.

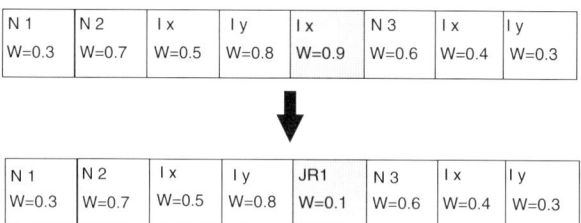

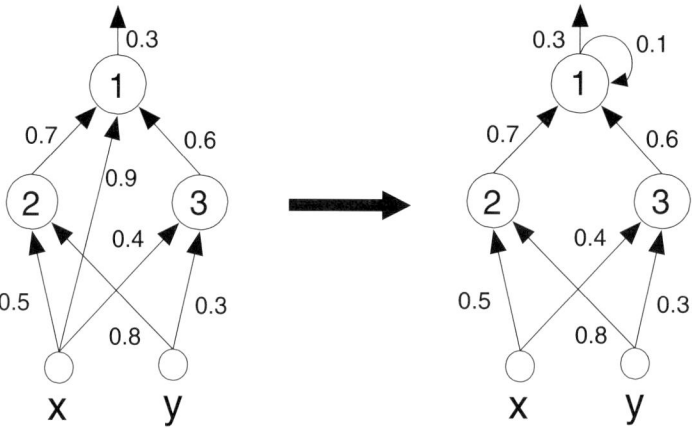

Fig. 5.5. An example of structural mutation. The structural mutation deleted the input connection to N1 and added a self-recurrent connection at its place.

crossover was introduced by Stanley and Miikkulainen [29] and has been incorporated into EANT. An example of the crossover operator under which the linear genome is closed is shown in Figure 5.6.

The structural selection operator that occurs at a larger timescale selects the first half of the population to form the next generation. New structures that are introduced through structural mutation and which are better according to the fitness evaluations survive and continue to exist. Since sub-networks that are introduced are not removed, there is a gradual increase in the complexity of structures along the evolu-

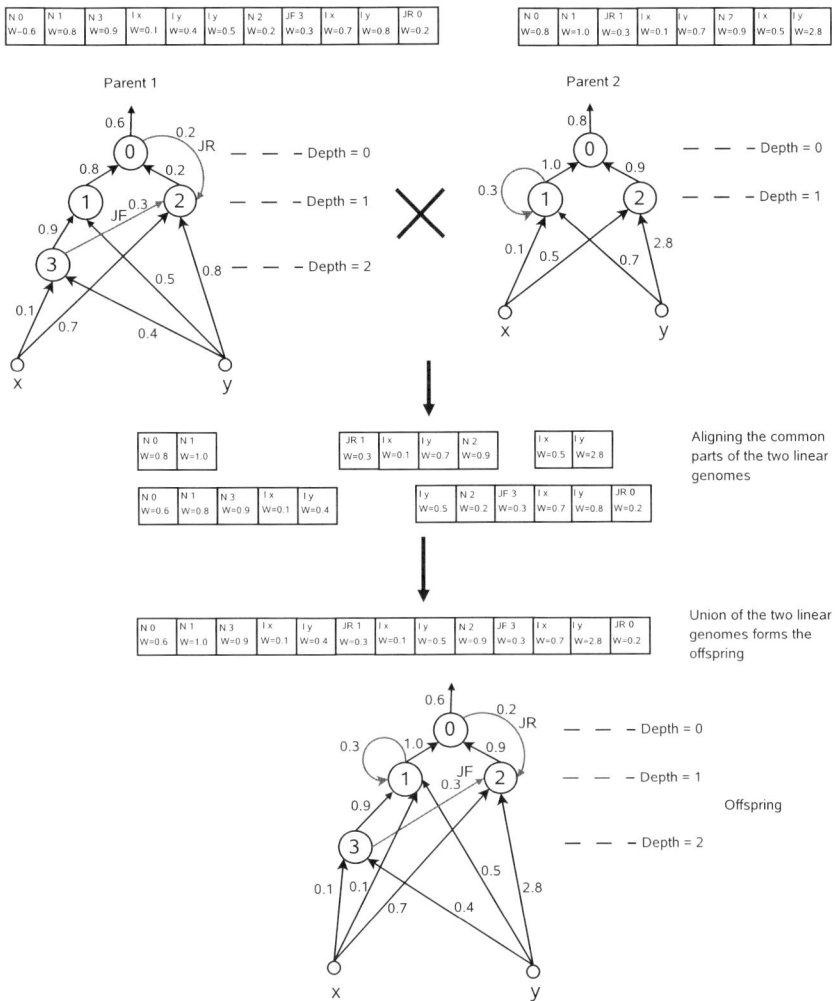

Fig. 5.6. Performing crossover between two linear genomes. The genetic encoding is closed under this type of crossover operator since the resulting linear genome maps to a valid phenotype network. The weights of the genes of the resulting linear genomes are inherited randomly from both parents.

tion. This allows EANT to search for a solution starting from a structure of minimum complexity and developing it further without the need to specify the required network size beforehand.

5.3.4 Structural Exploitation: Search for Optimal Parameters

In the exploitation step, EANT optimises the weights (and possibly, other parameters) of the networks, i.e. it *exploits the existing structures*. This is accomplished by an evolutionary process that occurs at smaller timescale. This process uses parametric mutation as a search operator. Parametric mutation is accomplished by perturbing the weights of the controllers according to the uncorrelated mutation in evolution strategy or evolutionary programming [7].

5.3.5 Related Work: Evolving Neural Networks

Until recently, only small neural networks have been evolved by evolutionary means [33]. According to Yao, a main reason is the difficulty of evaluating the exact fitness of a newly found structure: In order to fully evaluate a *structure* one needs to find the optimal (or, some near-optimal) *parameters* for it. However, the search for good parameters for a given structure has a high computational complexity unless the problem is very simple *(ibid.)*.

In order to avoid this problem most recent approaches evolve the structure and parameters of the neural networks simultaneously. Examples include EPNet [34], GNARL [1] and NEAT [29].

EPNet uses a modified backpropagation algorithm for parameter optimisation (i.e. a local search method). The mutation operators for searching the space of neural structures are addition and deletion of neural genes and connections (no crossover is used). A tendency to remove connections/genes rather than to add new ones is realised in the algorithm. This is done to counteract the "bloat" phenomenon (i.e. ever growing networks with only little fitness improvement; also called "survival of the fattest" [7]).

GNARL is similar in that is also uses no crossover during structural mutation. However, it uses an EA for parameter adjustments. Both parametrical and structural mutation use a "temperature" measure to determine whether large or small random modifications should be applied—a concept known from simulated annealing [20]. In order to calculate the current temperature, some knowledge about the "ideal solution" to the problem, e.g. the maximum fitness, is needed.

The author groups of both EPNet and GNARL are of the opinion that using crossover is not useful during the evolutionary development of neural networks [1, 34]. The research work underlying NEAT, on the other hand, seems to suggest otherwise. The authors have designed and used the crossover operator described in section 5.3.3 above. It allows to produce valid offspring from two given neural networks by first aligning similar or equal subnetworks and then exchanging differing parts. Like GNARL, NEAT uses EAs for both parametrical and structural mutation. However, the probabilities and standard deviations used for random mutation are constant over time. NEAT also incorporates the concept of speciation, i.e. separated sub-populations that aim at cultivating and preserving diversity in the population [7, chap. 9].

5.4 Combining EANT with CMA-ES

5.4.1 Motivation

During and after its development in the recent years EANT was tested on simple control problems like pole balancing where is has shown a very good performance and convergence rate—that is, it learns problems well with only few evaluations of the fitness function. However, problems like pole balancing are relatively simple. For instance, the neural network found by EANT to solve the double pole balancing problem without velocity information only has 1 hidden neuron. The new task, visuo-motor control, is much more complex and therefore required some improvements to EANT on different levels.

In order to study the behaviour of EANT on large problems we have implemented visuo-motor control simulators both for 6 DOF and 3 DOF control problems with 16/6 and 10/3 network in-/outputs, respectively. As a *fitness function F* for the individual networks N we used again the negative RMS of the remaining image errors, as defined in (5.1) above. This means that fitness takes on negative values with 0 being the optimal solution. Our studies were carried out on a small Linux PC cluster with 4 machines that each have 2 CPUs running at 3 GHz. This parallelisation was necessary because of the significant amount of CPU time required by our simulation. One evaluation of the fitness function in the 6 DOF case (58,677 robot movements and image acquisitions) takes around 1 second. In the 3 DOF case ("only" 1023 robot movements) the evaluation is of course considerably faster, however, parallelisation is still very helpful.

For our experiments we have set the following EANT parameters:

- population size: 20 individuals for exploration, $7\,n$ for exploitation, n being the size of the network
- structural mutation: enabled with a probability of 0.5
- parametric mutation: enabled; mutating all non-output weights
- crossover: disabled
- initial structure: minimal; 1 gene per output, each connected to all inputs

The results from our initial studies have shown that EANT does develop structures of increasing complexity and performance. However, we were not satisfied with the speed at which the performance (fitness) improved over time.

5.4.2 Improving the convergence with CMA-ES

In order to find out whether the structural exploration or the structural exploitation component needed improvement we took intermediate results (individuals with 175–200+ weights) and tried to optimise these structures using a different optimisation technique. Since our problem is highly non-linear and multi-modal (i.e. it has multiple local optima) we needed to use a global optimisation technique, not a local one like backpropagation, which is usually equivalent to a stochastic gradient descent method and therefore prone to get stuck in local minima. For our re-optimisation tests we used a global optimisation method called "CMA-ES" (Covariance Matrix Adaptation Evolution Strategy) [10] that is based on an evolutionary method like the one used in EANT's exploitation. CMA-ES includes features that improve its convergence especially with multi-modal functions in high-dimensional spaces.

One important difference between CMA-ES and the traditional evolutionary optimisation method in EANT is in the calculation of the search area for sampling the optimisation space by individuals. In EANT, each parameter in a neural network carries with it a learning rate which corresponds to a standard deviation for sampling new values for this parameter. This learning rate is adapted over time, allowing for a more efficient search in the space: parameters (e.g. input weights) that have not been changed for a long time because they have been in the network for a while are assumed to be near-optimal. Therefore their learning rate can be decreases over time, effectively reducing the search area in this dimension of the parameter space. New parameters (e.g. weights of newly added connections), on the other hand, still require a large learning rate so that their values are sampled in a larger interval. This technique is closely related to the "Cascaded Learning" paradigm presented by Fahlman and Lebiere [8]. It allows the algorithm to concentrate on the new parameters during optimisation and generally yields better optimisation results in high-dimensional parameter spaces, even if a relatively small population is used.

In EANT, the adaptation of these search strategy parameters is done randomly using evolution strategies [7]. This means that new strategy parameters may be generated by mutation and will then influence the search for optimal network parameters. However, one problem with this approach is that it may take a long time for new strategy parameters to have an effect on the fitness value of the individual. Since adaptation is random the strategy parameter may have been changed again by then, or other changes may have influenced fitness. Therefore evolution strategies tend to work well only for evolutionary algorithms that work with large populations and/or over very many generations.

CMA-ES uses a method similar to the original evolution strategies concept. The sampling range of the parameters is also expressed by a standard deviation hyper-ellipsoid. However, it is not necessarily aligned with the coordinate axes (and hence, its axes identified with specific parameters). Instead, it is expressed in a general covariance matrix which is adapted over time (leading to the letters "CMA", Covariance Matrix Adaptation) depending on the function values within the current population. Different to EANT's evolution strategies, the strategy parameters that define the hyper-ellipsoid are not adapted by random mutation. Instead, they are adapted at each step depending on the parameter and fitness values of current population members. CMA-ES uses sophisticated methods to avoid things like premature convergence and is known for fast convergence to good solutions even with multi-modal and non-separable functions in high-dimensional spaces *(ibid.)*.

Using CMA-ES, we improved the fitness of a network for the 6 DOF problem from -1.64 to a level between -1.57 and -1.35 in several experiments. This can be seen in Figure 5.7 where the fitness is plotted against evaluations of the fitness function (short: "fevals" for "function evaluations"). Each such experiment has taken up to 24,000 CMA-ES generations (456,000 fevals) which has taken slightly more than

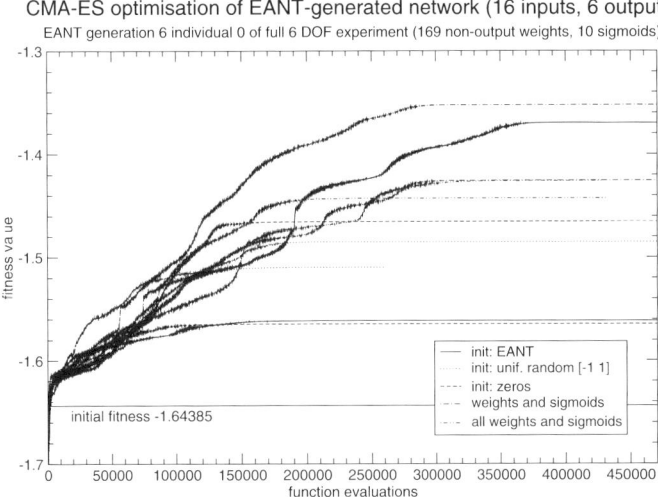

Fig. 5.7. Re-optimisation with CMA-ES of networks generated by EANT, 6 DOF

41 days to develop running on a single CPU. However, as can be seen in Figure 5.7, it should be noted that all of these experiments showed improvement over the original fitness in under 10 hours. Most of the CPU time was taken up by fevals but a small percentage also by CMA-ES internal calculations that—among other things—aim to reduce the total number of fevals needed for the optimisation. While these results show that the optimisation still needs a large amount of CPU time (at least in the 6 DOF case) the improvement in fitness was very significant. Experiments with different initialisations have shown that the convergence of CMA-ES does not depend much on the initial values of the parameters. The variance in the resulting fitness values for optimisations with the same initial values is also an indicator for the multi-modality of our problem, which stems, in part, from our definition of the fitness function as a sum of many functions.

These 6 DOF experiments are very expensive to run due to their enormous CPU usage. However, with only few experiments the results have only little statistical significance. Therefore we made further experiments with networks of similar size for the 3 DOF visuo-motor control scenario. In over 700 CMA-ES re-optimisation experiments we always achieved very similar results to the ones shown in Figure 5.7 and conclude that the parameter optimisation with CMA-ES really does usually give a significant improvement in fitness value.

Our experiments have shown that by optimising only the parameters of the networks that were generated by EANT their fitness can be considerably increased. This indicates that for networks of this size the exploitation part of EANT that optimises these parameters can and should be improved. Encouraged by our positive results with CMA-ES we have therefore *replaced the structural exploitation loop of EANT* by a new strategy that uses *CMA-ES as its optimisation technique*.

5.5 Experimental Evaluation

5.5.1 Experimental Setup

After the studies with 6 DOF visuo-motor control described in Section 5.4 we decided that the 3 DOF case with 1023 start poses will be difficult enough to test the new CMA-ES-based EANT and compare it to the original version. With the same setup as before, 10/3 in-/outputs and starting from minimal structures (3 output neurons, each connected to all 10 inputs) we started EANT again on 4 PCs, each with 2 CPUs running at 3 GHz. One master process was responsible for the exploration of new structures and distributed the CMA-ES optimisation of the individuals (exploitation of current structures) to slave processes. We used the same fitness function $F(N)$ as before for evaluating the individual networks N, in this case

$$F(N) = -\sqrt{\frac{1}{1023}\sum_{i=1}^{1023}\left(\frac{1}{4}\sum_{j=1}^{4}\left\|(y^\star)_{2j-1,2j}-(y_i)_{2j-1,2j}\right\|_2^2 + b(y_i)\right)}, \quad (5.3)$$

which means that fitness takes again on negative values with 0 being the optimal solution.

Up to 15 runs of each method have been made to ensure a statistically meaningful analysis of results. Different runs of the methods with the same parameters do not differ much; shown and discussed below are therefore simply the mean results from our experiments.

5.5.2 Parameter Sets

Following our paradigm to put as little problem-specific knowledge into the system as possible, we used the standard parameters in EANT and CMA-ES to run our experiments. Additionally we introduced CMA-ES stop conditions that were determined in a few test runs. They were selected so as to make sure that the CMA-ES optimisation converges to a solution, i.e. the algorithm runs until the fitness does not improve any longer. These very lax CMA-ES stop criteria (details below) allow for a long run with many function evaluations (fevals) and hence can take a lot of time to terminate. In order to find out how much the solution depends on these stop criteria additional experiments were made with a second set of CMA-ES parameters, effectively allowing only $\frac{1}{10}$ of the fevals and hence speeding up the process enormously. Altogether this makes 3 types of experiments:

1. the original EANT with its standard parameters;
2. the CMA-ES-based EANT with a large allowance of fevals; and
3. the CMA-ES-based EANT with a small allowance of fevals

The optimisations had the following parameters:

Original EANT

- initial structure: minimal; 1 neuron per output, each connected to all inputs
- up to 20 individuals allowed in the exploration of new structures (global population size)
- structural mutation: enabled with probability 50%; random addition of hidden neurons and forward connections enabled; recurrent connections and crossover operator disabled
- parametric mutation: enabled for non-output weights, probability 5%
- exploration: new hidden neurons connected to all inputs
- exploitation: 3 to 6 parallel optimisations of the same individual, adaptively adjusted according to current speed of increase in fitness (threshold: 5% fitness improvement during exploitation)
- exploitation population size $7n$ or $14n$, n being the size of the network; adaptation as before
- number of exploitation generations: 15 or 30; adapted as above

CMA-ES EANT, many fevals

- new hidden neurons connected to approx. 50% of inputs (which makes the search for new structures stochastic)
- always only 3 parallel optimisations of the same individual
- $4 + 3\log n$ CMA-ES individuals (equal to number of fevals per CMA-ES generation) when optimising n parameters
- CMA-ES stop criteria: improvement over previous 5,000 generations (iterations) less than 0.000001 or maximum standard deviation in covariance matrix less than 0.00005 or number of generations more than 100,000
- up to 2 optimisation results of the same individual may be kept, so that a single structure cannot take over the whole population in less than 5 generations (very unlikely; it has not happened)

All other parameters, especially the exploration parameters, remained the same as in the original EANT.

CMA-ES EANT, few fevals

The only change compared to the previous parameters is that all stop criteria of the CMA-ES optimisation are more strict by a factor of 10:

- CMA-ES stop criteria: improvement over previous 5,000 generations (iterations) less than 0.00001 or maximum standard deviation in covariance matrix less than 0.0005 or number of generations more than 10,000

Due to the nature of the stop criteria in both cases the number of generations in the CMA-ES optimisations varied strongly (from 2,696 to 100,000). Therefore a parallelisation scheme with dynamic load balancing was employed.

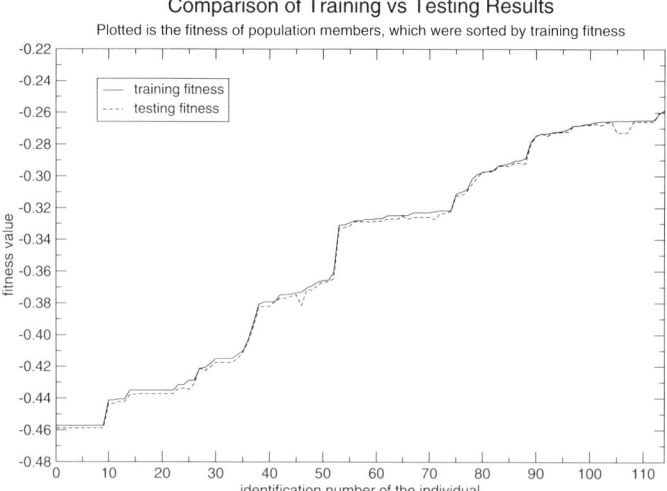

Fig. 5.8. Comparison Training vs. Testing Fitness Values

5.5.3 Training and Testing

In order to carry out a meaningful analysis of the neural networks trained by the EANT system we have generated a test set of 1023 visuo-motor control tasks. They are comparable with the 1023 tasks the system was trained on. In particular, the fitness value when not moving the robot is the same. However, the testing data require completely different robot movements. All 115 neural networks that were generated as intermediate results during one run of EANT were tested, without any change to them, on the testing data. Figure 5.8 shows a comparison of the resulting fitness values of these individuals, sorted by training fitness. It can be seen that the training and testing fitnesses are very similar indeed. The maximum deviation of testing fitnesses compared to training fitnesses is 2.738%, the mean deviation 0.5527% of the fitness value. From this follows that the neural networks developed with our technique did not just memorise the correct responses of the network but are capable of generalising to different, but compatible tasks.

5.5.4 Results

Figure 5.9 shows the development of the fitness value, plotted against the EANT exploration generation since this is the determining factor for the complexity of the networks. It can be clearly seen that our new version of EANT which uses CMA-ES in the exploitation converges much faster to networks with a good fitness. While the original EANT approach develops from around -0.490 to -0.477 in 11 generations both CMA-ES-based methods reach a value around -0.2 at that point.

The CMA-ES exploitation experiment with "many fevals" uses many more fevals per exploration generation than the EANT's original exploitation, resulting in longer

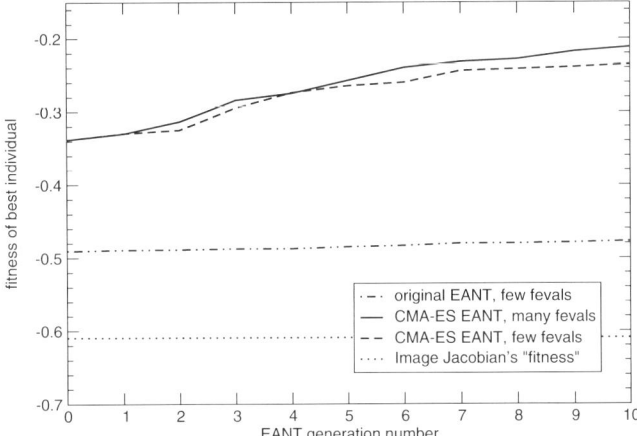

Fig. 5.9. Results from 3 DOF experiments: EANT and CMA-ES-based EANT

running times of the algorithm. However, running times of the "few fevals" variant uses about the same number of function evaluations as the original EANT. When comparing the resulting fitness values of these two variants one can see a difference of only about 10%. This indicates that the more strict stop criteria could be sufficient for the problem.

5.5.5 Discussion

Let us recall that the fitness values are (modulo $b(\cdot)$) the remaining RMS errors in the image after the robot movement. The value without moving the robot is -0.85. For comparison with the new methods we also calculated the fitness value of the traditional Image Jacobian approach. The robot movement was calculated using the (undampened) product of the Image Jacobian's pseudoinverse with the negative image error, a standard method [14]. The resulting fitness is -0.61. Why is this comparison meaningful? As in most optimisation techniques, both the Image Jacobian and our networks calculate the necessary camera movement to minimise the image error in *one* step. However, in practice optimisation techniques (which includes visuo motor control methods) usually multiply this step by a scalar *dampening factor* before executing it. This dampening of the optimisation step is independent of the nature of the model that was used to calculate it[6].

This comparison with the standard approach shows that our networks are very competitive when used for visuo-motor control. It can of course be expected that a non-linear model will be able to perform better than a linear model. However, it

---

[6]It is nevertheless useful to make it dependent on the correctness of the model, as it is done in *restricted step methods* [9].

should be taken into consideration that the Image Jacobian is an analytically derived solution (which is something we aim to avoid). Also, and more importantly, the Image Jacobian contained the exact distance (z coordinate) of the object from the camera. While this is easy to provide in our simulator in practice it could only be estimated using the image features.

The two types of experiments using CMA-ES have also shown that in our optimisation task CMA-ES is not very demanding when it comes to the number of fevals. The experiments with "few fevals" resulted in fitness values similar to those obtained with "many fevals" while keeping the CPU requirements about the same as the original EANT. Separate re-optimisation attempts with the original EANT exploitation that allowed for more fevals did not improve the performance of existing EANT individuals significantly. It can therefore be assumed that the main performance increase stems from the use of CMA-ES, not from a the CPU time/feval allowance.

To conclude, it can be clearly seen that the use of CMA-ES in EANT's exploitation results in better performance of neural networks of comparable size while not increasing the computational requirements. The performance of neural networks developed with our new method is also very much better than that of traditional methods for visuo-motor control.

5.6 Conclusions

Our aim was to develop neural networks automatically that can be used as a controller in a visuo-motor control scenario. At the same time, our second goal was to develop a method that would generate such networks with a minimum of predetermined modelling. To achieve this, we used and improved our own evolutionary method called *EANT*, *Evolutionary Acquisition of Neural Topologies*. EANT uses evolutionary search methods on two levels: In an outer optimisation loop called *structural exploration* new networks are developed by gradually adding new structures to an initially minimal network. In an inner optimisation loop called *structural exploitation* the parameters of current networks are optimised. EANT was used with a complete simulation of a visuo-motor control scenario to learn neural networks by reinforcement learning.

Initial experiments with a 6 DOF visuo-motor control scenario have shown that EANT is generally well suitable for the task. However, the convergence of the original EANT method needed to be improved. Tests with resulting networks have indicated that it is most useful to work on the exploitation of network structures. Re-optimisation of existing networks with an optimisation method called *CMA-ES*, *Covariance Matrix Adaptation Evolution Strategy* have shown a significant improvement in the controller's performance.

Based on these results the exploitation loop of EANT was replaced with a new strategy that uses CMA-ES as its optimisation algorithm. Experiments with this new method have shown much improved results over the original EANT method for developing a visuo-motor controller in the 3 DOF scenario. It could also be seen that varying the CPU time available to the CMA-ES-based parameter optimisation in the exploitation part by a factor of 10 did not significantly influence the performance of the resulting networks. Their performance is also very much better than that of the traditional approach for visuo-motor control.

Our experimental results show that the new EANT method with CMA-ES is capable of learning neural networks as solutions to complex and difficult problems. The CMA-ES based EANT can be used as a "black-box" tool to develop networks without being given much information about the nature of the problem. It also does not require a lot of parameter tuning to give useful results. The resulting networks show a very good performance.

Acknowledgements

The authors wish to thank Nikolaus Hansen, the developer of CMA-ES, for kindly providing source code which helped us to quickly start integrating his method into EANT.

References

[1] Peter J Angeline, Gregory M Saunders, and Jordan B Pollack. An evolutionary algorithm that constructs recurrent neural networks. *IEEE Transactions on Neural Networks*, 5:54–65, 1994.
[2] Wolfgang Banzhaf, Peter Nordin, Robert E Keller, and Frank D Francone. *Genetic Programming: An Introduction on the Automatic Evolution of Computer Programs and Its Applications*. Morgan Kaufmann, San Francisco, USA, 1998.
[3] Richard Ernest Bellman. *Adaptive Control Processes*. Princeton University Press, Princeton, USA, 1961.
[4] Andrea Beltratti, Sergio Margarita, and Pietro Terna. *Neural Networks for Economic and Financial Modelling*. International Thomson Computer Press, London, UK, 1996.
[5] Chris C Bissell. *Control Engineering*. Number 15 in Tutorial Guides in Electronic Engineering. CRC Press, Boca Raton, USA, 2nd edition, 1996.
[6] Wolfram Blase, Josef Pauli, and Jörg Bruske. Vision-based manipulator navigation using mixtures of RBF neural networks. In *International Conference on Neural Network and Brain*, pages 531–534, Bejing, China, April 1998.
[7] Ágoston E Eiben and James E Smith. *Introduction to Evolutionary Computing*. Springer Verlag, Berlin, Germany, 2003.
[8] Scott E Fahlman and Christian Lebiere. The cascade-correlation learning architecture. Technical Report CMU-CS-90-100, Carnegie Mellon University, Pittsburgh, USA, August 1991.
[9] Roger Fletcher. *Practical Methods of Optimization*. John Wiley & Sons, New York, Chichester, 2nd edition, 1987.

[10] Nikolaus Hansen and Andreas Ostermeier. Completely derandomized self-adaptation in evolution strategies. *Evolutionary Computation*, 9(2):159–195, 2001.
[11] Koichi Hashimoto, editor. *Visual Servoing: Real-Time Control of Robot Manipulators Based on Visual Sensory Feedback*, volume 7 of *Series in Robotics and Automated Systems*. World Scientific Publishing Co., Singapore, 1994.
[12] Gilles Hermann, Patrice Wira, and Jean-Philippe Urban. Neural networks organizations to learn complex robotic functions. In *Proceedings of the 11th European Symposium on Artificial Neural Networks (ESANN 2003)*, pages 33–38, Bruges, Belgium, April 2005.
[13] Kurt Hornik, Maxwell B Stinchcombe, and Halbert White. Multilayer feedforward networks are universal approximators. *Neural Networks*, 2:359–366, 1989.
[14] Seth Hutchinson, Greg Hager, and Peter Corke. A tutorial on visual servo control. Tutorial notes, Yale University, New Haven, USA, May 1996.
[15] William R Hutchison and Kenneth R Stephens. The airline marketing tactician (AMT): A commercial application of adaptive networking. In *Proceedings of the 1st IEEE International Conference on Neural Networks, San Diego, USA*, volume 2, pages 753–756, 1987.
[16] Martin Jägersand. Visual servoing using trust region methods and estimation of the full coupled visual-motor Jacobian. In *Proceedings of the IASTED Applications of Control and Robotics, Orlando, USA*, pages 105–108, January 1996.
[17] Jae-Yoon Jung and James A Reggia. A descriptive encoding language for evolving modular neural networks. In *Proceedings of the Genetic and Evolutionary Computation Conference (GECCO)*, pages 519–530. Springer Verlag, 2004.
[18] Yohannes Kassahun and Gerald Sommer. Automatic neural robot controller design using evolutionary acquisition of neural topologies. In *19. Fachgespräch Autonome Mobile Systeme (AMS 2005)*, pages 259–266, Stuttgart, Germany, December 2005.
[19] Yohannes Kassahun and Gerald Sommer. Efficient reinforcement learning through evolutionary acquisition of neural topologies. In *Proceedings of the 13th European Symposium on Artificial Neural Networks (ESANN 2005)*, pages 259–266, Bruges, Belgium, April 2005.
[20] Scott Kirkpatrick, Charles Daniel Gelatt, and Mario P Vecchi. Optimization by simulated annealing. *Science*, 220(4598):671–680, May 1983.
[21] James W Melody. On universal approximation using neural networks. Report from project ECE 480, Decision and Control Laboratory, University of Illinois, Urbana, USA, June 1999.
[22] Tom M Mitchell. *Machine Learning*. McGraw-Hill, London, UK, 1997.
[23] David E Moriarty and Risto Miikkulainen. Evolving obstacle avoidance behavior in a robot arm. In *Proceedings of the Fourth International Conference on Simulation of Adaptive Behavior*, Cape Cod, USA, 1996.
[24] Arnold Neumaier. Complete search in continuous global optimization and constraint satisfaction. *Acta Numerica*, 13:271–369, June 2004.

[25] Apostolos-Paul Refenes, editor. *Neural Networks in the Capital Markets*. John Wiley & Sons, New York, Chichester, USA, 1995.
[26] Claude Robert, Charles-Daniel Arreto, Jean Azerad, and Jean-François Gaudy. Bibliometric overview of the utilization of artificial neural networks in medicine and biology. *Scientometrics*, 59(1):117–130, 2004.
[27] Raúl Rojas. *Neural Networks - A Systematic Introduction*. Springer Verlag, Berlin, Germany, 1996.
[28] James C Spall. *Introduction to Stochastic Search and Optimization: Estimation, Simulation, and Control*. John Wiley & Sons, Hoboken, USA, 2003.
[29] Kenneth O Stanley and Risto Miikkulainen. Evolving neural networks through augmenting topologies. *Evolutionary Computation*, 10(2):99–127, 2002.
[30] Robert R Trippi and Efraim Turban, editors. *Neural Networks in Finance and Investing*. Probus Publishing Co., Chicago, USA, 1993.
[31] Jean-Philippe Urban, Jean-Luc Buessler, and Julien Gresser. Neural networks for visual servoing in robotics. Technical Report EEA-TROP-TR-97-05, Université de Haute-Alsace, Mulhouse-Colmar, France, November 1997.
[32] Lee E Weiss, Arthur C Sanderson, and Charles P Neuman. Dynamic sensor-based control of robots with visual feedback. *IEEE Journal of Robotics and Automation*, 3(5):404–417, October 1987.
[33] Xin Yao. Evolving artificial neural networks. *Proceedings of the IEEE*, 87(9):1423–1447, September 1999.
[34] Xin Yao and Yong Liu. A new evolutionary system for evolving artificial neural networks. *IEEE Transactions on Neural Networks*, 8(3):694–713, May 1997.
[35] Michael Zeller, Kenneth R Wallace, and Klaus Schulten. Biological visuo-motor control of a pneumatic robot arm. In Cihan Hayreddin Dagli, Metin Akay, C L Philip Chen, Benito R Fernandez, and Joydeep Ghosh, editors, *Intelligent Engineering Systems Through Artificial Neural Networks. Proceedings of the Artificial Neural Networks in Engineering Conference, New York*, volume 5, pages 645–650. American Society of Mechanical Engineers, 1995.

6

Dimension reduction for performing discriminant analysis for microarrays

Sang Hee Lee[1], A. K. Singh[2], and Laxmi P Gewali[3]

[1] Health Data Insights, INC.
 2620 Regatta, Suite 208, Las Vegas, NV 89128
 coolshlee@gmail.com
[2] Department of Hotel Management
 University of Nevada, Las Vegas, NV 89154,
 aksingh@unlv.nevada.edu
[3] School of Computer Science
 University of Nevada, Las Vegas, NV 89154
 laxmi@cs.unlv.edu

Summary: Gene expression data from microarray has very high dimensionality, resulting in extremely large sample covariance matrices. In this paper, we investigate the applicability of the block principal components analysis and a variable selection method based on principal components loadings for dimension reduction prior to performing discriminant analysis on the data. In such cases, because of high correlations among variables, the Mahalanobis distances between clusters becomes very large due to ill-conditioning. . It is shown in this paper that the Mahalanobis distance is unreliable when the condition number of the covariance matrix exceeds 480,000 or the natural log of the determinant of the covariance matrix is less than -26.3.

6.1 Introduction

The combinatorial interaction of DNA fragments and proteins is monitored by array technologies, such as DNA arrays, via a predetermined library of molecular probes. DNA microarrays provide a snapshot of the level of expression of all the genes in the cell, which can be used to determine the role of a group of genes in diseases, or monitor the effect of drugs on gene expression [3].

One characteristic of gene expression data from microarray is the fact that a very large number of genes can be collected on a relatively small number of samples [7, 9, 19] In many practical situations, interest lies in dimension reduction and discrimination between groups of samples using gene expression data [2, 4, 8, 11, 14, 17, 18, 20, 22]. Because of high dimensionality of the sample covariance matrix, the variable selection methods that are based on Principal Components Analysis (PCA) need modification before they can be used. In this chapter, we use the method of Block PCA [16] and a variable selection method based on principal component loadings for dimension reduction. Block PCA is a method that groups all variables of the original data into a small number of blocks before performing PCA to make the analysis computationally feasible. Two grouping method are used in this chapter: one is the simple orderly grouping, and the other method is based on Partial Least Square Regression (PLSR) [25, 26]; to find sets of variables that are correlated. This chapter is only concerned with how to deal with large number of variables (gene expressions) in data sets from microarray; for other details of microarray data, please see [1]. The discriminant analysis [12, 15] procedure is then used on the selected variables. Due to the presence of high correlations among the original variables, discriminant analysis programs that are run on the original variables run into computational difficulties; for example, the discriminant analysis procedure of MINITAB may not run on such data, whereas the same procedure in SAS will produce results. On the data sets used in this chapter, the Mahalanobis distance between the clusters, however, turned out to be extremely large, which indicated the presence of ill-conditioning in the covariance matrix. In this chapter, we propose a method for dealing with this ill-conditioning. In order to investigate the effect ill-conditioning has on the Mahalanobis distance between clusters, we used the well-known Hilbert matrix. We computed the effect of a small perturbation on the Mahalanobis distance between two points, assuming the covariance matrix to be the Hilbert matrix. It appears, from these calculations, that the Mahalanobis distance is unreliable when the condition number of the covariance matrix exceeds 480,000 or the natural log of the determinant of the covariance matrix is less than -26.3. A further reduction in dimensionality was achieved by using the correlation matrix. A SAS macro was developed to perform Block PCA, followed with variable selection, for dimension reduction.

6.2 Methodology

Principal Component Analysis (PCA) is one of the most commonly used tools to reduce dimensionality in multivariate data [12, 15]. The major objective of PCA is to reduce the p elements of the data matrix X to a small number while discarding very little relevant information [10]. All p variables of X_{pxl} are required to explain total variability in the data set $X_1, X_2, X_3, ... X_n$. In most situations, however, only a small number of linear combinations of the p variables (components) are needed to explain most of this variability. The k principal components (PCs) can then replace the original data, and be used as inputs to further statistical analyses. Geometrically, PCs are new coordinate systems obtained from the original system of axes. The new axes are directions of maximal variability. PCs depend solely on the covariance matrix $\Sigma_{p \times p}$ (or the correlation matrix $\rho_{p \times p}$), and are obtained by performing eigenanalysis of the covariance matrix $\Sigma_{p \times p}$ (or the correlation matrix $\rho_{p \times p}$). If the covariance matrix $\Sigma_{p \times p}$ is used for PCA, then $\rho_{p \times p}$ is factored as [12]:

$$\Sigma_{p \times p} = P \wedge P^r$$

6 Dimension reduction for performing discriminant analysis for microarrays 119

where P is the matrix of eigenvectors of Σ, $P = [e_1, e_2, e_p]$, and $(\lambda_1, e_1), (\lambda_2, e_2), \cdots, (\lambda_p, e_p)$, are the eigenvalue-eigenvector pairs of Σ and $\wedge$ is the is the diagonal matrix of eigen values: $\wedge = diag(\lambda_1, \lambda_2, \cdots, \lambda_p)$. The arguments of the eigenvectors are referred to as loadings. The i-th Principal Component is given by $PC_i = Y_i = e_i^T X$, and the values of PC computed for data at hand are called *scores*.

Jolliffe [13] suggests three methods to reduce the number of variables. We will use one among the three: select one variable with each of the first m PCs, namely the variable not already chosen with the highest coefficient in absolute value in each successive PC. These k variables are retained, and the remaining $k^* = p - k$ deleted. However, when we have large numbers of gene expressions, the derivation of the principal components involves computing a covariance matrix (or correlation matrix) with high dimensionality. It is computationally intense; often the limitation of resources may hinder the analysis.

Block PCA

Liu et al. (2002) [16] proposed the modified *PCA* called Block Principal Components Analysis (**Block PCA**). The first step of Block PCA is to group the original variables into several blocks of variables. PCA computation and selections of the first few leading principal components, which will explain a large percentage of variability in the data matrix, is done for each block. We then combine the selected variables from each block and examine them to see if the number of variables selected is sufficiently small. If it is still too large, we conduct principal component analysis again with the selected variables and perform the selection process using the new eigenvectors.

A brief description of Block PCA [16] is given below:

Let the $n \times p$ data matrix $\underline{X}'$ be divided into $\underline{X}'_j = [\underline{X}_1, \underline{X}_2, \cdots, \underline{X}_k]$ where n is the sample size, p is the total number of variables, and p_i is the dimentionality of vector $\underline{X}_j$, with $p_1 + p_2 + \cdots + p_k = p$.

The covariance matrix Σ of $\underline{X}'$ can be partitioned as:

$$\Sigma = \begin{pmatrix} \Sigma_{11} & \cdots & \Sigma_{1k} \\ \Sigma_{12} & \cdots & \Sigma_{2k} \\ \cdots & \cdots & \cdots \\ \Sigma_{k1} & \cdots & \Sigma_{kk} \end{pmatrix}$$

Define $PC_j^* = \underline{E}_j^T \underline{X}_j$, where $(\lambda_i, \underline{e}_i) = $ (eigenvalue, eigenvector) pair for Σ_{jj}. Then $\underline{E}_j = (\underline{e}_{j1}, \cdots, \underline{e}_{j p_k})$, $j = 1, \cdots k$ and
$\underline{E}_j^T \Sigma_{jj} \underline{E}_j = diag(\lambda_{j1}, \cdots, \lambda_{j p_k})$, $\lambda_{j1} \geq \cdots \lambda_{j p_k}$.

Let $Q = diag(\underline{E}_1, \cdots, \underline{E}_k)$ and define $Y = Q^T \underline{X} = (PC_1^T, \cdots, PC_k T)^T$ a random vector combining all 'block' principle components, then

$$\sum_{i=1}^{p} Var(Y_i) = \underline{\Omega} = Q^T \Sigma Q = \begin{pmatrix} \lambda_1 & \underline{E}_1^T \Sigma_{12} \underline{E}_2 & \cdots & \underline{E}_1^T \Sigma_{1k} \underline{E}_k \\ \cdot & \cdot & \cdots & \cdot \\ \cdot & \cdot & \cdots & \cdot \\ \underline{E}_k^T \Sigma_{k1} \underline{E}_1 & \underline{E}_k^T \Sigma_{k2} \underline{E}_2 & \cdots & \lambda_k \end{pmatrix}$$

Note that $trace(\underline{\Omega}) = trace(\Sigma)$, because $\underline{\Omega}$ and Σ have the same eigenvalues. Hence the p principal components of $\underline{Y}$ are identical to those of $\underline{X}$.

The above mathematical derivation from Liu et al. (2002)s [16] tells us that the definition of blocks does not affect the results of PCA. Gouping the variables into blocks according to their correlation is recommended, since PCA performed on correlated variables will typically result in maximum reduction in dimensionality. First, we adopt the concept of the Block PCA to analyze the gene expression data sets; however, for the sake of simplicity, we divide the set of variables into B blocks containing an equal number of variables (B ranged from1 to 16). Second, we follow the authors recommendation and the correlation of the data is taken into consideration. This was done using the Partial Least Square Regression [25, 26] method, which is briefly explained below.

Partial Least Squares as a Tool for Forming Blocks of Variables

Partial Least Squares (PLS) regression is a multivariate statistical method which extracts a majority of the information present in the predictor variables (X block) that is related to the dependent variables (Y block). PLS was introduced as an econometric prediction method [24], and later applied to spectrometric calibration problems [26]. PLS has also been used to forecast streamflows based upon Pacific and Atlantic Ocean sea surface temperatures [23].

In multiple linear regression (MLR), if the number of predictors X exceeds the number of observations, one can get a model that fits the sample data well, but will give a poor prediction for new data due to over-fitting. In such cases, one can first perform a principal components analysis (PCA) of X, and then perform MLR of Y on the PC-scores. This method of regression is called the principal components regression (PCR). PCR is based on the spectral decomposition of $X^T X$. In PLS, the latent factors of X that have the maximum correlation with Y are computed by performing the singular value decomposition of $X^T Y$.

If X and Y denote the matrices of predictors and dependent variables, respectively, then PLS fits a bilinear model of the form

$$\underline{Y} = t_1 \underline{q}_1 + t_2 \underline{q}_2 + \cdots + t_a \underline{q}_a + \underline{F},$$

$$\underline{X} = t_1 \underline{p}_1 + t_2 \underline{p}_2 + \cdots + t_a \underline{p}_a + \underline{E}$$

or

$X = TP' + E$ and $Y = TQ' + F$

where T is the score matrix, P, Q are loading matrices, and E, F are residual matrices. This can be expressed as:
$T = XW =$ an orthogonal matrix.

where W is a matrix of coefficients whose columns are the PLS factors which are linear combinations of the independent variables. Successive PLS factors are computed so as to minimize the residuals in E and simultaneously to have high squared covariance with a single Y variate (in the case of PLS1) or a linear combination of multiple Y variates (in the case of PLS2). Cross-validation is used to determine the correct number of latent variables (factors) to include in the PLS model.

Our goal here is to form blocks of variables that are highly correlated. We will use PLS in the following manner to achieve this goal: 1) Select one variable arbitrarily (say $X1$). Run a PLS with X1 as the dependent variable and the rest of the Xs as the independent variables. 2) Examine the factor loadings and calculate the mean and the variance of the absolute values of the loadings. Let l_i be a loading of an ith variable, where $i = 2, \cdots, p$. Set $\bar{l} = \frac{\sum_{j=2}^{p} |l_i|}{p-1}$, and s = standard deviation of $|l_2|, |l_3|, \cdots, |l_p|$. Select any X_j with $|l_j| > \bar{l} \pm s$. Then, the variable $X1$ and the set of selected variables whose loadings exceed one standard deviation form the first block of variables. 3) Repeat steps 1-2 with the remaining variables, until all the blocks have been formed. If the number of the remaining variables is small enough, these form the last block.

Discriminant Analysis

The goal of Discriminant Analysis (DA) is to separate distinct sets of objects, in our case, samples [12, 15]. With the data sets, we want to find out if that the gene expression values of X differ, to some extent, from the melanoma to the control group or from one kind of cancer to the other.

Ill-Conditioning of Covariance Matrix

In the discriminant analysis step, the Mahalanobis distances between groups are calculated using the covariance matrix. However, the gene expression data typically is highly correlated and the covariance matrix gets highly ill-conditioned which causes unreliable distances being reported by software packages such as SAS. An ill-conditioned matrix is a matrix whose condition number is too large. To explain the ill-conditioning, we will introduce two definitions here [5, 6].

Definition 1: The matrix norm is the real-valued function $||A||$ of the matrix A defined by $||A|| = sup_{||x||=1} ||Ax||$, where $||x||$ = vector norm of the vector x.

One example of a vector norm is the Euclidean norm: $||x|| = sqrt(x^T x)$.

Definition 2: The condition number of a nonsingular matrix A is defined as:

$$\kappa(A) = ||A|| \cdot ||A^{-1}||$$

Suppose we have an approximate solution $\tilde{X}$ of $\mathbf{AX} = \mathbf{b}$, where $\mathbf{A}$ is nonsingular. The residual vector then can be defined as $\mathbf{r} = \mathbf{b} - \mathbf{A}\tilde{X}$. Intuitively, we infer that if $||\mathbf{r}||$ is small, then $||\mathbf{X} - \tilde{\mathbf{X}}||$ would be small as well. Since $\mathbf{b} = \mathbf{AX}$, then $\mathbf{X} - \tilde{X} = A^{-1}r$. Using a result related to the natural matrix norm [5], we obtain $||\mathbf{X} - \tilde{\mathbf{X}}|| \leq ||\mathbf{A}^{-1}|| \, ||\mathbf{r}||$ Using the definition of the condition number, the previous inequality then becomes: $||\mathbf{X} - \tilde{\mathbf{X}}|| \leq \kappa(\mathbf{A}) \frac{||\mathbf{r}||}{||\mathbf{A}||}$. For any nonsingular matrix $\mathbf{A}$ and natural norm $||.||, \mathbf{1} = ||\mathbf{I}|| = ||\mathbf{AA}^{-1}|| \leq ||\mathbf{A}^{-1}|| \, ||\mathbf{A}|| = \kappa(\mathbf{A})$. Matrices with condition numbers near 1 are said to be well-conditioned. The condition number is basically a measure of stability or sensitivity of a matrix to numerical operations. In other words, the results of computations on an ill-conditioned matrix are not to be trusted.

An Illustration of Effect of Ill Conditioning on Mahalanobis Distance

The Hilbert matrices are known to be ill-conditioned. The elements of the Hilbert matrix Hp of order p are given by:

$$\begin{pmatrix} 1 & \frac{1}{2} & \cdots & \frac{1}{p} \\ \frac{1}{2} & \frac{1}{3} & \cdots & \frac{1}{p+1} \\ \cdots & \cdots & \cdots & \cdots \\ \frac{1}{p} & \frac{1}{p+1} & \cdots & \frac{1}{2p-1} \end{pmatrix}$$

Table 6.1 shows the condition number (Hp) of the Hilbert matrix for $p = 3, 4,, 11$, computed in the R programming language. The R is a free statistical software which is available at www.R-project.org. Clearly, the Hilbert matrix is heavily ill-conditioned for $p \geq 5$.

Table 6.1. Condition number (Hp) and $ln(|Hp|)$ of the Hilbert matrix

p	κ(Hp)	Natural Log of the Determinant
3	524	-7.677864
4	15,514	-15.615240
5	476,607	-26.309450
6	14,951,059x	-39.766210
7	475,367,357	-55.988580
8	15,257,575,673	-74.978430
9	493,154,000,000	-96.736950
10	16,024,730,000,000	-121.264800
11	521,668,600,000,000	-148.560300

The statistical distance or Mahalanobis distance of point $\underline{x}^T = (x_1, x_2, \cdots, x_p)$ from the mean vector $\underline{\mu}^T = (\mu_1, \mu_2, \cdots, \mu_p)$ in the p-dimensional real vector space is defined by $d_\Sigma(\underline{x}) = (\underline{x} - \underline{\mu})^T \Sigma^{-1} (\underline{x} - \underline{\mu})$, where Σ is the covariance matrix of $\underline{x}^T = (x_1, x_2, \cdots, x_p)$.

Mahalanobis distance is also used as a measure of dissimilarity between two random vecotrs $\underline{x}^T = (x_1, x_2, \cdots, x_p)$ and $\underline{y}^T = (y_1, y_2, \cdots, y_p)$ of the same probability distribution, and is defined by $d_\Sigma(\underline{x}, \underline{y}) = (\underline{x} - \underline{y})^T \Sigma^{-1} (\underline{x} - \underline{y})$, where Σ is the covariance matrix of the common distribution.

Mahalanobis distance is used for determining similarity of an unknown sample set to a known one. It differs from the Euclidean distance as it takes into account the correlations of the data set. Mahalanobis distance is scale-invariant, i.e., it does not depend on the units of measurements.

Let $\Sigma p = Hp$, the p-dimensional Hilbert matrix, $x^T = (1,1,1,\cdots,1)$ and $y^T = (2,2,2,\cdots,2)$ Suppose the first point $x^T = (1,1,1,\cdots,1)$ is perturbed by a small amount δ: $x_1^T = (1+\delta,1,1,\cdots,1)$ The Mahalanobis distances between pairs of points (x,y) and $(x1,y)$ are:

$$D = (\underline{x}-\underline{y})^T H_p^{-1}(\underline{x}-\underline{y})$$

$$D_1 = (\underline{x}_1-\underline{y})^T H_p^{-1}(\underline{x}_1-\underline{y})$$

Table 6.2 shows the change $Diff = |D-D1|$ and percentage change = $100|D-D1|/\delta$ when S is the Hilbert matrix of order $p = 3,4,,11$.

Tables 6.3 shows that the relative change in Mahalanobis distance exceeds 10 percent when $p \geq 5$ or $(\kappa(A) \geq 476607)$, which may be considered to be unacceptable for most applications.

Table 6.2. Change in D for a small perturbation $(\delta = 0.0001)$ in x

p	κ	D	D1	Diff	per-cent Change
3	524.1	9	8.9994	0.0006	6
4	15,513.7	16	16.0008	0.0008	8
5	476,607.3	25	24.999	0.001	10
6	14,951,059.0	36	36.0012	0.0012	12
7	475,367,357.0	49	48.9986	0.0014	14
8	15,257,575,673.0	64	64.0016	0.0016	16
9	4.93E+11	80.99995	80.99815	0.0018	18
10	1.60E+13	99.99834	100.0003	0.00196	19.6
11	5.22E+14	120.9622	120.9601	0.0021	21

6.3 Results

In order to illustrate the variable selection method based upon Block PCA, two data sets were used: the Cutaneous Malignant Melanoma data set and the cDNA Microarray Data of the NCI 60 Cancer Cell Lines. These data sets are published and are available at the NIH web site [21].

The Cutaneous Malignant Melanoma data set contains 8037 gene expression from 38 gene expression profiles (or samples). There are 7 control samples and 31 Melanoma samples. The Melanoma samples are divided into two groups: 19 Melanoma Primary Cluster and 12 Melanoma Non-Clustered. We labelled the control group as control, melanoma primary cluster group as Cluster, and melanoma non-clustered as Non-Cluster for analysis purposes. This gives us a 38×8037 matrix for the first data set, with 38 cases or samples, and 8037 variables.

The data set of the NCI60 Cancer Cell Lines contains 9,706 gene expressions of 60 cells from nine types of cancer. For simplicity, three types of cancer, colorectal (7 cell lines), leukemia (6 cell lines), and renal (8 cell lines) will be studied. We removed some gene expressions and some samples which had a large number of missing values. This resulted in 3890 gene expressions. The second data set is a 21 × 3890 matrix, with 20 cases or samples, and 3890 variables.

The PCA with all data of the first set is not executable because of hardware limitations when calculating 8037*8037 correlation matrixes, whereas the second one is small enough to do the complete PCA. We tried several recent high-end personal computers (with 2-3 gigabyte memory) to do the PCA on the first data set and failed. Instead of using all the data, the first data set was divided into three subsets and the PCA was performed on each subset. We selected about 33 variables from each subset using the method which Jolliffe introduced [13] and combined those selected variables into one subset. SAS applications including SAS BASE, SAS/STAT, and SAS macro were used to perform PCA here. The dimensionality was reduced from 8037 to 110. The Discriminant Analysis was then performed on this set of 110 variables. The standard statistical discriminant procedure of SAS was used and the result showed that the gene expressions are well classified into groups (Table 6.3), whereas other software packages like Minitab failed to perform the analysis with the error message that the data is highly correlated.

Table 6.3. The Result of Discriminant Analysis showing Percentages of Correct Classification with 110 data (Number of Observations and Percent Classified into Groups)

>From Group	Cluster	Control	Non-Cluster	Total
Cluster	19	0	0	19
	100.00	0.00	0.00	100.00
Control	0	7	0	7
	0.00	100	0.00	100.00
Non-Cluster	0	0	12	12
	0.00	0.00	100.00	100.00

Because of the error message mentioned above, the correlation matrix of 110 data was inspected. We discarded several variables which were highly correlated with one another and further reduced the number of variables to 22. With the final subset of 22 variables, we got the same result as Table 6.3, i.e., and the gene expressions fell into the right groups. However, when we examined the distances between groups, the distances between the groups using 110 data (Table 6.4) are excessively large compared to those using the 22 variables (Table 6.5).

The main purpose of the Block PCA or PCA is that we find the best subset of all variables which can explain the total variance of the original data. The two factors we consider are: 1) the computer time to run the code and 2) ill-conditioning. Table 6.6 shows the processing time of the Block PCA on the first data set. This may vary depending on the machine and the version of software used. Work in this chapter was performed on a personal computer which is configured with 512 Mb memory and 3

GHz Pentium 4 processor and SAS version 9. From the result, any block with less than 2000 variables will be small enough to ignore the time factor.

Table 6.4. The Distances between Groups with 110 data Pooled Covariance Matrix Information. Covariance Matrix Rank = 35, Natural Log of the Determinant of the Covariance Matrix = -1347. (Number of Observations and Percent Classified into Groups)

Group	Cluster	Control	Non-Cluster
Cluster	0	673451624	454861330
Control	673451624	0	455198887
Non-Cluster	454861330	455198887	0

Table 6.5. The Distances between Groups with 110 data Pooled Covariance Matrix Information Covariance Matrix Rank = 22, Natural Log of the Determinant of the Covariance Matrix = -39.88773. (Generalized Squared Distance to Group)

Group	Cluster	Control	Non-Cluster
Cluster	0	14.5	19.6
Control	14.5	0	13.9
Non-Cluster	19.6	13.9	0

Table 6.6. The Processing Time of the Block PCA (B = number of blocks, p = number of variables)

	B=2 ($p \approx 4000$)	B=3 ($p \approx 3000$)	B=4 ($p \approx 2000$)	B=5 ($p \approx 1000$)
Time in Step1	1.5 - 2 hours	25 - 30 minutes	4 - 6 minutes	around 30 seconds
Num of Variables in Step1	74	110	148	294
Num of Variables in Step2	32	34	32	37

We performed the Block PCA on each data set. The number of blocks used (B) varied from 2 to 16 for the first data, and 1 to 10 for the second data. After the discriminant analysis was performed using the gene expressions selected through Block PCA, the genes from the first data set fell into one of three groups (Control, Melanoma-clustered, and Melanoma-Non-clustered) without any mis-classification error. The classification of the second data set, NCI60, was also 100 percent successful.

The difference between Block PCA using PCA loadings and Block PCA with PLS loadings lies in the grouping method. When we group variables into blocks, the former one uses loadings from PCA, whereas the latter uses the loading from PLS. The steps described above are programmed using SAS.

The first data set was used to illustrate this method. After PLS, there are 7 blocks formed. Each block has a different number of variables and the last block consisted of 1242 variables. Within a block, the variables are considered to be highly correlated. We performed PCA seven times on the variables of 7 blocks and selected variables in the same manner as with Block PCA.

Discriminant Analysis was executed on the selected variables and we verified that the successful classification was achieved. Therefore, we conclude that Block PCA with PLS is a good grouping method.

Ill-Conditioning in Discriminant Analysis

Example 1: The variable selection method using Block PCA was used on the Cutaneous Malignant Melanoma data set (n = 38, p = 8067) with 38 samples and 8067 variables. In the following table, B represents the number of blocks, when performing Block PCA and p1 is the number of variables selected for performing discriminant analysis (DA). The software package SAS was used for Block PCA and DA. Table 6.4 shows the natural log of the determinant of S (the pooled covariance matrix) and the condition number. The general trend shown in Table 6.4 is that as the number of the block increases, the condition number of the pooled covariance matrix becomes larger. Thus, we may conclude that grouping the total variables into many blocks is unwise. Table 6.5 shows the Mahalanobis distance when the number of blocks is 4 and 11.

The distances between the groups from 11 blocks are much larger when compared to those from 4 blocks. In the previous section, we considered that a relative change in Mahalanobis distance exceeding 10% is unacceptable for most applications. Furthermore the condition number at that level is 476607 (Hilbert matrix with p=5) and the natural log of the determinant is -26.309. Therefore, the criterion for finding a better subset is either: 1) if the condition number of a subsets pooled covariance matrix is lower than 476,607 or 2) if its natural log is less than -26.309. Applying this criterion, we chose that the subsets from 2 blocks or 3 or 4 blocks are good sets. However, if we form only two blocks, i.e., we group all variables into two blocks, each block has around 4000 variables. Hence the time for performing PCA on each block (Table 6.6) needs to be considered. Thus the subsets of 3 blocks and 4 blocks are the best choices.

The variable selection method using Block PCA was used on the NCI 60 Cancer Cell Lines (n = 21, p = 3890). Table 6.9 shows the natural log of the determinant of S (the pooled covariance matrix) and the condition number. The DA was performed using SAS and the p1 variables were selected using Block PCA. It can be seen from Table 6.6 that the pooled covariance matrices obtained from Block PCA with $B \geq 4$ are highly ill-conditioned. This explains the extremely large distances (Table 6.8) between clusters obtained from DA when $B \geq 4$. Applying the same criterion about

6 Dimension reduction for performing discriminant analysis for microarrays   127

Table 6.7. Values of ln(|Σ|) and the Condition Number as a function of Number of Blocks (B)

B	Covariance Matrix Rank	Condition Number	Natural Log of the Determinant of the Determinant of the
2	32	54,165	-42.31987
3	34	6,498	-42.36532
4	32	122,515	-42.86877
5	35	52,789,329	-62.41880
6	35	87,209,220	-70.87111
7	35	102,843,488	-36.49157
8	35	106,665,260	-63.83255
9	35	212,873,664	-33.74519
10	35	4,430,929,463	-72.65356
11	35	579,492,118	-95.54235
12	35	2,224,810	-68.20560
13	35	24,748,368	-80.46257
14	35	6,192,211,188	-61.40031
15	35	41,889,084	-52.61295
16	35	32,420,105	-80.53878

Table 6.8. The Distances between Groups: 4 Blocks vs. 11 Blocks

	From Group	Cluster	Control	Non-Cluster
B=4	Cluster	0	32.8	180.4
	Control	32.8	0	115.7
	Non-Cluster	180.4	115.7	0
	From Group	Cluster	Control	Non-Cluster
B=11	Cluster	0	45826014	33708004
	Control	45826014	0	27341961
	Non-Cluster	33708004	27341961	0

the ill-conditioning and the time factor we considered with the previous data, the good subsets are 2 blocks and 3 blocks.

With this data, we examined how the ill-conditioning of the covariance matrix affects the Mahalanobis distance between groups. Two subsets are chosen for this test: the subsets from two blocks and five blocks, for which the condition numbers are 436 and 9085088, respectively. The value of one variable from each subset is changed by a very small amount; the actual value tested was 0.00071566. Table 6.10 demonstrates the resulting changes. The difference of the distance from colorectal to leukemia in the subset of 2 blocks is only 0.00707, whereas the difference in the subset of 5 blocks is 14681.

6.4 Conclusion and Recommendations

Microarray technique enables us to analyze a huge amount of gene expressions data. Its major application lies in oncology: classifying gene expressions into normal or

Table 6.9. Values of ln(|Σ|) and the Condition Number

B	p1	Covariance Matric Rank	Condition Number	Natural Log of the Determinant of the Covariance Matrix
1	13	13	55	-18.35762
2	16	16	436	-26.55781
3	17	17	415	-37.11519
4	20	18	6,564	-65.69217
5	20	18	9,085,088	-73.98421
6	19	18	14,143	-59.68438
7	20	18	67,622	-67.69106
8	20	18	1,992,384	-72.71837
9	19	18	602	-52.10573
10	20	18	9,012.0450	-71.41885

Table 6.10. The differences of the Mahalanobis distances

Value of Variable that was perturbed	B=2		
	From Group	Colorectal Leukemia Renal		
The Original Value = 0.032232507	Colorectal	0 122.13286 20.88958		
	Leukemia	122.13286 0 202.36609		
	Renal	20.88958 202.36609 0		
	From Group	Colorectal Leukemia Renal		
The New Value = 0.031516841	Colorectal	0 122.13993 20.88740		
	Leukemia	122.13993 0 202.37101		
	Renal	20.88740 202.37101 0		
Value of Variable that was perturbed	B=5		
	From Group	Colorectal Leukemia Renal		
The Original Value = 0.410715666	Colorectal	0 40108573 74502376		
	Leukemia	40108573 0 223912721		
	Renal	74502376 223912721 0		
	From Group	Colorectal Leukemia Renal		
The New Value = 0.41	Colorectal	0 40093892 74514741		
	Leukemia	40093892 0 223899455		
	Renal	74514741 223899455 0		

diseased or into different types of cancer. However, since the number of variables we can get from mircroarrays is very large, the high dimensionality of the data is the main difficulty in performing accurate statistical analysis. This chapter describes an approach to maneuver past this difficulty. Principal Component Analysis (PCA) is one of the most common tools used to reduce dimensionality. Thus, PCA is chosen as a tool for reducing the dimensionality of the data set being considered, however, the data set is sometimes too big to perform PCA on the whole data. From our experience, if the number of variables exceeded 4000, performing PCA itself is problematic. The data set we analyzed in this chapter has 8067 variables. Since the number of variables in this data exceeds 4000, we expected that it would be impossible to perform PCA on the entire data set. Several attempts on several computer platforms using varied software such as SAS, Minitab, or R verified our assumption. We even attempted discriminant analysis directly on the whole data and did not get any result after 24 hours of computation. Block Principal Component Analysis (Block PCA) which was introduced by Liu et al. (2002) [16] was used to overcome this problem. Block PCA is a method that groups the variables into several blocks before performing PCA and executes PCA on the variables of each block. Hence, the formation of blocks becomes an important step in the process. Two grouping methods were taken. The first way is a simpler way. We divide the set of all variables into B blocks, each consisting of an equal number of variables. The first data set was divided into 2 blocks (around 4000 variables per block) through 16 blocks (around 500 variables). When using 2 blocks, PCA was executed 3 times; 2 times per block and one for the selected variables from each block. In the same sense, the 16 blocks need 17 PCA iterations. Though the number of iterations for 16 blocks is near 6 times larger than that of the 2 blocks, the time for PCA on the former is much shorter than on the latter. The number of variables in a block is the key in terms of the time factor; therefore, only the time factor is considered, which is at that moment an important consideration, formation of a block with a small number of variables is the ideal goal. When performing discriminant analysis on the selected set of variables, care must be taken so that Mahalanobis distances reported by software are not overly inflated due to ill-conditioning. We have developed a method for dealing with this problem.

References

[1] Alberts, B., Johnson, J., Lewis, J., Raff, M., Roberts, K., and Walter, P. (2002). Molecular Biology of the Cell, Garden Science Publishing, London.

[2] Antoniadis, A., Lambert-Lacroix, S., and Leblanc, F. (2003) Effective Dimension Reduction Methods for Tumor Classification Using Gene Expression Data. Bioinformatics, 19, 563-570.

[3] Baldi, T. and Hatfield, G.W. (2002). DNA Microarrays and Gene Expressions. Cambridge University Press, U.K.

[4] Bolshakova, N., Azuaje, F., and Cunningham, P (2004) An Integrated Tool for Microarray Data Clustering and Cluster Validity Assessment. Bioinformatics, 21, 451-455.

[5] Burden, L. R.and Faires, J. D. (1997) Numerical Analysis. 6th edition. Brooks/Cole.
[6] Chapra, S. C. and Canale, R. P. (2006) Numerical Methods for Engineers. 5th edition. McGraw-Hill.
[7] Chen, Y., Radmacher, M., Simon, R., Ben-Dor, A., Yakhini. Z., Dougherty, E., and Bittner, M. (2000) Molecular Classification of Cutaneous Malignant Melanoma by Gene Expression Profiling Nature 406: 536-540.
[8] Draghici, S. (2003) Data Analysis Tools for DNA Microarray Chapman and Hill/CRC.
[9] Duggan D. J., Bittner M., Chen Y., Meltzer P., and Trent JM. (1999). Expression Profiling using cDNA Microarrays Nat Genet. Jan;21(1 Suppl):10-4. 1999.
[10] Farnham I. M., Stetzenbach K. J., Singh A. K., and Johannesson K. H. (2000) Deciphering Groundwater Flow Systems in Oasis Valley, Nevada, Using Trace Elenment Chemistry, Multivariate Statistics, and Geographical Information System Mathematical Geology, Vol.32 No. 8.
[11] Golub T.R., Slonim D. K., Tamayo P., Huard C., Gaasenbeek M., Mesirov J. P., Coller H., Loh M. L., Downing J. R., Caligiuri M. A., Bloomfield C. D., and Lander E. S. (1999) Molecular Classification of Cancer: Class Discovery and Class Prediction by Gene Expression Monitoring. SCIENCE VOL 286.
[12] Johnson, R.A. and Wichern, D. W. (2002) Applied Multivariate Statistical Analysis. 5th edition. Prentice Hall.
[13] Jolliffe, I. T. (1972) Discarding Variables in a Principal Component Analysis Applied Statistics, 21, 160-173; (1986) Principal Component Analysis, Springer-Verlag
[14] Jones, N. C. and Pevzner, P. A. (2004) An Introduction to Bioinformatics Algorithms (Computational Molecular Biology) The MIT Press.
[15] Kachigan, S. K. (1991) Multivariate Statistical Analysis 2nd edition. Radius.
[16] Liu, A., Zhang, Y., Gehan, E., and Clarke. R. (2002) Block Principal Component Analysis with Application to Gene Microarray Data Classification. Statist. Med. 21:3465-3474.
[17] Liu Z., Chen D., Bensmail H., and Xu Y. (2005) Clustering Gene Expression data with Kernel Principal Components Journal of Bioinformatics and Computational Biology Vol. 3, No. 2 2005: 303-316.
[18] Miyano, S., Mesirov, J., Kasif, S., Istrail, S., Pevzner, P., and Waterman, M. (2005) Research in Computational Molecular Biology : 9th Annual International Conference, RECOMB 2005, Cambridge, MA, USA, MAY 14-18, 2005, Proceedings, RECOMB 2005 Springer.
[19] Mount, D. W. (2001) Bioinformatics: Sequence and Genome Analysis Cold Spring Harbor Laboratory Press.
[20] Nguyen D. V. and Rock D. M. (2001) Tumor Classification by Partial Least Squares Using Microarray Gene Expression Data. Bioinformatics, Vol. 18 no. 1 2001:39-50.

[21] NIH Web Site: Cutaneous Malignant Melanoma data Lines: http://dc.nci.nih.gov/dataSets cDNA Microarray Data of the NCI 60 Cancer Cell: http://discover.nci.nih.gov
[22] Qin J., Darrin P. L., and Noble W. S. (2003) Kernel Hierarchical Gene Clustering From Microarray Expression Data. Bioinformatics, Vol. 19 no. 16 2003:2097-2104.
[23] Tootle, G., Singh; A. K.; Piechota, T.; Farnham, I. (in press). Long Lead-time Forecasting of U.S. Streamflow using Partial Least Squares Regression. ASCE Journal of Hydrologic Engineering.
[24] Wold, H. (1966). Estimation of Principal Components and Related Models by Iterative Least Squares. Multivariate Analysis, (P. R. Krishnaiah, ed.), 391-420. New York: Acedemic Press.
[25] Wold S. (1978) Cross-Validatory Estimation of the Number of Components in Factor and Principal Components Methods. Technometrics, 20:397-405
[26] Wold S., Geladi K., and Ohman L. (1987) Multi-way Principal Components and PLS analysis. Journal of chemometrics, 1: 41-56

7

Auxiliary tool for the identification of genetic coding sequences in eukaryotic organisms

Vincenzo De Roberto Junior[1] Nelson F. F. Ebecken[2] and Elias Restum Antonio[3]

[1] COPPE/Federal University of Rio de Janeiro, Ilha do Fundao, Centro de Tecnologia, B 100 C.P. 68506, CEP 21945-970, Rio de Janeiro droberto@medilabsistemas.com.br
[2] COPPE/Federal University of Rio de Janeiro, Ilha do Fundao, Centro de Tecnologia, B 100 C.P. 68506, CEP 21945-970, Rio de Janeiro nelson@ntt.ufrj.br
[3] COPPE/Federal University of Rio de Janeiro, Ilha do Fundao, Centro de Tecnologia, B 100 C.P. 68506, CEP 21945-970, Rio de Janeiro eliasra@medilabsistemas.com.br

Summary: The genome needs interpretation to obtain useful information. This process goes through many phases, including the gene finding problem.
This manuscript describes the development of a new tool that helps solving this problem. The software recognizes coding regions with a user-friendly interface. The main goal is to increase the prediction rate for the gene finding problem.
The system is based on a gene model and combines the weight-position matrix technique with the flexibility of artificial neural networks in classification problems. The performance was compared to many other tools (Fgenes, GeneID, Genie, HMM-Gene, SNB and Grail 2) and showed effective in the solution of the proposed problem.

7.1 Introduction

The conclusion of several sequencing projects, principally the human genome project started in 2003, provides a considerable amount of data, apparently without any meaning, that needs to be processed appropriately in order to obtain useful genetic information. This processing includes several phases, where the first one corresponds to the analysis of the DNA (deoxyribonucleic acid) sequences with the purpose of recognition of the diverse component areas of this molecule.

Among these areas, the most important for the process of cellular protein synthesis are known as genes, resulting in the gene finding problem.

This work tries to improve the performance of the prediction rate for some of these problems, and the main objective is to create an auxiliary tool for the identification of coding areas and the principal genetic structures in eukaryotic organisms. The main purposes of the developed tool are:

• To predict the genetic structure from the genetic sequence;

- To find exons in nucleotide groups with single exons or multi-exons.

For the creation of this system it was necessary to develop a gene finding technique. The first step of this methodology is to define what will be interpreted by the tool as a gene.

The next step to solve this problem is the definition of the method to be used in each stage of the gene model. The main aspect of this new model is the use of neural networks with inputs based on the probabilities of hexamers for the detection of coding areas.

Section 7.2 describes the main methods and tools used for the prediction of genes. In the next section, the main challenges regarding the data characteristics are defined. The evaluation measures for the techniques are described in section 7.4. The proposed model, description of the tool, results and discussion, are described in sections 7.5, 7.6 and 7.7 respectively.

7.2 The main gene finding programs

In the last twenty years, a great deal of effort has been spent on the solution of the problem of the identification of genes, an effort that has resulted in a great number of methods that allow the identification of the genes in a given sequence of DNA.

Gene-finding strategies can be grouped into three major categories [1]:

- Comparative methods

  This method is one of the oldest for the identification of genes. Its principle is based on the tendency of the component bases of coding areas to be preserved along the genetic evolution. This tendency is due to the great relationship that exists between the functionality of a gene and the sequence of bases that constitutes it. In this method, similar areas are sought among the sequences under study and the sequences of a known database. With the growth of databases of genes and proteins, the use of this approach has become more interesting.

  The biggest advantage of this method is that if a similar sequence is found, the function of the new sequence is suggested, together with the function of the new gene. If the search is accomplished at the level of amino acids instead of nucleotides, an additional advantage is the sensitivity to the "noise" caused by, for example, neutral mutations (mutations that modify the nucleotide but don't modify the amino acid) or natural selection.

  When discovered sequences don't exist in the database used for comparison, this method has the disadvantage of producing a small amount of information, usually useless. Another problem occurs when primary databases are used, as these can contain mistakes, resulting in the research heading in the wrong direction.

- Content-based methods (statistical)

  The core of many gene recognition algorithms are the code measures (statistics). The aggregation of the measures of an area can form a mask to find exons, introns and other genetic areas. These measures have a long and rich history, and in the work of Fickett & Tung (1992) [2] they are synthesized and appraised.

These measures correspond, basically, to functions that calculate a number or vector (in agreement with some statistical criterion) that allow one to determine the probability of the subsequences inside of a window belonging to a genetic structure. Despite having been used widely, these statistical methods present a series of disadvantages. These include the fact that the accuracy of their results decreases as the size of the window gets smaller and, for most of the measures, the optimized size of their windows is larger than the mean size of the present exons in vertebrate genes.

Some examples of these code measurements are:
– Used codons
   A vector with 64 elements giving the frequencies of the 64 possible codons.
– Hexamer
   Frequency in a window of all of the hexamers (6 nucleotides).
– Used aminoacids
   A vector with 21 elements giving the frequencies of the 20 possible amino acids and the terminal codon.
– Used diaminoacids
   A vector with 441 elements giving the frequencies of all the possible dipeptides (including aminoacids and terminal codon).
– Composite [f(b,i)]
   For each base b = A,C,G,T and the position of the tested codon i=1,2,3, f(b,i) is the frequency of b in the position i.

- Site-based methods
  The focus of this strategy is the verification of the presence or absence of specific sequences, patterns or consensus. Usually, the sequences of the sites involved in gene determination are degenerate or badly defined, impeding the clear distinction between the parts of the sequence that really participate in the process of synthesis of proteins from the parts apparently without function. Some examples of these sites are:
  – TATA-box
     The TATA box is a consensus sequence in the promoter region of several eukaryotic genes (about 70% of them have this sequence). The promoter specifies the position where the transcription begins.
  – GC Box and CCAAT Box
     Besides the TATA box, other consensus sequences are necessary for the correct and efficient transcription of a gene, for example CAAT box and GC box. These elements are frequently found in areas about 40 to 100 nucleotides above the site at the beginning of the transcription in eukaryotic beings.
     The GC boxes are constituted by sequences GGGCGG which are related to most of the constituent genes (genes always expressed, with no need of regulation). CAAT boxes are formed by sequences GGNCAATCT.
  – Poly A
     Most of the eukaryotic RNAs are altered so as to contain a poly A tail at its extremity. There are nearly 200 adenines (A) in this tail.

Derived from the methods above are a series of computational systems known as tools for the prediction of genes, and their main objective is to discover the probable location of the genes present in a sequence, besides other information related to them (for instance, the ribbon where the gene is, the exons that compose them, etc).

Nowadays, the main tools of prediction of genes are GenScan [3] [4] and HMMGene [5]. GenScan uses a semi-Markov model type, that is formulated as a state of explicit duration of an HMM (Hidden Markov Model) of the type described by Rabiner (1989) [6]. In summary, the model works as a "grammatical analysis" generator. HMMgene predicts the whole gene of a certain sequence of DNA starting from an HMM, generated to maximize the probability of success of a prediction.

Other several tools were developed. Some of them are described below:

- GRAIL

  GRAIL [7] [8] is the oldest technique used for the prediction of genes. It was the first method developed for this which was really used.

  This tool is based on neural networks techniques, and, nowadays, has three versions: GRAIL 1, GRAIL 1a and GRAIL 2. GRAIL 1 uses a neural network to recognize a potential coding area of fixed size without using additional information such as initial and final codons.

- FGENES [9]

  FGENES (FindGENES) is the multiple gene prediction program based on dynamic programming. It uses discriminant classifiers to generate a set of exon candidates.

- Fgenesh [9]

  Fgenesh is an HMM-based gene-finding program with an algorithm similar to Genie [10] and Genscan [3] [4]. The difference between Fgenesh and analogous programs is that in the model of gene structure, site terms (suchas splice site or start site score) have some advantage over content terms (such coding potentials), reflecting a biological significance of the sites.

- GeneID

  The current version of GeneID [11] looks for exons based on measures of code potential. The original version of this program uses a system based on rules to examine supposed exons and to group the "most probable gene" for the sequence. GeneID uses a weight-position matrix to evaluate if an extension of the sequence represents a splice site (acceptor or donor) or not, an initialization codon or an ending codon. Once this evaluation has been made, models of supposed exons are built.

- MZEF

  This prediction method is based on the technique of quadratic discriminant analysis (QDA) [12].

- Genie

  Genie [10] uses a generalized HMM (GHMM) with distributions of states of associated arbitrary size in the model The system is described so as to allow each state to be determined and trained separately, and new states can be easily added.

- GeneParser

  GeneParser [13] [14] uses a different technique to identify supposed introns and exons. Instead of predetermining candidate areas of interest, this program computes the punctuation scores of all of the "subintervals" of the submitted sequences. Once each subinterval is scored, a neural network is used to determine whether each subinterval contains an initial exon, internal exon, final exon or intron.
- Morgan

  Morgan [15] is a system for the prediction of genes in sequences of vertebrate DNA. This system combines the techniques of decision trees, dynamic programming and Markov Chains.
- GeneMark.hmm

  GeneMark.hmm [16] was initially developed for the search of genes in bacteria, and it was modified for the detection of genes in eukaryotic organisms. This program uses a HMM of explicit duration like Genie and GenScan.
- SpliceMachine [17]

  SpliceMachine recognizes splice sites based on information position, composition and extracted codons of candidates for splice sites. The key of this technique is the model LSVM (linear support vector machines - separates two classes by one hyperplane). LSVM was based on the technique of SVM [18] [19], and is a fast classifier of candidate sites.
- TwinScan [20]

  TwinScan is a direct extension of the prediction program GenScan. The difference is the extension of GenScan to enable the exploration of similarities found between two homologous sequences.
- SNB [21]

  This method uses simple naive Bayesian networks for the combination of multiple gene predictors.

There are other tools like SGP2 [22] [23], DGSplicer [24], JIGSAW [25] and SpliceScan [26] involved in the gene finding problem.

7.3 Data characteristics

One of the great challenges of gene prediction is the data characteristics that are treated in these techniques.

The main characteristics are:

7.3.1 Data volume

The data volume is an important point in the analysis. This is increasing quickly in the course of time due to technological progress and the great interest in the area. Nowadays, GenBank [27] stores about 63 billion bases, with the human species being the most sequenced (12 billion bases in GenBank).

This amount of data is due to the length of a species' genome, that is big. In addition, the need to store several beings' genomes and the large amount of information related to them causes the increasing in the database.

7.3.2 Information consistency

Regarding the consistency of the stored information, we can separate the databases in two kinds:

- The primary databases
  Results of experimental data that were published with some interpretation, in which there was not a careful analysis of this data in relation to others published previously. GenBank, EMBL and PDB are examples of primary databases.
- The secondary databases
  Databases in which there are a compilation and interpretation of the input data so that they can be obtained as more representative and interesting data. These are adjusted databases, such as SWISS-PROT and TrEMBL.

Usually, the secondary databases are smaller than the primary ones due to delay in the compilation and interpretation of the data. However, the data contained is less subject to error (the error rate of a primary database is estimated as 1 for each 10.000 of bases) [1].

7.3.3 Stored information

The molecular biology databases used can be classified according to the biological information that is stored [28]. They mainly consist of:

- Nucleotide sequences and their annotations;
- Sequences of proteins and their annotations;
- Proteins and information about their respective functions;
- Secondary or tertiary structures of the molecules of proteins;
- Taxonomy (classifications of the living organisms);
- Bibliography in the area of molecular biology (papers, journals, periodicals and so on).

7.3.4 Database format

Another characteristic of molecular biology databases is the variety of formats used for information storage. There is no standard format for these databases, therefore, each database provider follows its own format or in some cases uses commercial databases, for example, GSDB (Genome Sequence Database - Sybase).

As well as the data storage format used in public databases, several applications used in molecular biology additionally have their own format.

7.4 Accuracy measures

The accuracy measures are used to evaluate the results of a prediction, and therefore, they have great importance in the verification of the execution of the tools of gene finding.

The group of accuracy measures proposed by Burset and Guigó (1996) [29] is nowadays used as the "pattern" or standard in the gene finding area. These metrics are divided into two levels: nucleotide and exon.

7.4.1 Nucleotide level

At this level, the accuracy of the prediction of a sequence is measured by comparing the value predicted with the true value codified for each nucleotide along the tested sequence. This approach is the more thoroughly used for the evaluation of the coding areas and in the methods for the prediction of gene structure.

The basic measures are:

- Nucleotides codings correctly predicted as codings (true positives, TP);
- Nucleotides no codings correctly predicted as no codings (true negatives, TN);
- Nucleotides codings predicted as no codings (false negatives, FN);
- Nucleotides no codings predicted as codings (false positives, FP).

Figure 7.1 shows an example of these measures.

The sensitivity (Sn) and specificity (Sp) measures are the two more widely used. Usually, the sensitivity and the specificity are defined as:

$$Sn = \frac{TP}{(TP+FN)} \qquad (7.1)$$

$$Sp = \frac{TP}{(TP+FP)} \qquad (7.2)$$

Sn is the proportion of coding nucleotides that were predicted correctly, and Sp is the proportion of coding nucleotides that are really codings. These metrics can be rewritten as:

$$Sn = P(F(x) = c | x = c) \qquad (7.3)$$

$$Sp = P(x = c | F(x) = c) \qquad (7.4)$$

Where x represents the current state of a certain nucleotide (c for coding and n for no coding), and F(x) is the condition predicted for this nucleotide.

7.4.2 Exon level

At this level, the measures of accuracy of the prediction compare the predicted exons and the true exons along the tested sequence.

To measure the sensitivity (ESn) and the specificity (ESp) for exons the following equations are used:

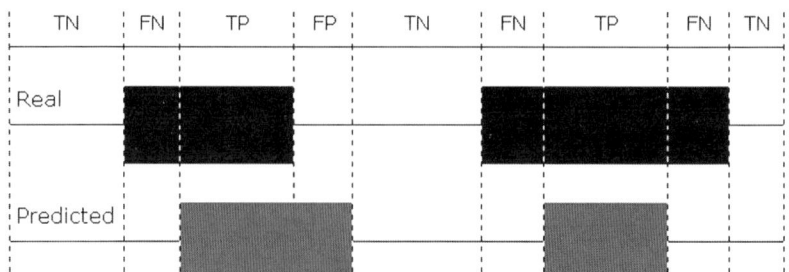

Fig. 7.1. Example of the measures in nucleotides level

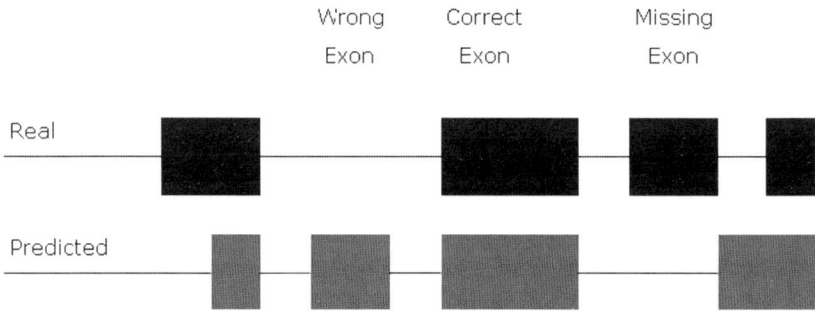

Fig. 7.2. Example of measures in exon level

$$ESn = \frac{Number\ of\ correct\ exons}{Number\ of\ actual\ exons} \tag{7.5}$$

$$ESp = \frac{Number\ of\ correct\ exons}{Number\ of\ predicted\ exons} \tag{7.6}$$

Thus, the sensitivity is the proportion of real exons in a tested sequence that were predicted correctly and the specificity is the proportion of exons that were predicted correctly.

At this level two another measures are important: missing exons (ME) and wrong exons (WE). The equations for ME and WE are:

$$ME = \frac{Number\ of\ missing\ exons}{Number\ of\ actual\ exons} \tag{7.7}$$

$$WE = \frac{Number\ of\ wrong\ exons}{Number\ of\ predicted\ exons} \tag{7.8}$$

ME is the proportion of real exons without overlapping with the predicted exons and WE is the proportion of exons predicted without overlapping with real exons.

7.5 Gene model

The creation of a tool for the prediction of genes needs the definition of what will be considered as a gene and, for such, a model will be created as described in Figure 7.3, in which the structures and their possible orders are identified within gene.

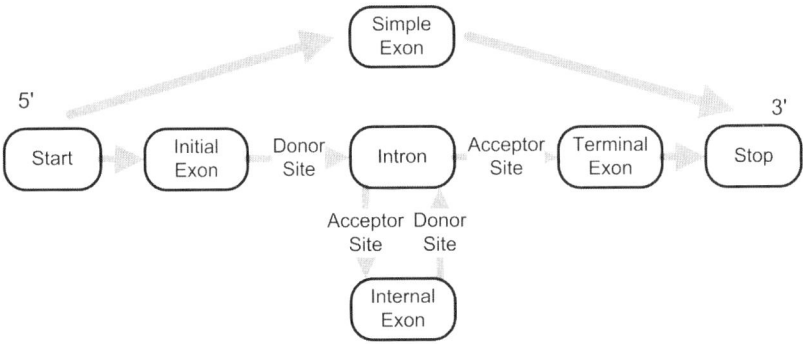

Fig. 7.3. Gene model

The defined genetic structures in the proposed model are:

- Start (start codon)
  Start site of gene translation.
- Simple Exon
  It models the situation in which the gene doesn't have introns.
- Initial Exon
  Exon after the beginning site.
- Internal Exon
  Exon among introns.
- Terminal Exon
  Exon before the terminal site.
- Intron
  Area no coding among exons.
- Intergenic Region
  Non-coding area among genes. In this model, any area not translated before the initial exon and after the terminal exon will be considered as an intergenic area.
- Donor splice site
  Area located between the end of an exon and the beginning of an intron. There are no simple exons and terminal exons at this site.
- Acceptor splice site
  Area located between the beginning of an exon and the end of an intron. There are no simple exons and terminal exons at this site.
- Stop codon
  Site where the translation of a gene is finished.

With the objective of solving the problem of prediction of coding area, a model was used for each structure defined as coding. This model doesn't make the distinction between introns and intergenic areas.

7.5.1 Data selection

Data selection is a stage of great importance in the gene finding problem. As demonstrated by Claverie (1997) [30], a gene finding tool predicts with a good degree of accuracy only the organisms for which it was developed and those that are evolutionarily "close".

Because of these issues, one organism was chosen for the construction of a training and validation database. Only the sequences containing relevant information to the problem were used.

The organism chosen for the training and the validation of the technique was *Drosophila melanogaster* (fruit fly), that is used to develop tests for a database with 2.9 Mbp.

7.5.2 The model for the discovery of coding areas

The new model proposed to identify coding areas (simple exon, initial exon, internal exon and terminal exon) was based on neural networks, since this technique is recognized as a great solution for classification problem solving. The first step for this model was to create the database for the training and validation. This database was developed with combinations of coding and non-coding areas with the same size of the chosen window. The window initially tested has 42 bp. This choice is due to the fact that this size corresponds to the smallest exon predicted correctly by the most of existent tools.

Another important point for the definition of this model is the determination of the neural network input. The proposed model uses hexamers information in this layer. This choice is due to the fact that in many systems for the prediction of genes, information on these polymers is the main information used in the algorithm. Tests accomplished by Burge (1997) [3] in his work show that the hexamer is the main source of information for the discovery of coding areas.

With this choice, the next stage consists in deciding the way the hexamers will be codified. There are $4096(4^6)$ hexamers and it is impracticable to use the codification without algebraic dependency, as each hexamer would need 4096 inputs in the neural network. For example, a neural network that was mentioned with a window of 42 bp (37 hexamers) would have 151552 inputs. The solution was to treat each hexamer as one single neural network input.

In the proposed model, each hexamer was represented as the normalized amount of its existence in the desired position (weight-position matrix). This punctuation was calculated starting from the training group and uses for any input sequence in the neural network. Therefore, the calculated value in the weight-position matrix is the neural network input, for example, the ACTAGT hexamer in position 2 (second neural network input) is 0.134.

Areas with some chance of being coding areas were tested, since at least one hexamer should have its punctuation different from 0.

The next step was the definition of the amount of neurons and the exit code of the neural network output. A neuron, which has as exit the information of being a coding area or not, is used in this layer.

Afterwards, the type of neural network used was chosen. As this is a classification problem, the network that was chosen was totally interlinked using the algorithm of learning backpropagation. The activation function used was the hyperbolic tangent.

Neural networks with different amounts of bases in the input layer and with several amounts of neurons in the hidden layer were appraised, and, in the case of the model based on the backpropagation algorithm, networks with one and two hidden layers were tested too. One neural network was created for each type of coding area to be predicted. Figure 7.4 shows an example of the backpropagation networks tested supposing an input of 43 bp.

Another challenge is the overlapping of the structures. The chosen solution was to accept only the structures that fit in the gene model described previously.

The gene probability is an important piece of information to be defined. This probability can be defined as a measure that denotes the chance of the tested sequence (or subsequence) to be a coding area. The neural network output was used as the probability of the gene. Several probabilities were tested to verify their influence in the final result.

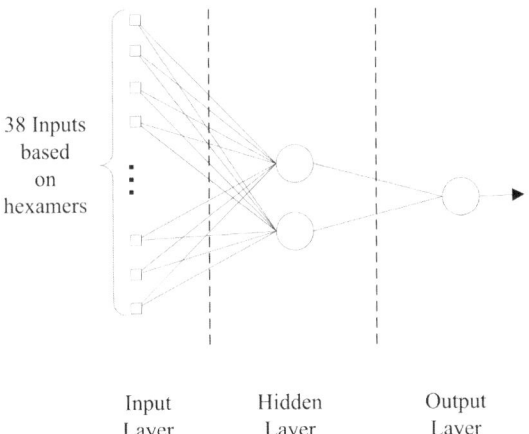

Fig. 7.4. Example of backpropagation neural network tested for coding areas

7.6 ExonBR system

The objective of this section is to describe the techniques used for the development of the new tool for the discovery of coding areas, denominated ExonBR (Exon Brazil). This system is not yet available, but will be distributed to the scientific community in a near future.

This system works for all organisms and was divided into two modules. These were:

- Training Module
  The training module is responsible for the training of the neural networks involved in the process of detection of the coding area. The final result of this module is one database with the values of neural network inputs based on the hexamer, input size and the resulting weights of its training.

- Test Module
  This module allows the user to use a database already created for the search of coding areas in one sequence.

The training module can be divided into the following subsystems:

- Syntactic Analyzer
  This subsystem allows the analysis of a file in the FASTA format or GenBank format [27], in this case CDS field is analyzed. It looks for important information for the training. The analyzed data are:
  – Position of the coding areas in the locus;
  – Kind of coding area (simple exon, initial exon, terminal exon or internal exon);
  – Invalid sequences.
- Statistical Analyzer
  The task of the statistical analyzer is to generate the information on the hexamer to form the neural network input.
  For such, a matrix with 4096 lines with the amount of columns equal to the neural network input is generated with the position information of each hexamer. This data is stored for the training and used in the test module.
- Database Generator
  In this stage, the training validation database is created. Coding sequences in the rate of 90 The repeated sequences are removed. This information is included in the neural network input that is based on the hexamer probability. This is done with the purpose to not leading the neural network to learn a set of specific sequences, allowing a better generalization. A group with the same amount of non-coding sequences is created and inserted randomly in the training and validation database.
  Non-coding sequences randomly created should have a chance of being a coding sequence (in the statistical matrix it should have at least one hexamer with the

chance of being a coding region).

After the creation of the database, it is mixed up.

- Pre-processing

  Sequences with all input values equal to zero are discarded, and the data are prepared for input in the neural network (the hexamers are converted in agreement with the weight-position matrix).

- Neural Network

  This module performs the neural network training using the backpropagation algorithm and the input based on the weight-position matrix discovered previously. Some modifications were implemented for the best operation of the tool. These were:

  – "Intelligent" learning rate, in other words, after an amount of time without change in the error rate or divergence in the learning process, the learning rate is decreased automatically.

  – Continuous verification of the error rate and of the amount of time with the objective of verifying the training of the network.

  The results of this stage are the weights and the neural network architecture trained. Several networks should be tested for searching the best performance. ExonBR tests many neural networks varying the amount of inputs and neurons in the hidden layer.

- Post-processing

  In this stage the tests are performed for the validation of the technique in the suggested locus.

  The result of this stage is the acceptance or not of the new data for the composition of the base of trained species.

The test module can be divided into the following subsystems:

- Pre-processing

  This accomplishes the adaptation of the data for input into the neural network in agreement with the species selected in the species database.

- Neural Network

  The objective of this neural network is to apply the chosen data on the sequence that is being analyzed. This stage uses the weight-matrix position, weights and neural network architecture discovered in the training stage. The result of this stage is the information where the coding areas are located.

- Post-processing

  The task of this stage is to accomplish the necessary adjustments for the display of the coding areas, in agreement with what was specified by the user.

These states are shown in Figure 7.5.

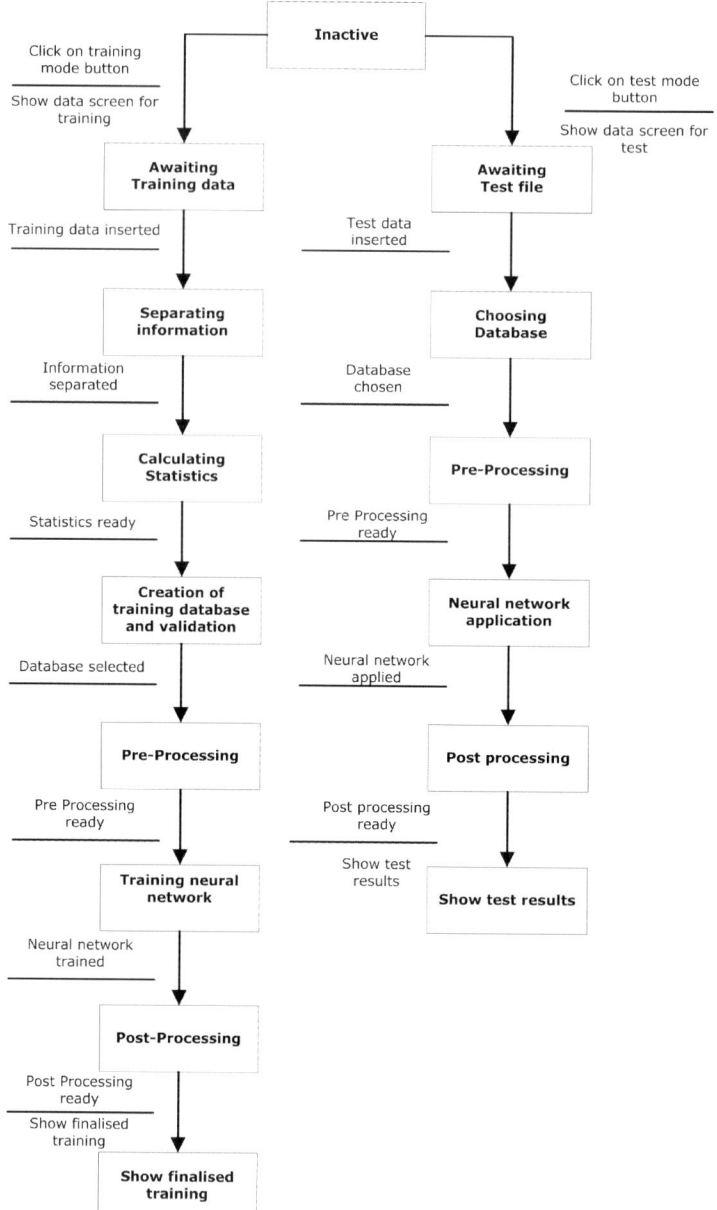

Fig. 7.5. Diagram of ExonBR system

7.7 Results and conclusion

The tests were accomplished using the database created for the validation of the methodology. The metrics suggested by Burset and Guigó (1996) [24] were applied for the evaluation of this tool performance, since these measures are considered to be a standard in the area of gene prediction.

The system developed during this work will be compared to the main genetic discovery programs on the market used for *Drosophila melanogaster*. These are:

- Fgenes
- GeneID
- Genie
- HMMGene
- SNB
- GRAIL 2

This comparison was made through the measurement of the performance of each tool in relation to the validation database.

Table 7.1 describes the results for *Drosophila melanogaster*. The tools selected for comparison were chosen because they showed better results for this organism, except for Grail 2, that was selected for the neural network performance comparison.

Table 7.1. Results

Program	Sp	Sn	ESn	ESp	ME	WE
ExonBR	0.98	0.97	0.95	0.87	0.03	0.08
FGenes	0.89	0.77	0.65	0.49	0.11	0.32
GeneID	0.86	0.83	0.58	0.34	0.21	0.47
Genie	0.96	0.92	0.68	0.53	0.05	0.20
SNB	0.97	0.93	0.94	0.84	0.04	0.13
GRAIL 2	0.91	0.83	0.18	0.11	-	-

The best neural network architectures and the threshold in the output layer that characterized a coding area are described in Table 7.2.

Table 7.2. Neural networks architectures

	Bp	Hidden Layer	Thresold (output)
Internal Exons	48	17	0.85
Initial Exons	40	3	0.85
Terminal Exons	42	3	0.85

From the results, we can note that for each type of coding area we have one different neural network (input window and amount of neurons in the hidden layer), and this is due to the fact that each area has different characteristics, with information verified by several gene detection tools. The neural networks vary, also, in agreement with the studied species.

The new neural network based on punctuation hexamers was shown effective for the problem of coding area prediction, both at the nucleotides level and at the exons level. Their results are comparable to the best gene-finding programs. The main advantage of this technique is the newness in the combination of the weight-position matrix information with the flexibility of the neural network in classification problems. However, this technique needs considerable computational power at its training stage, as the bigger the group used, the bigger the computational need. This problem can be reduced by breaking up the training group and creating network overlaps. Several tests should be done until the ideal network is found for a locus of a certain species.

Another problem of this technique is the difficulty of prediction for coding areas smaller than the achieved window, but this problem is faced by all the prediction techniques.

This methodology has the advantage of good performance, as well as giving the freedom to the specialist for the creation of his own group of bases. The initial objectives of this tool were reached.

Radial basis function networks can also be another approximation choice. As with other architectures, most training algorithms for this kind of neural network are concerned with parameter optimization, while topology configuration is still an open question. Applying genetic algorithms to the topological definition of RBF networks usually results in excellent solutions, but the associated computational cost is excessive. Perhaps an hybrid algorithm, as the genetic orthogonal least squares algorithm could be usefull [31].

Future work can be done to improve the performance of this tool, such as the need for computational power and for the discovery of other areas around the coding areas.

References

[1] Baxevanis A D, Ouellette B F F (2001) Bioinformatics: A practical guide to the analysis of genes and proteins., 2nd ed., Ed. Wiley-interscience

[2] Fickett J W, Tung C S (1992) Assesssment of protein coding measures Nucleid Acids Res 20:6441

[3] Burge, C (1997) Identification of Genes in Human Genomic DNA, Thesis Stanford University

[4] Burge C, Karlin S (1997) Prediction of complete gene structures in human genomic DNA J. Mol. Biol. 268:78–94

[5] Krogh A (1997) Two methods for improving perfomance of an HMM and their application for gene-finding ISBM 1997 pp. 179-186, AAAI Press, Menlo Park, CA
[6] Rabiner L R (1989) A tutorial on Hidden Markov Models and selected applications in speech recognition Proc. IEEE 77(2):257–285
[7] Uberbacher E C, Mural R J (1991) Locating protein-coding regions in human DNA sequences by a multiple sensor-neural network approach Proceedings of the National Academy of Sciences of the U.S.A. 88:11261–11265
[8] Mural R J, Einstein J R, Guan X, Mann R C, Uberbacher E C (1992) An artificial intelligence approach to DNA sequence feature recognition Trends Biotech. 10:67–69
[9] Salamov A A, Solovyev V V (2000) Ab initio Gene Finding in *Drosophila* Genomic DNA Genome Research 10:516–522
[10] Kulp D, Haussler D, Reese M G, Eeckman F H (1996) A generalized hidden Markov model for the recognition of human genes in DNA, In Proceedings of the Fifth International Conference on Intelligent Systems for Molecular Biology, pp. 134–142, AAAI Press, Menlo Park, CA
[11] Guigo R, Knudsen S, Drake N, Smith T F (1992) Prediction of gene structure Journal of Molecular Biology 226:141–157
[12] Zhang M Q (1997) Identification of protein coding regions in the human genome by quadratic discriminant analysis Proc. Natl. Acad. Sci. 94:565–568
[13] Snyder E E, Stormo G D (1993) Identification of coding regions in genomic DNA sequences: an application of dynamic programming and neural networks Nucleic Acids Res. 21:607–613
[14] Snyder E E, Stormo G D (1997) Identification genes in genomic DNA sequences. DNA and Protein Sequence analysis, M.J. Bishop and C.J.Rawlings, eds. (New York: Oxford University Press), p. 209–224
[15] Salzberg S L, Delcher A, Fasma K, Henderson J (1998) A decision tree system for finding genes in DNA J. Comp. Biol. 5:667–680
[16] Lukashin A V, Borodovsky M (1998) GeneMark.hmm: The new solutions for gene-finding Nucleic Acids Res. 26:1107–1115
[17] Degroeve S, Saeys Y, De Baets B, Rouze P, Van De Peer Y (2005) SpliceMachine: predicting splice sites from high-dimensional local context representations Bioinformatics 21(8):1332–1338
[18] Boser B, Guyon I, Vapnik V N (1992) A training algorithm for optimal margin classifiers. In: Proc. COLT (Haussler, D., ed.), ACN Press, Pittsburgh, PA, p. 144-152
[19] Vapnik V N (1995) The Nature of Statistical Learning Theory. Springer-Verlag, Berlin
[20] Korf I, Flicek P, Duan D, Breant M R (2001) Integrating genomic homology into gene structure prediction Bioinformatics 1:S1–S9
[21] Pavlovic V, Garg A, Kasif S (2002) A Bayesian framework for combining gene predictions Bioinformatics 18:19–27
[22] Parra G, Agarwal P, Abril J F, Wiehe T, Fickett J W, Guigo R (2003) Comparative gene prediction in human and mouse Genome Research 13(1):108–117

[23] Guigo R, Dermitzakis E T, Agarwal P, Ponting C P, Parra G, Reymond A, Abril J F, Keibler E, Lyle R, Ucla C, Antonarakis S E, Brent M R (2003) Comparison of mouse and human genomes followed by experimental verification yields an estimated 1,019 additional genes Proc. Nat. Acad. Sci. 100(3):1140–1145
[24] Chen T, Lu C, Li W (2005) Prediction of splice sites with dependency graphs and their expanded bayesian networks Bioinformatics 21(4):471–482
[25] Allen J E, Salzberg S L (2005) JIGSAW: integration of multiple sources of evidence for gene prediction Bioinformatics 21(18):3596–3603
[26] Churbanov A, Rogozin I B, Deogun J S, Ali H (2006) Method of predicting Splice Sites based on signal interactions Biology Direct 2006:1–10
[27] Genbank (2006) NCBI-GenBank Flat File Release 135.0 ftp://ftp.ncbi.nih.gov/genbank/gbrel.txt
[28] Ashburner, M, Goodman N (1997), Informatics – Genome and Genetics Databases In: Current Opinion in Genetics & Development 7:750–756
[29] Burset M, Guigo R (1996) Evaluation of Gene Structure Prediction Programs Genomics 34:353–367
[30] Claverie J M (1997) Computational methods for the identification of genes in vertebrate genomic sequences Human Molecular Genetics 1997 6(10) Review:1735–1744
[31] Barreto A M S, Barbosa H J C, Ebecken N F F(2006) GOLS-Genetic Orthogonal Least squares algorithm for training RBF networks Neurocomputing 69:2041–2064

8

Language engineering and information theoretic methods in protein sequence similarity studies

A. Bogan-Marta[1,3], A. Hategan[2], and I. Pitas[3]

[1] University of Oradea, Department of Computers, Universtatii No1, 410087, Oradea, Romania, `alinab@uoradea.ro`
[2] Tampere University of Technology, Institute of Signal Processing, Korkeakoulunkatu 1, P.O. Box 553, FIN-33101, `andrea.hategan@tut.fi`
[3] Aristotle University of Thessaloniki, Department of Informatics, Artificial Intelligence and Information Analysis Laboratory, Box 451,Thessaloniki, Greece, `pitas@aiia.csd.auth.gr`

Summary: The representation of biological data as text information opened new perspectives in the evolution of biological research. Many biological sequence databases are providing detailed information about sequences allowing investigations like searches, comparison, the establishment of relations between different sequences and species. The algorithmic procedures used for data sequence analysis are coming from many areas of computational sciences. Within this book chapter, we are bringing together a diversity of language engineering techniques and those involving information theoretic principles in analyzing protein sequences from similarity perspective. After we are proposing a state of the art in the subject, presenting a survey of the different approaches identified, the attention is oriented to the two methods we experimented. The description of these methods and the experiments performed open discussions addressed to the interested reader that may think about new ideas of improvement.

8.1 Introduction

Proteins are essential molecules to sustain life in all of the organisms. A normal development and function of an organism depends on the normal function of all proteins. Thus the first question to be asked about a newly discovered protein is "What is its function?". The function of a protein is highly correlated with its three dimensional shape. Currently the most reliable way to determine the three dimensional shape of a given protein is by wet laboratory techniques, such as X-ray crystallography and nucleic magnetic resonance (NMR). However, these methods are money and time consuming, taking even months or years to complete and also prone to human errors [1]. All the 3D structures that have been experimentally determined are kept in the Protein Data Bank (PDB) [2] and as of April 2007 there are 42861 structures. On the other hand, the number of protein sequences that are produced each year is growing and so is the gap between the number of proteins for which the function was experimentally determined and the number of proteins for which the function is still unknown. A highly curate repository for protein sequences is the Swiss-Prot protein knowledge database [3] which contains 264492 entries as of April 2007. Thus, a useful tool in helping to decrease the gap between the number of proteins with experimentally determined function and the number of proteins with unknown function, would be the prediction of protein function from its amino acid sequences. It is likely that the predictive methods will never replace completely the wet lab techniques. Still, they may help in providing a starting point for the experimental methods, thus reducing the time and cost necessary to perform the wet lab experiments. Moreover, predicting the protein structure from protein sequence will help understanding the sequence-structure-function relationship and in the future it might contribute to designing new proteins with desired functionalities by changing their three dimensional structure.

One common way to predict the function of a protein based on its amino acids sequence is to find the family to which the new protein belongs. Using the information from the already annotated proteins in the family, one can then predict the protein's function. A protein family contains homologous proteins, i.e. proteins that have a common ancestor. To directly explore if two proteins have a common ancestor we should have available all the fossil records of all intermediate forms. Because this information is not available, we have to use the current available information, i.e. the amino acid sequences. Therefore, to infer if two proteins are homologous we need a method to quantify the similarity of the two proteins based on their amino acid sequences. If the two sequences share a certain degree of similarity and it is proven that the similarity is significant (i.e. it is hard to obtain such a degree of similarity by chance), it is likely that the two sequences are homologous and then their alignment becomes a powerful tool for evolutionary and functional inference [4], [5].

Classical methods for measuring the similarity of two protein sequences [6], [7] use a scoring system and an alignment algorithm to compute the alignment score that it is used to quantify the similarity of the sequences compared. The alignment algorithm basically tries to find the optimal sequence of operations like insertions, deletions and substitutions that can transform one sequence into the other, given a scoring system. The alignment score is the sum of the individual scores for each pair of amino acids in the resulted alignment. When the alignment is created, some amino acids might be aligned with the symbol "-". Including this symbol in the alignment is needed to specify what amino acids are deleted or inserted. The substitution operation is used to specify positions in the alignment where identical or similar amino acids are aligned. In Figure 8.1 are presented three alignments of a region of the human alpha globin protein sequence and their resulted alignment score, under a very simple scoring system [4]. In this scoring system, the score for a pair of identical amino acids is 2, the score for a pair of similar amino acids, i.e. amino acids with the same chemical properties, is 1 and the score for a pair of different amino acids is -1. The middle row of each alignment shows by letters the positions in the alignment where are identical amino acids, by "+" the positions where are similar amino

Let s(identity) = 2; s(similar) = 1; s(gap) = -1

```
HBA_HUMAN  GSAQVKGHGKKVADALTNAVAHVDDMPNALSALSDLHAHKL
           G+ +VK+HGKKV  A++++++AH+D++ +++++LS+LH  KL    S1 = 47
HBB_HUMAN  GNPKVKAHGKKVLGAFSDGLAHLDNLKGTFATLSELHCDKL


HBA_HUMAN  GSAQVKGHGKKVADALTNAVAHV---D--DMPNALSALSDLHAHKL
           ++ ++++H+ KV   + +A  ++             +L+ L+++H+ K    S2 = 12
LGB2_LUPLU NNPELQAHAGKVFKLVYEAAIQLQVTGVVVTDATLKNLGSVHVSKG


HBA_HUMAN  GSAQVKGHGKKVADALTNAVAHVDDMPNALSALSD----LHAHKL
           GS+ + G +   +D L  ++ H+ D+  A +AL D     ++AH+    S3 = 18
F11G11.2   GSGYLVGDSLTFVDLL--VAQHTADLLAANAALLDEFPQFKAHQE
```

Fig. 8.1. Example of three possible sequence alignments of a region of the human alpha globin protein and three other proteins. The scoring system used gives the score 2 for a pair of identical amino acids, the score 1 for similar amino acids and -1 for different amino acids. The middle row of each alignment shows by letters the positions in the alignment where are identical amino acids, by "+" the positions where are similar amino acids and by space the positions where is a mismatch. The resulted alignment scores are S1, S2 and S3.

acids and by space the positions where is a mismatch. The first alignment has the greatest alignment score because the second sequence in the alignment is a region of the human beta globin protein sequence. The second alignment, even if it has the smallest score, it is a biologically meaningful alignment because the two proteins are evolutionary related and have the same three dimensional structure and function. The last alignment, even if it has a greater alignment score than the second one, is not a biologically meaningful alignment [4]. After we obtain the alignment score of two protein sequences we have to assess the statistical significance of the score, in order to be able to make some conclusions about their evolutionary relationship.

Despite the maturity of the developed methods for sequence similarity detection such as FASTA [6] and BLAST [7], the derivation of new similarity measures is still an active research area. The interest is actually renewed, due to the continuous growth in size of the widely available proteomic databases. This calls for alternative cost-efficient algorithmic procedures, which can reliably quantify protein similarity, without resorting to any kind of alignment. Apart from efficiency, a second specification of equal importance for the establishment of similarity measures is the avoidance of parameters that need to be set by the user (a characteristic inherent in the majority of the well known methodologies) [8], [9]. It is often the case with the classical similarity approaches that the user faces many difficulties in the choice of a suitable search algorithm, scoring matrix or function as well as a set of optional parameters, whose optimum values correspond to the most reliable similarity.

If we think that the similarity of two sequences is actually the amount of information shared by them, then we can use information theoretic methods, such as Kolmogorov complexity to quantify the similarity of the given sequences. The

Kolmogorov complexity deals with quantifying the information in individual sequences and in this context, the similarity of the sequences can be seen as the extent to which the two sequences are redundant with respect to each other. Such methods can be very useful when comparing very long sequence like the proteomes of different organisms. The proteome sequence is the collection of all the protein sequences in a given organism. In such applications, the classical methods that involve aligning the two sequences will fail. The comparison of organisms based on their proteome sequences can be a useful tool for comparing organisms with very different morphological and physiological characteristics and finally inferring their evolutionary relationships.

While DNA, RNA and proteomic sequences have their *language* and implicitly a *vocabulary* in textual representation, it is not a surprise the implication of language engineering in protein similarity studies. Language engineering techniques assume the application of knowledge of language to the development of computer systems that can predict, recognize, understand, interpret and generate human language in all its forms. The cooperation between researchers from these disparate fields is facilitated through the use of analogies. More precisely, the analogy between words and their meaning in speech and language processing on one side and the mapping between biological sequences to biological functions on the other, has proven useful. Some reviews of diverse applications of linguistic approaches and information theory principles to computational biology can be found in references [10], [11], [12].

Within this book chapter, we want to emphasize the potential of language engineering techniques and those involving information theoretic principles in analyzing protein sequences from similarity perspective. First, we are formulating a framework of the different approaches identified, presenting a survey of the state of the art in the subject. After, the attention is focused on two methods we experimented arguing why they may become promising strategies in comparing sequences of proteins. We end the chapter with discussions regarding the main aspects involved in these two new methods letting open the challenge for their improvement.

8.2 A survey of language engineering and information theoretic methods for protein sequence similarity

The fact that protein sequences from all different organisms can be treated as texts written in a universal language where the alphabet consists of 20 distinct symbols (the amino acid codes), opens the perspective of adapting many techniques from language and text processing to bioinformatics. The mapping of a protein sequence to its structure, functional dynamics and biological role then becomes analogous to the mapping of words to their semantic meaning in natural languages. This analogy is exploited in many applications that use statistical language modeling and text processing techniques for the advance of understanding biological sequences. Furthermore, the information content stored in biological sequences suggests the use of information theoretic methods in bioinformatics. They provide measures and methods for the evaluation and quantification of biological sequence information useful to a large diversity of proteomic investigations. In this section, we present some interesting techniques for protein sequence similarity detection based on linguistic approaches and information theoretical measures applied exclusively on primary structure of proteins which are sequences made of amino acids.

8.2.1 Protein sequence similarity based on linguistic techniques

Many research groups on computational biology are closely cooperating with those on speech and language processing or with people with experience in this area. They are exploring techniques from computational linguistics on biological sequences for a large diversity of purposes. Interested exclusively in protein sequence similarity, we observed that the applied linguistic methods are oriented even to the textual description attached to biological sequences in a data storage or to the protein sequences themselves. Here we bring together some of these methods and each one has the merit of adding new perspectives in sequence similarity analysis.

Similarity due to regions as index terms in information retrieval

Highly *conversed* regions in biological sequences implies that the corresponding subsequences are not exactly the same but only similar and it is assumed that many times, these regions are more conserved in biological meaning. In [13], a new technique for comparing pairs of biological sequences based on small patterns associated with highly conversed regions on some protein sequences is proposed. This similarity express the relatedness between the compared sequences through their groups of conversed regions. A first step for this new strategy is the grouping of amino acids into different sets according to their similarity based on a scoring matrix like BLOSUM 62 [14] and then assigning to each set a unique code. Two amino acids are considered similar if they have a positive score in BLOSUM 62. While this matrix is a symmetric one, if the amino acid a is similar to b then b is also similar to a. The similarity between amino acids is not transitive so that the organization of amino acids in few similarity groups was not possible. It means that if amino acids b and c are similar to a then b and c don't have to be similar with each other. So, twenty such similarity groups are created and each one get a unique code symbol. The original sequence is transformed into a coding sequence that contains the corresponding codes for each amino acid. Using a sliding window of length 4 over the codified sequence, for each such subsequence all possible combinations are generated, based on the created similarity groups. These combinations are stored as records for each 4 length pattern. Once all the short patterns are found it is defined the *Pattern(p)* as the set of all patterns contained in a protein sequence p. These patterns are used analogous to the text index terms in information retrieval. The new pattern-based similarity measure which we want to underline, that is a quantitative measure of the common information shared by two sequences, is calculated using one of the two following scores:

$$S_1(p_1,p_2) = c \times |Match(p_1,p_2)|/(|Pattern(p_1)|+|Pattern(p_2)|), \qquad (8.1)$$

where $Match(p_1,p_2)$ is the set of patterns shared by sequences p_1 and p_2 and c is a constant, normalizing factor used when the length of the proteins is ignored, or

$$S_2(p_1,p_2) = c \times Match(p_1,p_2)|/ \\ (|Pattern(p_1)|+|Pattern(p_2)|) - |Length(p_1)+Length(p_2)|, \qquad (8.2)$$

when the two protein-sequences are required to have the same length. This algorithm serves as a basic module for applications like phylogenetic analysis, protein clustering and protein secondary structure prediction. Even if the data storage may grow due to the patterns generated, the coding mechanism and the indexed patterns reduces the number of candidates to be checked. This criterion may be considered while protein features are more associated with small groups of amino acids than with individual amino acids. Most of the linguistic investigations on small subsequences of proteins are oriented to the finding similar subsequences, regions or motifs with biological importance than to methods that use them for protein sequence similarity detection. Such an example is in [15] where a protein is considered as a sequence composed of its domains and the extra information is available from "context" (the presence of other words before and after the word in question).

Semantic similarity measures

Many repositories of biological sequences may have a large amount of annotation associated with their entries. This ranges from semi-structured data, such as species information, to unstructured free text descriptions [16], [17]. An ontology provides a set of vocabulary terms that label domain concepts. These terms should have definitions and be placed within a structure of relationships, the most important being the "is-a" relationship between *parent* and *child* and the "part-of" relationship between *part* and *whole*. In analogy, bioinformatic ontologies provide a mechanism for capturing a community's view of a domain in a sharable form accessible by humans and also computationally amenable [16]. The Gene Ontology (GO) (http://www.geneontology.org/goa) is one of the most important ontologies within the bioinformatics community [18]. It comprises three different aspects that hold terms describing the molecular function, biological process and cellular component for a gene product(i.e. proteins). The terms are represented as nodes within a Directed Acyclic Graph (DAG) connected by relationships represented as edges. By providing a standard vocabulary across biological resources such as SWISS-PROT and InterPro annotated protein databases, this kind of shared information, offered by the annotation procedure, enables query across the databases. One way to interrogate these databases would be to ask for proteins which are *semantically similar* to a query protein. Semantic similarity is a concept whereby a set of documents or terms within term list are assigned a metric (i.e. a distance) based on the likeness of their meaning. The semantic distance suggested in [19] is characterized by the assumption that in the Directed Acyclic Graph (DAG) the further GO terms, the less related they are. An important drawback of this approach is that all the semantic links are of equal weight. That's why the information-theoretic metrics have the merits of compensating with heterogeneity in the taxonomy. A measure for the information content shared by two nodes is presented in [20]. Here, the common information shared by two nodes is represented by their common ancestors (called *least common subsumer*, LCS) assuming that the more information two terms share, the more similar they are. Following the notations from [16], the information content of the shared parents of the two terms is expressed by (8.3), where $S(c_1,c_2)$ is the set of parental concepts shared by both c_1 and c_2. The measurements introduced below are considered to be relevant and are based on the information content of each term. It is expressed as a probability which is defined as the number of times each term or any of its child terms occurs in the corpus (the relative frequency). As GO allows multiple parents for each concept, two terms can share parents by multiple paths. Here is taken the minimum $p(c)$ called *probability of the minimum subsummer* p_{ms}, if there is more than one shared parent:

$$p_{ms}(c_1,c_2) = min_{s \in S(c_1,c_2)}\{p(c)\}. \tag{8.3}$$

The similarity measure proposed in [21] uses only the information content of the shared parents. While p_{ms} can vary in the range [0,1], this measure varies between infinity (for very similar concepts) to 0. In practise, for terms actually present in the corpus, the maximum value of this measure is defined by $-\ln(1/t) = \ln(t)$, where t is the number of occurrences of any term in the corpus:

$$sim(c_1,c_2) = -\ln p_{ms}(c_1,c_2). \tag{8.4}$$

A second similarity measure uses both the information content of the shared parents and that of the query terms [22]:

$$sim(c_1,c_2) = \frac{2 \times [\ln p_{ms}(c_1,c_2)]}{\ln p(c_1) + \ln p(c_2)}. \tag{8.5}$$

In this case, as $p_{ms} \geq p(c_1)$ and $p_{ms} \geq p(c_2)$, its value varies between 1 (for similar concepts) and 0.

The similarity measure (8.6) involves the semantic distance which is the inverse similarity [23]. It uses the same terms as (8.5) but not in the same relation type:

$$dist(c_1,c_2) = -2\ln p_{ms}(c_1,c_2) - (\ln p(c_1) + \ln p(c_2)). \tag{8.6}$$

According to [16], this $dist(c_1,c_2)$ can give arbitrarily large values, although, in practice it has a maximum value of $2\ln(t)$ (for t previously defined). Experiments show that sequence similarity obtained with these measures is most tightly correlated (or inversely correlated in the case of distance measure) with the molecular function aspect of GO. One important aspect in these semantic similarity approaches is the number of terms annotated for each protein sequence. When a protein is annotated with more than one term these measures are combined. About the performance, it depends on the size and different aspects of the GO and none of these measures are having advantages over the others while each one is having its strengths and weaknesses. New methods derived from these similarity measures are proposed and tested in research works that use also Gene Ontology concepts [24]-[26].

Language techniques for protein sequence relations

Advances in proteomic sequencing have made available amino acid compositions of thousands of proteins. Knowing the three dimensional shape of the protein, that means knowing the relative positions of each of the atoms in space, would give information on potential interaction sites in the protein. This fact renders possible the analysis or inference of the protein function and establish relations between sequences.

Extracting protein interaction relationships from textual repositories, prove to be useful in generating novel biological hypotheses. Scientists often use textual databases to ascertain further information about specific biological entities such as proteins. Using a natural-language processing tool, in [17] is realized a rule-based analysis to retrieve textual data in order to find similar proteins, with the similarity expressing the notion of common functional attributes. With relevant abstracts of known functionally related proteins, and a modified existing natural language processing tool able to extract protein interaction terms, were obtained functional information about the proteins involved in experiments.

A method used in text processing which is able to **capture semantic relations** between words using global information extracted from a large number of documents rather than comparing the simple occurrences of words in two documents is Latent Semantic Analysis (LSA). This method is based on Singular Value Decomposition (SVD) [27]. It identify words in a text that address the same topic or are synonymous, even if such information is not explicitly available. This is an extremely useful approach in natural language processing to generate summaries, compare and classify documents, generate thesauri and further more for information retrieval [28], [29]. In biological context, the goal of LSA is to find in a collection of documents the most thematically similar documents with a new, unseen one. For a simplistic description, one assumes that we are dealing with a matrix where columns are representing documents and rows are the words from a vocabulary. Thus, the information in a document is represented in terms of its constituent words. Due to the differences in document lengths each word count is normalized by the length of the document where it occurs and the total count of the words in the corpus. This representation of words and documents is called Vector Space Model (SVM) [30] and it does not recognize synonymous or related words. Such kind representations may suffer from the peaking phenomenon because the features are usually very large and noise data may be introduced. Excepting when a thesaurus is available and word counts of similar terms can be merged, the LSA may be applied. It means that singular value decomposition (SVD) is performed and three matrices are obtained. Two of them are left and respectively right singular matrices and the other one have its terms in decreasing order of magnitude along the main diagonal. Us ually only the top r dimensions whose magnitude is over a threshold are considered for further processing.

So far, the three matrices product leads to a compression of data. For document vectors given as columns in the SVM matrix, they can be compared to each other using a similarity measure such cosine similarity . This cosine similarity is the cos of the angle between two vectors and is one when the two are identical and zero when they are completely ortogonal/different. The document with maximum cosine similarity to the given document is the one most similar to it. Detailed description of LSA method and cosine similarity may be read in [28]-[32].

The success of SVM methods respectively LSA depends on the feature set used to represent each protein. In remote homology detection of proteins it is assumed that documents are protein sequences and the words are different patterns, motifs, conserved regions in a protein, n-grams (all sets of amino acids of fixed length n) [33]. Analogous to document classification, word-document matrix is constructed using the weight of each *word* in the documents and the LSA model is applied in order to decrease the original dimension of protein vectors. Also, using words from PubMed abstracts, LSA in association with vector space model is applied on biomedical literature in order to find functional themes. On this way a successful method for protein family prediction based on literature analysis is tested in [34]. In a procedure for protein association discovery LSA is used for automatically extraction and determination of associations among proteins from biomedical literature [35]. Such a tool has notable potential to automate database construction in biomedicine, instead of relying on experts' analysis.

Even if our interest was mainly on protein similarity methods using the primary structure of proteins, we observed language techniques that use the implication of secondary structure elements in establishing structural similarity relations between proteins. Thus, the determination or prediction of the protein structure from the amino acid sequences has secured an important place both in experimental and computational areas of research. Since LSA captures conceptual relations in a text based on the word distribution in documents, it is used to capture secondary structure propensities (tendencies) in protein sequences using different vocabularies [27]. All the refereed works report successful results in using the latent semantic analysis but it is easy to observe the computational complexity involved in constructing the word-document matrix and reducing its rank for large amount of data.

A **combination of statistics and information theory** notions are in Hidden Markov Models (HMM) applications used for speech recognition systems. The mathematical method of HMM has found also considerable applications in biological sequence analysis especially for sequence alignment. Durbin et al. [4] have made a large description of the methods in biological sequences that apply this concept. Tools like Pfam [36], InterPro [37] or Sequence Alignment and Modeling System (SAM)[4] are successfully using it in sequence analysis and comparison. Existing a large literature on this subject here we do not insist more on these approaches.

Language technologies often use word n-grams as features that refer to sequential occurences of words in a text. In biological sequences, the best equivalent of human words is not known [38] so that n-grams usually describe short sequences of

---

[4]http://www.soe.ucsc.edu/compbio/sam.html

nucleotides or amino acids of length n. In BLAST algorithm [7] this notion is used to enhance the computational efficiency at the initial step of sequence searching. However, n-grams have proven to be useful in a number of other bioinformatics area. We are continuing to discuss about this concept in the 3-rd Section, where is introduced a similarity measure based on statistical n-gram evaluation.

8.2.2 Sequence similarity based on information theoretic methods

In many biological applications we are interested to quantify the similarity of a pair of sequences and to state to what extent one sequence is redundant with respect to the other, i.e. the information content in one is repeated in the other. Kolmogorov complexity theory, known also as algorithmic information theory, deals with quantifying the information in individual sequences. Algorithmic information theory has been introduced independently, with different motivations, by R.J. Solomonoff, A.N. Kolmogorov and G. Chaitin, between 1960-1966. Kolmogorov complexity of a sequence can be defined in an elegant way as the length of the program needed to be run for recovering the sequence on an universal computer. However, one of the important results of the theory tells that Kolmogorov complexity is non-computable, which makes it necessary to resort to approximations, when the concept is used in practice. In many instances the evaluation of Kolmogorov complexity needed in various definitions of similarity is based on the simpler notion of codelength of a compressed sequence, as provided by one of the general use compressors (like Lempel-Ziv or Burrows-Wheeler compressors). Several similarity distances based on approximates of the Kolmogorov complexity have been shown to perform well in different applications such as: language and authorship recognition [39], plagiarism detection [40], [41], language tree and genome phylogenetic trees reconstruction [39], [42]-[47], phylogeny of chain letters [48] or protein sequence classification [49].

The Kolmogorov complexity $K(x)$ of a sequence x is the length of the shortest binary program that outputs x on an universal computer and can be thought as the minimal amount of information necessary to produce x. The conditional Kolmogorov complexity, $K(x|y)$, is defined as the length of the shortest binary program that computes x when y is given as input, using an universal computer [50].

The problem of an absolute information distance metric between two individual objects was studied in [51] in terms of Kolmogorov complexity, which resulted in defining the information distance as the length of the shortest binary program that can transform either object into the other. Because the program is the shortest it has to take into account any redundancy between the information required to obtain x starting from y, or, to obtain y starting from x. It has been shown in [51] that the information distance equals:

$$I_D(x,y) = \max\{K(x|y), K(y|x)\} \quad (8.7)$$

up to an additive $O(\log \max\{K(y|x), K(x|y)\})$ term. $I_D(x,y)$ satisfies the metric properties up to an additive finite constant.

The problem with $I_D(x,y)$ is that it measures the absolute information between the two objects without taking into account their lengths. For example, if we have two very long strings that differ only in 100 bit positions that would represent about 0.001% of their length, we want to call them very similar; while if we have two other much shorter strings that differ also in 100 bit positions, but this represents about 90% of their length, we want to call the strings very dissimilar. However, the quantities $I_D(x,y)$ may be close to 100 in both cases, making it difficult to evaluate the similarity/dissimilarity in these cases of notably different length of sequences.

To overcome this problem, the first attempt to a normalized distance was introduced in [42]. The normalized similarity distance aims to provide a relative similarity between the objects: when the distance is 0 the objects under investigation are maximally similar and when the distance is 1 the objects are maximally dissimilar.

The normalized distance introduced in [42] was based on the property that the algorithmic mutual information between two objects $I(x,y) = K(x) - K(x|y)$ is symmetric, $I(x,y) = K(y) - K(y|x)$ within an additive logarithmic factor [52], yielding the following formula for the similarity distance of two sequences:

$$d(x,y) = 1 - \frac{K(x) - K(x|y)}{K(xy)} = 1 - \frac{K(y) - K(y|x)}{K(xy)} \qquad (8.8)$$

where $K(xy)$ represents the Kolmogorov complexity of the concatenated strings. It has been shown in [43], that this distance is a metric, i.e. it has the following properties: (a)-positivity $d(x,y) > 0$ for $x \neq y$; (b)-identity $d(x,x) = 0$; (c)-symmetry $d(x,y) = d(y,x)$ and (d)-triangle inequality $d(x,y) \leq d(x,z) + d(z,y)$.

In the paper [45], the authors introduced the normalized information distance "mathematically, more precise and satisfying" than the previous one:

$$d_i(x,y) = \frac{max\{K(x|y^*), K(y|x^*)\}}{max\{K(x), K(y)\}} \qquad (8.9)$$

where, for any string v, the notation v^* specifies the shortest binary program to compute v. There is an intuitive interpretation of this distance: if $K(y) > K(x)$ then $d_i(x,y) = \frac{K(y) - I(x,y)}{K(y)} = 1 - \frac{I(x,y)}{K(y)}$, where $I(x,y) = K(y) - K(y|x)$ is the algorithmic mutual information. It follows that $1 - d_i(x,y)$ is the number of bits of information that is shared between the two strings per bit of information of the string with most information. It is shown that the normalized information distance is a metric and it is universal up to a certain precision.

The problem with the normalized information distance is that its generality comes with the price of noncomputability, because it is expressed in terms of $K(x), K(y), K(x|y)$, and $K(y|x)$, which are noncomputable quantities. To overcome this problem, the normalized compression distance was introduced in [45], that uses a real-world reference compressor C to approximate Kolmogorov complexity:

$$NCD(x,y) = \frac{C(xy) - min\{C(x), C(y)\}}{max\{C(x), C(y)\}} \qquad (8.10)$$

where $C(xy)$ denotes the compressed size of the concatenated sequences, $C(x)$ denotes the compressed size of x and $C(y)$ denotes the compressed size of y. It has been shown in [47] that if the compressor satisfies simple regularity conditions, then $NCD(x,y)$ is a similarity metric. The performance of the normalized compression distance was tested in [47] for applications in different areas such as: genomic, music, language, handwriting, combination of objects from different domains, etc.

One of the most useful applications of the normalized compression distance is the comparison of two different genomes/proteomes and the study of the evolution of a group of species. Traditional phylogeny studies based on individual genes depend on the multiple alignment of the given gene shared by all the organism in the study. The problem with constructing phylogenetic trees based on individual genes is that different genes yield different trees. As the complete genomes for more and more organisms become available, the study of evolution based on the genome is more attractive. Any method based on multiple alignments will provide too many results to be combined when full genomes are involved, and the aggregation of partial results to infer a similarity measure has no straightforward solution.

To take full advantages of the normalized compression distance, it turns out that we need a very efficient compressor in order to have a powerful tool in genomic and proteomic sequence similarity studies. Several algorithms for the compression of biological sequences have been proposed with varying degree of success. While the compression of DNA sequences was carefully studied in the last decade, less is known about the compressibility of protein sequences. The main reason is that compression of DNA sequences was shown to be successful from its first attempts in the early 90's. That attracted many research groups to compete in capturing in the best way the regularities present in DNA sequences [53]-[58]. Unexpectedly, the compression of protein sequences attracted less research, a possible reason being the fact that the first elaborate report on this topic was negative: in a 1999 paper [59] at Data Compression Conference an authoritative opinion was expressed in the negative, the statement making the title being: "Protein is incompressible". Although several plausible schemes have been tried in [59], including making use of the statistical description by substitution probabilities, the compression results by using these mutational processes were not better than the results by using only memory models of small order, leading to the conclusion that proteins are incompressible. In 2004, a report [46] was published, in which the compressibility of protein sequences is revealed in a scheme making use of substitution probabilities. The main feature of the scheme was the adaptivity in estimating the substitution probabilities, in that only the substitution statistics collected over regions where these statistics will improve the description length, when compared to the raw model or to a simple memory model, were used. The positive conclusion regarding the compressibility of protein sequences was drawn in [46] from the significant improvement of the compression results over the results reported in [59]. In Section 8.4 we present our algorithm for protein sequences compression and how it can be used to estimate the Kolmogorov complexity and then to compute the similarity of the given sequences.

8.3 Statistical language modeling method for sequence similarity

As we already mentioned in the previous sections, the mapping of a protein sequence to its structure, functional dynamics and biological role becomes analogous to the mapping of words to their semantic meaning in natural languages. This analogy can be valorized by applying statistical language modeling and text classification techniques for the advance of biological sequences understanding. Different than linguistic concepts used for protein sequence similarity detection presented before, here we give attention to the identification of Gramar/Syntax rules that could reveal systematic information of high importance for biological and medical sciences.

8.3.1 Theoretical concepts

There are various kinds of language models that can be used to capture different aspects of regularities in natural language like latent semantic analysis, contrext free grammars that counts on word distribution in documents or sentence-level sintactic structures and document level semantic content [60], [61]. Markov chains are generally considered important concepts for building language models assuming that the observation of a word w_k at a position k in a given text depends only upon its immediate n predecessor words $w_{k-n} \ldots w_{k-1}$. The resulting stochastic models, usually referred as n-grams, constitute heuristic approaches for building language grammars. Nowadays n-gram language modeling has gained high popularity biological sequence analysis due to its simplicity and efficiency [38], [62]. In statistical sequence analysis proposed in [63], n-gram distribution was found to be characteristic of organisms as evidenced by the ability of simple unigram models to distinguish organisms. Also, the marked variation in n-gram distribution across organisms and the identification of organism-specific phrases suggests that different organisms utilize different *vocabularies*. In analogy to word n-gram analysis this linguistic structure results in powerful models for prediction, topic classification and information extraction in biological sequences. For protein secondary structure prediction, Liu et al. [64] proves that the use of context sensitive vocabulary improve the accuracy prediction of secondary structure over the common n-gram, which indicates that the context information is very important in protein structures formation. Segmenting the protein amino acid sequence according to its secondary structure is assumed to be analogous to the problem of topic segmentation in [65]. The method considers the building of an n-gram language model for each topic and compare their performance in predicting the current amino acid in order to determine whether a border in transmembrane helix occurs at the current position. For protein classification, on counts of n-grams, it is applied a Decision Three and Naive Bayes classifier [66]. There are also works in computational biology that are successfully using this n-gram concept even if it is out of the linguistic meaning. As example, the similarity is highlighted through the matching concept at a local similarity. For that, it is used a distance concept defined to measure the level of hits between the compared sequences so that the focus is on near perfect matching for many queries in protein database [67].

Closely related with the design of models for textual data are algorithmic procedures for validating them. Apart from the justification of a single model, they can facilitate the selection of the specific one (among competing alternatives), most faithfully representing the available data. Entropy is a key concept in this procedure. In general, its estimation is considered to provide a quantification of the information in a text and has strong connections to probabilistic language modeling [68]. As described in [69] and [70], the entropy of a random variable X defined over a domain $\aleph$, and having a probability density function, $P(X)$ is defined as:

$$H(X) = -\sum_{X \in \aleph} P(X) \log P(X). \qquad (8.11)$$

For the case where a written sequence $W = w_1, w_2, \ldots, w_{k-1}, w_k, w_{k+1}, \ldots$ is treated as a language model L based composition with the consecutive n elements of the sequence symbolized as w_1^n and called n-gram, the entropy may be estimated as follows:

$$\hat{H}(X) = -\frac{1}{N} \sum_{W^*} Count(w_1^n) \log_2 p_L(w_1^n \mid w_1^{n-1}), \qquad (8.12)$$

where the variable X has the form of an n-gram, $X = w_1^n$ and $Count(w_1^n)$ is the number of occurrences of w_1^n. The summation runs over all the possible n-length combinations of consecutive w_i, i.e. set $W^* = \{(w_1, w_2, \ldots, w_n), (w_2, w_3, \ldots, w_{n+1}), \ldots\}$ and N is the total number of n-grams in the investigated sequence. The second term in the summation (8.12) is the conditional probability that relates the n-th element of an n-gram with the preceding n-1 elements. Following the principles of maximum likelihood estimation (MLE)[69], it can be expressed by using the corresponding relative frequencies:

$$\hat{p}\left(w_1^n \mid w_1^{n-1}\right) = \frac{Count(w_1^n)}{Count(w_1^{n-1})}. \qquad (8.13)$$

According to a general definition, the cross-entropy between the actual probability distribution of a data $P(X)$, and the probability distribution $Q(X)$ estimated from a model, is defined as:

$$H(X, Q) = -\sum_{X \in \aleph} P(X) \log Q(X). \qquad (8.14)$$

Two important aspects involved in this approach are: first, the cross-entropy of a stochastic process, measured by using a model, is an upper bound on the entropy of the process (i.e. $H(X) \leq H(X, Q)$) [69], [70]; second, as mentioned in [71], between two given models, the more accurate is the one with the lower cross-entropy. The above entropic estimations are the basis for building the protein similarity measure, described in the sequel.

8.3.2 Method description

Choosing a hypothetical protein sequence WASQVSENR, in the 2-gram modeling, the available "words" are WA AS SQ QV VS SE EN NR, while in the 3-gram representation the words are WAS ASQ SQV QVS VSE SEN ENR. Based on the frequencies of these words (estimated by counting), the entropy of a n-gram model can be readily estimated by (8.12). This measure is indicative about how well a specific protein-sequence is modeled by the corresponding n-gram model. While this measure could be applied to two distinct proteins (and help us to decide about which protein is better represented by the given model), the outcomes cannot be used for a direct comparison of the two proteins. This shortcoming is leading to a corresponding cross-entropy measure, in which the n-gram model is first built based on the word-counts of one protein sequence Y and then used in sequence X, contrasting the two proteins. Thus, the information content between two proteins X, Y is expressed via the formula:

$$E(X,Y) = - \sum_{alw_1^n \in X} P_X(w_1^n) \log P_Y(w_1^n \mid w_1^{n-1}). \tag{8.15}$$

The first term $P_X(w_1^n)$ in the above summation refers to the reference protein sequence X, i.e. it results from counting the words of that specific protein. The second term, $\log P_Y(w_1^n \mid w_1^{n-1})$, refers to the sequence Y based on which the model has to be estimated (i.e. it results from counting the words of this protein). The variable w_1^n ranges over all the words (that are represented by n-grams) of the reference protein sequence.

8.3.3 Protein similarity search

The essential point of this approach is that the unknown query-protein (e.g. a newly discovered protein) as well as each protein in a given database (containing annotated proteins with known functionality, structure etc.) are represented via n-gram encoding and the above introduced similarity is utilized to compare their representations. Here two different ways are devised using n-gram similarity for efficient proteomic database searches. The most straightforward implementation is called hereafter as *direct method*. A second algorithm, called the *alternating method*, was devised in order to cope with the fact that the proteins to be compared might be of very different length. The implication of this aspect is observable in the ratio value between the number of words from the reference sequence involved in computing the similarity score and the total number of words in the particular sequence which is involved in the probability $P_X(w_1^n)$. The experimentation with both methods and the comparison of their performances gives the opportunity to check the sensitivity of the proposed measure to the sequences length.

Direct method:
Let Sq be the sequence of a query-protein and $\{S\} = \{S_1, S_2, \ldots S_N\}$ be the given protein database. The first step is the computation of the '*perfect*' score (PS) or '*reference*' score for the query-protein. This is done by computing $E(S_q, S_q)$ using the

query-protein both as reference and model sequence in equation (8.15). In the second step, each protein S_i, $i = 1,\ldots,N$, from the database serves as the model sequence in the computation of a similarity score $E(S_q, S_i)$, using the same equation (8.15) with the query-protein serving as the reference sequence. In this way, N similarities are computed $E(S_q, S_i)$, $i = 1,\ldots,N$. Finally, these similarities are compared against the perfect score PS. By computing the absolute differences $D(S_q, S_i) = |E(S_q, S_i) - PS|$, the 'discrepancies' in terms of information content between the query-protein and the database-proteins are expressed. By these N measurements, we can easily identify the most similar proteins to the query-protein as those which have been assigned the lowest $D(S_q, S_i)$.

Alternating method:
The only difference with respect to the direct method is that, when comparing the query-protein with each database-sequence, the role of reference and model protein can be interchanged based on which of the two sequences is the shortest one, i.e. the shortest sequence plays the role of the reference sequence in (8.15). The rest of the steps (i.e. perfect-score estimation, ranking and selection) are the same as in the *direct method*.

8.3.4 Experimental results

The *n*-gram based methods proposed for measuring protein similarity were demonstrated and validated in some experiments described in detail in [9], [72], [73]. A first set of experiments were done over a sequence database containing 50 random protein sequences from NCBI public databaseand other 50 entries corresponded to proteins resulted from different mutations of the p53 gene. The mutations were selected randomly from the database we created using the descriptions provided by the International Agency for Research on Cancer[5] (IARC) Lyon, France. In order to provide the performance of the two variants, the similarity relation between all the possible pairs of sequences of the database is analyzed. Thus, it is expected that the mutated sequences will have a high degree of similarity. When validating protein-database searches we adopted an index of search accuracy derived from Receiver Operating Characteristic (ROC) curves [74], [75]. This index, is the ratio of the area under the ROC-curve in the plot of true positive versus false positive rates for different thresholds of dissimilarity. The interest was to obtain the values where the true positive rates reach 1 or a very close value to 1, for a small rate of false positives. In Table 8.1 are the values of false positive and true positive rates for different *n*-gram models, thresholds and both of the methods till maximum true positive rate is reached.

The same experiments are performed over a second database of sequences which is a set of 1460 proteins extracted from the current version (i.e. 1.67) of Astral SCOP[6] sequence resource database. >From the available corpus of data, only those families that contained at least 10 protein sequences were included in our database

---
[5]http://www.iarc.fr/p53/Somatic.html
[6]http://astral.berkeley.edu

Table 8.1. False positive rates (FPR) and true positive rates (TPR) for different n-gram models using both evaluation strategies.

n-gram	Thresholds	Direct Method		Alternating Method	
		FPR	TPR	FPR	TPR
2-gram	0.005	0.009	0.298	0.009	0.416
	0.1	0.106	0.698	0.118	0.849
	1.46	0.900	1.000		
3-gram	0.005	0.007	0.476	0.018	0.512
	0.1	0.256	0.701	0.250	0.834
	0.38	0.885	1.000	0.895	1.000
4-gram	0.005	0.005	0.527	0.005	0.612
	0.1	0.005	0.894	0.007	0.998
	0.25	0.175	1.000		

since it was dictated by the *precision* measure adopted for the evaluation. In this way, 31 different families unequally populated, were finally included in three sets that do not exceed 500 sequences. We recall here the fact that the annotation of our database follows the original annotation which relies on the biological meaning of similarity concept adopted for SCOP database. Therefore, it provides a 'ground-truth' for the attempted similarity measurements. The *precision* measure adopted as index of search accuracy, is the ratio computed by dividing the correctly classified number of protein sequences (identified by the algorithm as the 10 most similar ones) with 10 (the minimal number of sequences within a family). More specifically, each protein was treated as query and we measured the accuracy of the first 10 sequences identified within the set as the most similar to the query-protein. In Table 8.2, the precision scores provided by both of our approaches for different n-gram models have been included. It is worth mentioning that this new algorithmic strategy reaches (in the case of 4-gram modeling for the third set) a high performance. For the sake of completeness, we repeated the Precision-index measurements for the case that our search strategy was applied to the overall set of 1460 proteins. The computed values were not significantly different from the values corresponding to the three different sets, providing some further evidence about the robustness of the method and indicating that its performance scales well with the size of the database.

Table 8.2. The precision scores for similarity results obtained by similarity methods for 2,3,4-gram models for three data sets.

Set	Direct Method			Alternating Method		
	2-gram	3-gram	4-gram	2-gram	3-gram	4-gram
1	0.439	0.662	0.830	0.471	0646	0.823
2	0.446	0.650	0.874	0.439	0.605	0.860
3	0.534	0.865	0.931	0.574	0.828	0.919

8.3.5 Discussions

The results obtained by applying this strategy for measuring protein similarity gave us a good motivation to keep the attention on it. Considering the general dichotomy between "global" and "local" protein similarity measures, this new approach for sequence similarity belongs to the former category. The assumption is motivated by the fact that a global method for sequence similarity assumes the consideration of the whole content of the compared sequences while the local similarity methods are addressed only to subsections of the involved sequences.

The experimental results indicated the reliability of the algorithmic strategy for expressing similarity between proteins. The performance of the method improves with the order of the model up to 4. After the order of 5 due to the lack of data, the corresponding maximum likelihood estimates become unreasonably uniform and poor. Data sparsity is one of the problems encountered in statistical evaluation methods. Here no smoothing algorithm is considered while the predictability of amino acids in a protein structure is difficult to be established. For this stage of development of the similarity method the purpose was to keep only those events (unique n-length sequences) that may contribute with a positive value to the profile of the analyzed sequence.

It is easy to observe the ability of this approach to capture the regularities in protein sequences. The good performance of the 4-gram models may suggest the implication of some groups of amino acids repeats in characterization of protein sequences. This order of n value was also confirmed in other research works [64], [38]. For comparison of sequences having the same length, both methods (*alternative* and *direct*) performs similar. While this method performs well on long and very long sequences, at this stage of development, it may be suggested as a first search for long proteins in large databases of sequences. While the contribution of each n-gram event and sequences length are important in sequence similarity detection and maximum likelihood estimations are not enough for this purpose, a normalizing factor or an adequate strategy that increase this contribution aspect is desirable. In [73] is made a comparison of the performance of this method with that based on sequence alignment applied by Clustal W. The results are almost the same while the simplity and computational afficiency of the new method is evident. An important step forward in development of this method would be to consider the biological properties of amino acids. It can be easy observed that this method is exclusively based on statistical estimation of linguistic n-gram models but due to the conceptual simplicity and fast computation provided it may deserve attention for future developments.

8.4 Protein similarity detection based on lossless compression of protein sequences

The primary goal of a compression algorithm is to reduce as much as possible the size of a data set. For biological sequences, the study of their compressibility has a double value. The first one is a concrete, practical value, since storing or transmitting a sequence which was compressed leads to savings of computer resources and transmission costs. However, at the current compressibility rates obtained for DNA and proteins, these savings seem to be only marginally important. The second value, which is probably the most important one, is that of the statistical models uncovered by an efficient coding technique from the sequence to be compressed, models that can be subsequently used to measure the similarity of different sequences or for further statistical inference in various biological problems. The most useful application of protein similarity detection based on the compressibility of their sequences is the building of phylogenetic trees using the whole proteome of the given organisms. The proteome is the collection of all protein sequences in one organism.

8.4.1 Theoretical concepts

To define the relation or similarity of two proteome sequences, based on the average description length obtained by a given compressor, we introduce first the mutual information of two random variables X and Y that range over an alphabet $\mathcal{A}$. According to [76], the mutual information of two random variables is a measure of the amount of information one random variable contains about the other and is defined as:

$$I(X,Y) = H(X) - H(X|Y) = H(Y) - H(Y|X) \tag{8.16}$$

where $H(X)$ and $H(Y)$ are the entropies of X and Y defined by (8.11). $H(Y|X)$ is the conditional entropy of Y given X and is defined as the expected value of the entropies of the conditional distributions over the conditioning random variable [76]:

$$H(Y|X) = \sum_{x \in \mathcal{A}} p(x) H(Y|X = x) \tag{8.17}$$

Since the entropy is an idealistic measure of the average codelength for encoding a symbol generated by the source, it might be replaced by the implementable average codelength obtained by a compression algorithm to obtain a realistic evaluation of average codelengths or information content. Because the protein sequences are kept in text files, one might think that the classic algorithms for text compression could be used to compress such a file. Practically, these algorithms do not perform better than $\log_2 20 = 4.3219$ bits per symbol which is the cost for encoding a symbol without any modelling. The reason for this poor performance is that protein sequences obey other rules than human created text. It turns out that we need a specialized compressor for proteome sequences. Such a compressor, named *ProtComp* was introduced in [46]. Its main idea and its use in computing the similarity of two sequences is described in the next section.

8.4.2 ProtComp algorithm and its use in sequence comparison

One of the first attempts at compressing proteins [59], presented a negative result, claiming from title that proteins are incompressible. The authors proposed a scheme base on a sophisticated context algorithm, where not only the current context is used, but also similar contexts are used for prediction, the weighting of contexts being dependent on the mutation probabilities of amino-acids. However, their results were not better than the results obtained with simple, low order Markov models, which led them to the conclusion that the approximate repeats in protein can not provide statistically significant information to be exploited for compression. The main problem of this scheme is that the model used is based on the patternsfound in the immediate vicinity of the symbol that is to be encoded at a given moment and it ignores the redundancy of different regions of the proteome, that are the result of different biological phenomena such as gene duplication.

The *ProtComp* algorithm was developed with the purpose of extracting the regularities at the scale of full proteome, by searching for approximate repeats and adaptively estimate the amino acids substitution probabilities over the regions where the statistics will improve the description length of that region, when compared to the description length obtained by the raw model. The *ProtComp* algorithm can operate in *single* mode, when the input is a single proteome and the regularities are extracted based on this sequence; and it can operate also in *conditional* mode, when the input is composed of two proteomes, one that is encoded and one that is considered to be known and the regularities are extracted from both sequences.

ProtComp is a two pass algorithm. The goal of the first pass is to collect the substitution probabilities and the goal of the second pass is to encode the symbols. The proteome sequence that is to be encoded is split into non-overlapping blocks of same length and for each *current block* we look for that block in the sequence from the beginning until the current block, obtaining the greatest number of matches (the same amino acid in the same position) and we refer to it as a *regressor block*. When the algorithm operates in the conditional mode, the regressor block can be found in the conditioning proteome. In the first pass, the probability substitution matrix is collected for the symbols having the same rank in the current block and in its regressor block, but only for those pairs (current block, regressor block) for which the number of matches is greater than a given threshold. For each conditional distribution, obtained from each row of the substitution matrix, we design an optimal Huffman code [77]. All these optimal codes have to be transmitted to the decoder as a prefix of the encoded stream. In the second pass, we go through the proteome sequence and encode a block that have the number of matches greater than the threshold using the optimal codes built in the first pass. The rest of the blocks, for which the number of matches does not exceed the threshold, are encoded by arithmetic coding [78], using the statistics of an adaptive first order Markov model [79].

Inspired by the mutual information of two random variables $I(X,Y)$ (8.16), and using the average codelengths obtained by *ProtComp* algorithm, in [46] the similarity of two proteomes X and Y was defined as:

$$R(X,Y) = ProtComp(X) - ProtComp(X|Y) \quad (8.18)$$

where $ProtComp(X)$ is the average codelength obtained when the proteome X is encoded by *ProtComp* in the single mode and $ProtComp(X|Y)$ is the average codelength obtained when the proteome X is encoded by *ProtComp* in the conditional mode, i.e. when the proteome Y is given as input argument and is considered to be known. The value of $R(X,Y)$ will be close to *ProtComp*(X) when the two proteomes are very similar, because *ProtComp*$(X|Y)$ will tend to zero (if Y is already known and X is very similar to Y then the average codelength of encoding X knowing Y will tend to zero) and the value of $R(X,Y)$ will tend to zero when X and Y are maximum dissimilar (if X and Y are completely dissimilar or independent, than knowing Y does not help at all and the average codelength of encoding X knowing Y will tend to *ProtComp*(X)).

Using this measure of similarity of two proteomes a phylogenetic tree can be built for a given set of organisms. The building process of the phylogenetic tree consists at each step in computing the relatedness of all pairs of proteomes and the two proteomes that yield the maximum R are grouped, i.e. the two proteome sequences are concatenated and in the next step they form a new single proteome sequence. The process is repeated until only two proteome sequences are left.

The fact that plausible phylogenetic trees can be built using this measure of similarity means that the *ProtComp* algorithm manages to capture the biological meaningful features of the proteome sequences. Thus, a natural question arises, i.e. if the similarity measure defined based on the average codelength produced by *ProtComp* can be used to measure the similarity of two protein sequences, which are of much shorter length than a whole proteome. Using a slightly different version of *ProtComp* algorithm, the similarities of two protein sequences can be defined in a similar way to (8.18), such that the resulted codelength can be seen as the sum of substitution scores over the similar parts of the proteins and can be compared to alignment scores obtained by classical algorithms for sequence comparison.

A modified version of the *ProtComp* algorithm and its use in defining a measure of similarity for pairs of proteins was presented in [80]. Because the goal now is to compare pairs of proteins in different organisms, the substitution matrix is not collected for each pair of proteins, because there is not enough statistics at this level and only the cost of transmitting the matrix may be greater than the cost of encoding the whole sequence of amino acids. Then, for each pair of organisms, a substitution frequency matrix is collected at the proteome level and the associated Huffman codes are used to compute the similarity of proteins from that organisms.

Following the same idea as in the original *ProtComp* algorithm, for a given pair of proteins, the protein to be encoded is first compressed using the statistics of its own sequence and then is conditionally encoded using the statistics of the other sequence. The similarity of the two proteins is given by the difference in the encoding costs. The protein to be encoded is also split in non-overlapping blocks of a certain length. In the first case, the regressor block is searched only in the already seen sequence and in the second case, the regressor is searched also in the other protein. The pair of blocks having the number of matches greater than a fixed threshold are encoded conditional on their regressor using the Huffman codes designed at the proteome level, while the blocks with less number of matches than the threshold are encoded in clear using $\log_2(20)$ bits/amino acid. Using this method to encode the amino acids in the blocks with number of matches less than the threshold has an interesting interpretation when computing the similarity of the two proteins.

Let $X = x_1,\ldots,x_{N_x}$ be the protein which is to be encoded and $Y = y_1,\ldots,y_{N_y}$ the conditioning protein. For each block $x^k = x_{(i-1)k+1},\ldots,x_{(i-1)k+L}$, where L is the length of the block, a regressor block is found $r_p^k = r_1,\ldots,r_L$ where depending on the value of p we have two cases: $r_1,\ldots,r_L = x_t,\ldots,x_{t+L-1}$ if $p = 1$, which means that the regressor is found before the current block in the protein sequence which is to be encoded, or $r_1,\ldots,r_L = y_t,\ldots,y_{t+L-1}$ if $p = 2$, which means that the regressor is found in the other protein. If $p = 1$, then $t \leq (i-2)k+L$ and if $p = 2$, then $t \leq N_y$. The similarity of the two proteins X and Y is given by $R(X,Y)$ (8.18), where *ProtComp* is modified to work with short sequences. Let $N_b = \lfloor \frac{N_x}{L} \rfloor$ be the number of non-overlapping blocks in the protein X and let $\mathcal{L}(a|b)$ be the encoding cost of a given block a when the regressor block b is given. Then (8.18) becomes:

$$R(X,Y) = \sum_{k=1}^{N_b}[\mathcal{L}(x^k|r_1^k) - \mathcal{L}(x^k|r_p^k)] =$$

$$= \sum_{i=1}^{N_{b1}}[\mathcal{L}(x^i|r_1^i) - \mathcal{L}(x^i|r_p^i)] +$$

$$+ \sum_{j=1}^{N_{b2}}[\mathcal{L}(x^j|r_1^j) - \mathcal{L}(x^j|r_2^j)] =$$

$$= \sum_{j=1}^{N_{b2}}[\mathcal{L}(x^j|r_1^j) - \mathcal{L}(x^j|r_2^j)] \qquad (8.19)$$

where N_{b1} is the number of blocks for which the number of matches is less then the fixed threshold and N_{b2} is the number of blocks for which at least in the conditional case the number of matches is greater than the fixed threshold. Because the sum of the encoding costs over the blocks that do not have the number of matches greater than the threshold is the same even the protein is conditionally encoded or not, is zero, we can further write (8.19) as:

$$R(X,Y) = \sum_{i=1}^{N_{b21}}[L\log_2(20) - \mathcal{L}(x^i|r_2^i)] +$$

$$+ \sum_{j=1}^{N_{b22}}[\mathcal{L}(x^i|r_1^i) - \mathcal{L}(x^i|r_2^i)] \qquad (8.20)$$

where N_{b21} is the number of blocks for which only in the conditional case the number of matches exceeds the fixed threshold and N_{b22} is the number of blocks for which in both cases the number of matches is greater than the fixed threshold. It turns out that our method to define the relatedness of two proteins is in fact a measure of the local similarities of the two proteins because the regions where the proteins are not similar are discarded.

8.4.3 Experimental results

To assess the ability of the *ProtComp* algorithm to help on finding similarities at a macro scale, i.e. at proteome level, as well at a micro scale, i.e. at the protein level, two experiments were done in [46] and [80].

In the first experiment, the goal was to build a phylogenetic tree, to see if the similarity measure (8.18) can manage to capture regularities at the full proteome level. To do this, seven organisms for which the phylogentic tree was built previously at the genome level [42], were used. The proteome sequences for the following organisms have been used: *Archaeoglobus fulgidus* (AF), *Escherichia coli K-12 MG1655* (EC), *Pyrococcus abyssi* (PA), *Pyrococcus horikoshii* (PH), *Haemophilus influenzae Rd* (HI), *Helicobacter pylori 26695* (HP1) and *Helicobacter pylori, strain J99* (HP2). The first step in building the tree is to compute the similarity between all the proteomes and the results are presented in Table 8.3. Because the similarity measure is not symmetric in practice, we pick the proteomes having the highest sum $R(X,Y) + R(Y,X)$ as being the most related, so that for the first step $HP1$ and $HP2$ are the most related. For the next step, $HP1HP2$ is treated as a single proteome and we have to compute the relatedness between this new proteome and all the others. In the second step, the most related proteomes will be *PA* and *PH*, in the third step *EC* and *HI*, in the fourth step *PAPH* and *AF*, in the fifth step *HP1HP2* and *ECHI* and finally, *HP1HP2ECHI* and *PAPHAF*. The final phylogenetic tree, that is the same as in [40], is presented in Figure 8.2.

Table 8.3. The similarity between all the proteomes in the first step of the phylogenetic tree building.

	AF	EC	PA	PH	HI	HP1	HP2
AF		0.01	0.11	0.10	0.01	0	0
EC	0		0	0	0.29	0.03	0.03
PA	0.14	0.01		1.51	0.01	0	0
PH	0.13	0.01	1.52		0	-0.01	0
HI	0.01	0.78	0.01	0		0.07	0.07
HP1	0.01	0.09	0	0	0.08		**2.22**
HP2	0.01	0.09	0	0	0.08	**2.26**	

In the second experiment, the goal was to test if the similarity measure (8.18) can be used to capture regularities at the protein level, i.e. to detect related proteins. To do this, for different pairs of organisms two data sets were chosen: the positive control data set, i.e. all the orthologous proteins in the two organisms and the negative control data set, i.e. all pairs of proteins in the positive set, except the orthologous pairs. For the positive data set the similarity measure should yield values as big as possible, while for the negative control data set, the similarity measure should yield values close to zero.

In [81] the authors studied if standard substitution matrices, like BLOSUM [14] are appropriate for comparison of sequences with non-standard amino acid

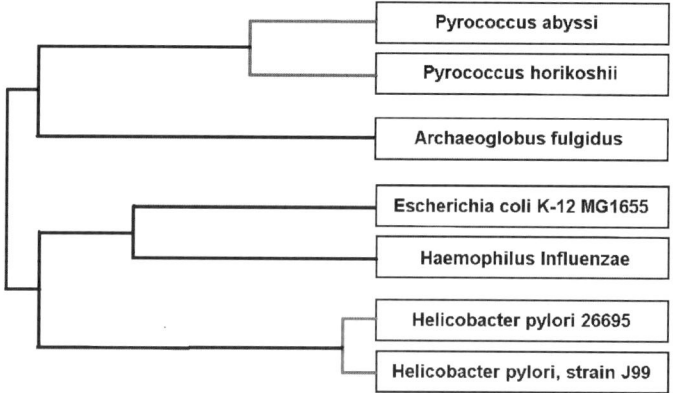

Fig. 8.2. The resulted phylogenetic tree

composition. They argue that in most commonly used substitution matrices, the substitution score is in the form of log-odds ratio of the target frequencies and of the background frequencies, derived from accurate alignments of closely related proteins. These matrices are then appropriate for comparison of protein sequences for which the amino acid composition is close to the background frequencies used to construct them. Unfortunately, the standard substitution matrices are also used when comparing protein sequences with very different background frequencies. To overcome this problem, a method for adjusting the implicit target frequencies of the substitution matrix used for comparison was presented. They show that composition specific substitution matrix adjustment is useful for comparing compositional biased proteins, including those of organism with nucleotide bias and therefore with codon bias composition.

To test the ability of the similarity measure (8.18) we used the same data set as in [81] where three pairs of organisms with very biased AT or GC genomes were used. The three pairs of organisms considered are: (i) *Clostridium tetani* (AT-rich) and *Mycobacterium tuberculosis* (GC-rich) with contrasting strong biases; (ii) *Bacillus subtilis* and *Lactococcus lactis* both with relatively unbiased genomes; and (iii) *Mycobacterium tuberculosis* and *Streptomyces coelicolor* with strong biases in the same GC direction. For each pair of organisms there is one positive control and one negative control data set. The optimal Huffman codes used by *ProtComp* algorithm are built at the proteome level of the organism for which the proteins are compared.

The results for the positive control data set, for each pair of organisms are listed in Table 8.4. In this table, the values in the columns denoted by "Relatedness" are computed with (8.20), while the others are taken from [81]. In the fourth column, for each pair of organisms, is listed the mean of the local alignment bit scores obtained when using a scaled version of the BLOSUM 62 substitution matrix for comparing the orthologous proteins. In the fifth and sixth columns are listed the median change in bit scores with respect to BLOSUM 62, when using composition-adjusted BLOSUM 62 matrices. For the composition-adjusted BLOSUM 62 matrices, the background frequencies were adjusted for proteome frequencies (the column denoted by

"Organism") and for the frequencies of the two sequences considered (the column denoted by "Sequence"). In the last two columns are presented: the median changes in bit score when using (8.20) to compute the local similarity score with respect to the values obtained when using the scaled version of the BLOSUM 62 substitution matrix and the median changes in bit score when using (8.20) to compute the local similarity score with respect to the values obtained when composition adjusted BLOSUM 62 matrices with background frequencies adjusted for the frequencies of the two sequences compared.

For the negative control data set, the only values that can be reported are the mean of the local alignment bit score for the three pair of organisms, because the number of sequences compared for each pair of organisms is quite big and the original paper [81] did not report the local alignment bit score for all protein comparisons, when using the scaled version of BLOSUM 62 matrix or compositional adjusted BLOSUM 62 matrices. The third column contains the mean bit score obtained when comparing the unrelated protein pairs using the scaled version of the BLOSUM 62 substitution matrix and the last column presents the mean bit score when comparing the unrelated pairs of proteins using (8.20). From the results presented for the positive control data set in Table 8.4 and the results presented for the negative control data set in Table 8.5, it can be concluded that the similarity measure computed based on the codelength obtained by the modified version of the *ProtComp* algorithm, does not artificially increase the local similarity score, because for the two pairs of organisms for which it yields a bigger median change in the bit score for the positive data set, it also yields a smaller mean bit score for the negative control data set.

Table 8.4. The relatedness computed for the orthologous pairs of proteins in the three pairs of organisms.[1] Values taken from [81].[2] Values computed with (8.20).

Sequence pairs	Organisms compared	No. of sequences	Mean BLOSUM 62 bit score	Median change in bit score with respect to BLOSUM 62			Median change in bit score with respect to Sequence Relatedness [2]
				Organism [1]	Sequence [1]	Relatedness [2]	
Related	C.tetani and M.tuberculosis	40	68.3	+1.6	**+2.3**	+0.6	-3.5
	B.subtilis and L.lactis	37	59.8	+1.1	+2.1	**+10.9**	+7.5
	M.tuberculosis and S. coelicolor	34	58.6	+1.4	+2.7	**+4.6**	+1.79

8.4.4 Discussions

The similarity measure of two sequences $R(X,Y)$ computed based on the estimated information shared by the sequences using the *ProtComp* algorithm, is able to operate at a macro scale, by comparing proteome sequences and at a micro scale, by comparing protein sequences. The results show that the *ProtComp* algorithm manages to capture the biological meaningful patterns of protein sequences and it proves that certainly there are regularities in the protein sequences that can be exploited in order to compress protein sequences. This conclusions are in deep contrast with

Table 8.5. The mean bit score for the unrelated pairs of proteins in the three pairs of organisms.[1] Values taken from [81].[2] Values computed with (8.20).

Sequence pair	Organism compared	No. of sequences	Mean bit score	
			BLOSUM 62[1]	Relatedness[2]
Unrelated	C. tetani and M. tuberculosis	1,560	**16.7**	17.05
	B. subtilis and L. lactis	1,332	15.7	**12.26**
	M. tuberculosis and S. coelicolor	1,122	16.4	**14.33**

the conclusions in [59] were the authors stated from the title that "Protein is incompressible". Since *ProtComp* was introduced in 2004, some other algorithms such as *XM* (expert model) [82] were introduced. This algorithm is based on estimating the probability of each symbol to be encoded based on the information gained from the already encoded symbols. The algorithm was mainly developed for DNA sequences, for which the alphabet contains only four symbols, but it can be adjusted to encode also protein sequences. The results obtained whit this algorithm are only marginally better than the results obtained with *ProtComp* algorithm for the data set that was first used in [59]. They do not present results for the more complete data set that was introduced in [46]. We can conclude that after almost three years since *ProtComp* algorithm was introduced, it is still one of the top algorithms for protein sequence compression.

8.5 Conclusions

This chapter is conceived as a collection of methods for protein similarity analysis that are using concepts and techniques from language engineering applications and information theory field. We have presented the considered methods in subsections based on the predominance of the notions, techniques and data involved in analysis. It is not a singular case when linguistic structures are evaluated with metrics from information theory field, e.g. the similarity measures mentioned for Gene Ontology terms. Due to the encouraging results obtained in practice, the methods reviewed or introduced here may claim the attention of researchers in bioinformatics to the textual analysis of biological sequence descriptions. Even if they do not perform at this stage at their full potential, further development is possible, making them alternative and efficient similarity methods for sequence alignment. Each of the methods we are dealing with has found a similarity procedure that serves to a well defined scope and they are tightly connected to the input data format. When natural language processing methods are used, they need the biological description of sequences in order to extract sequence relationships. For that, it is shown that a rule based investigation tool from natural language processing could be adapted to capture protein interaction relationships from textual repositories. Index terms, largely used in information retrieval field, have their application in sequence similarity detection using conversed regions or secondary structure attributes. In order to capture the relations between protein sequences new techniques may be developed or other largely known, like LSA, SVM, can be applied. Gene Ontology is a particular way of data description allowing semantical similarity search for a query protein. For statistical language modeling the Hidden Markov Models and n-gram concepts are used in order to find good alignments of sequences respectively to find the predictability of a natural language. Their application in biological sequences is made especially for sequence alignment and predictability of sequences in large proteome analysis. Known as algorithmic information theory, Kolmogorov complexity deals with quantification of the information in individual sequences. With applications that perform well in language and authorship recognition and phylogeny of chain letters, it is also successfully applied for genome phylogenetic trees reconstruction or protein sequence classification. In addition to these approaches, from linguistic and information theoretical field, the two newly introduced methods in this chapter are bringing their contribution to the investigated area. The main aspects that characterize these new methods and may help the reader in concluding and suggesting ideas for further development are shortly pointed below.

- Behind the relatively good performance of the new statistical method for protein sequence similarity, provided by the high scores in validation procedures stays the amino acid distribution and the order of n-gram models aspects, already remarked in [63], [64].
- An advantage over the alignment methods for sequence similarity is the reduced complexity of algorithms, their implementation, no need of additional parameters or the choose of optimal algorithms in order to perform the sequence comparison or evaluation.
- At this stage of development, the method is based only on statistical evaluation of linguistical n-gram models but working with biological information as amino acid properties or secondary structure characteristics the level of accuracy may be considerably improved.
- We are considering that one of the main contribution to the improvement of this method is the use of a normalization factor or a suitable procedure able to put more weight on the contribution of all the n-gram events participating to the sequence content evaluation.
- *ProtComp* algorithm can be used to quantify the similarity of amino acid sequences, at a macro scale by comparing *proteome* sequences and at a micro scale by comparing *protein* sequences.
- The main benefit of quantifying the similarity of two sequences using the *ProtComp* algorithm is that it can be used in comparing very long sequences like the proteomes of different organisms. In this task, classical methods that quantify the similarity of two sequences using an alignment algorithm will fail. The comparison of different organisms using their proteome sequence is important because early methods for comparing and building a phylogentic tree for a group of organisms, used only one protein that was found in all given organisms. The

problem with this approach is that we don't know which protein should be used in such a task and of course that choosing different proteins yields different trees. It is obvious that using the whole set of proteins is more appropriate.
- The sensitivity of the similarity measure based on the *ProtComp* algorithm, can be improved by using some extra information about the amino acids such as if they belong to a certain secondary structure region.

Many strategies originally developed for linguistic and information theoretical field found their application in biological knowledge discovery. They come to add more color to the panoramic view of protein sequence similarity detection and we let the reader to evaluate and appreciate each of the methods. Here we tried to inform about their application in protein sequence similarity detection and to introduce for discussions and future perspectives two new methods.

References

[1] Metfessel BA and Saurugger PN (1993) Pattern recognition is the prediction of protein structural class. In: Proceedings of the Twenty-Sixth Hawaii INternational Conference on System Science 1:679–688

[2] Berman HM, Westbrook J, Feng Z, Gilliland G, Bhat TN, Weissig H, Shindyalov IN,BournePE (2000) The Protein Data Bank. Nucleic Acids Research (28):235–242

[3] Boeckmann B, Bairoch A, Apweiler R, Blatter MC, Estreicher A, Gasteiger E, Martin MJ, Michoud K, O'Donovan C, Phan I, Pilbout S, Schneider M (2003) The SWISS-PROT protein knowledgebase and its supplement TrEMBL in 2003. Nucleic Acids Res. 31:365–370

[4] Durbin R, Eddy S, Krogh A, Mitchison G (1998) Biological Sequence Analysis: probabilistic models of proteins and nucleic acids. Cambridge University Press

[5] Koonin EV and Galperin MY (2002) Sequence-Evolution-Function Computational approaches in comparative genomics. Kluwe, Boston

[6] Pearson WR and Lipman DJ (1988) Improved tools for biological sequence comparison. PNAS 85(8): 2444–2448

[7] Altschul SF, Gish W, Miller W, Myers EW and Lipman DJ (1990) Basic local alignment search tool. J Mol Biol 215(3):403–410

[8] G.J. Barton, (1996) Protein Sequence Alignment and Database Scanning. M.J. E. Sternberg (eds), IN: Protein Structure Prediction - a practical approach, IRL Press at Oxford University Press

[9] Bogan-Marta A, Laskaris N, Gavrielides M, Pitas I, Lyroudia K (2005) A novel efficient protein similarity measure based on n-gram modeling. In: IEEE, IEE Second International Conference on Intelligence in Medicine and Healthcare 122–127

[10] Ganapathiraju M, Balakrishnan N, Reddy R, Klein-Seetharaman J, (2005) Computational Biology and Language. Ambient Intelligence for Scientific Dis-

covery, Springer-Verlag Berlin Heidelberg, Lecture Notes in Computer Science LNAI 3345:25–47
[11] Searls DB (2002) The Language of Genes. Nature 420(6912):211-7
[12] Bolshoi A (2003) DNA Sequence Analysis Linguistic Tools: Contrast Vocabularies, Compositional Spectra and Linguistic Complexity. Appl. Bioinformatics 2(2):103–12
[13] Wu K-P, Lin H-N, Sung T-Y and Su W-L (2003) A new Similarity Measure among Protein Sequences. IEEE Computer Society Bioinformatics Conference (CSB'03) Proceedings 347–352
[14] Henikoff S and Henikoff JG (1992) Amino acid substitution matrices from protein block. In: Proceedings of the National Academy of Science USA 89(22):10915–10919
[15] Lachlan Coin, Alex Bateman, and Richard Durbin (2003) Enhanced protein domain discovery by using language modeling techniques from speech recognition, Proc Natl Acad Sci U S A 100(8): 4516–4520
[16] Lord PD, Stevens RD, Brass A and Goble CA (2003) Semantic similarity measures as tools for exploring the gene ontology. In: Pacific Symposium on Biocomputing, PubMed 601–612
[17] Sarkar I, Rindflesch T (2002) Discovering Protein Similarity using Natural Language Processing, Proc AMIA Symp :677-81
[18] The Gene Ontology Consortium (2001) Creating the gene ontology resource: design and implementation. Genome Res 11(8):1425–33
[19] Rada R, Mili H, Bicknell E, Blettner M (1989) Development and application of a metric on semantic nets. IEEE Transactions on Systems Management and Cybernetics, 19(1):17–30
[20] Lord PW, Stevens RD, Brass A, Goble CA. (2003) Investigating semantic similarity measures across the Gene Ontology: the relationship between sequence and annotation, Bioinformatics Vol. 19(10):1275–1283
[21] Resnik P (1995) Using information content to evaluate semantic similarity in a taxonomy. IJCAI 448–453
[22] Lin D (1998) An information-theoretic definition of similarity. In Morgan Kaufman (EDS) Proc 15th International Conf. on Machine Learning. San Francisco, CA 296–304
[23] Jiang JJ and Conrath DW (1998) Semantic similarity based on corpus statistics and lexical taxonomy. In: Proc.of International Conference on Research in Computational Linguistics
[24] Resnik P (1999) Semantic Similarity in a Taxonomy: An Information-Based Measure and its Application to Problems of Ambiguity in Natural Language." Journal of Artificial Intelligence Research, 11:95-130
[25] Schlicker A, Domingues FS, Rahnenführer J, Lengauer T (2006) A new measure for functional similarity of gene products based on Gene Ontology, BMC Bioinformatics 7: 302
[26] Guo X, Shriver CD, Hu H, Liebman MN (2005) Semantic similarity-based validation of human protein-protein interactions, Computational Systems Bioinformatics Conference :149–150

[27] Ganapathiraju MK, Klein-Seetharaman J, Balakrishnan N and Reddy R (2004) Characterization of Protein Secondary Structure. Application of latent semantic analysis using different vocabularies. IEEE Signal Processing Magazine 78–86
[28] Bellegarda J (2000) Exploiting latent semantic information in statistical language modeling. In: IEEE Proceedings 88(8):1279–1296
[29] Landauer T, Foltx P and Laham D (1998) Introduction to latent semantic analysis. Discourse Processes 25:259–284
[30] Salton G, Wong A, and Yang CS (1975) A Vector Space Model for Automatic Indexing. Communications of the ACM, 18(11)613–620
[31] Haley D, Thomas P, Nuseibeh B, Tailor J, Lefrere P (2003) E-assesment using Lantent Semantic Analysis, Electronic Workshops in Computing, LeGE-WG
[32] Yuan Y, Lin L, Dong Q, Wang X, Li M (2005) A Protein Classification Method Based on Latent Semantic Analysis, Engineering in Medicine and Biology Society, 2005. IEEE-EMBS 27th Annual International Conference : 7738–7741
[33] Dong Q, Wang X, Lin L (2005) Application of latent semantic analysis to protein remote homology detection, Bioinformatics Advance Access published online, Bioinformatics, doi:10.1093/bioinformatics/bti801
[34] Maguitman AG, Rechtsteiner A, Verspoor K, Strauss CE, Rocha LM (2006) Large-Scale Testing of Bibliome. Informatics Using Pfam Protein Families, In: Pacific Symposium on Biocomputing 11:76-87
[35] Tueyu F, Mostafa J, Seki K (2003) Protein association discovery in biomedical literature, Proceedings of the 3rd ACM/IEEE-CS joint conference on Digital libraries :113-115
[36] Finn RD, Mistry J, Schuster-Böckler B, Griffiths-Jones S, Hollich V, Lassmann T, Moxon S, Marshall M, Khanna A, Durbin R, Eddy SR, Sonnhammer ELL, Bateman A (2006) Pfam: clans, web tools and services, Nucleic Acids Research, 34 Database issue D247-D251
[37] Mulder NJ, Fleischmann W, Kanapin A, Apweiler R (2006) InterPro as a new tool for complete genome analysis: An example of comparative analysis, Biofizika 51(4):656-660
[38] Ganapathiraju, M., V. Manoharan, et al. (2004) BLMT: Statistical Sequence Analysis using N-grams Applied Bioinformatics 3(2-3): 193-200
[39] Benedetto D, Caglioti E, and Loreto V (2002) Language trees and zipping. Physical Review Letters 88(4):048702
[40] Chen X, Francia B, Ming L, McKinnon B and Seker A (2004) Shared information and program plagiarism detection. IEEE Transactions on Information Theory 50(7):1545–1551
[41] Grozea C (2004) Plagiarism detection with state of the art compression programs. In: CDMTCS Research Report Series
[42] Chen X, Kwong S, and Li M (1999) A compression algorithm for DNA sequences and its applications in genome comparison. In: Genome Informatics. Universal Academy Press, Tokyo
[43] Li M, Badger JH, Chen X, Kwong S, Kearney P, and Zhang H (2001) An information-based sequence distance and its application to whole mitochondrial genome phylogeny. Bioinformatics 17(2):149154

[44] Otu HH and Sayood K (2003) A new sequence distance measure for phylogenetic tree construction. Bioinformatics 19(16):2122–2130
[45] Li M, Chen X, Li X, Ma B, and Vitányi PMB (2004) The similarity metric. IEEE Transactions on Information Theory 50(12):3250–3264
[46] Hategan A and Tabus I (2004) Protein is compressible. In: NORSIG2005 1992–195
[47] Cilibrasi R and Vitanyi PMB (2005) Clustering by compression.IEEE Transactions on Information Theory 51(4):1523–1545
[48] Bennett CH, Li M, and Ma B (2003) Chain letters and evolutionary histories. Scientific American 288(6):76–81
[49] Kocsor A, Kertész-Farkas A, Kaján L, and Pongor S (2006) Application of compression-based distance measures to protein sequence classification: a methodological study. Bioinformatics 22(4):407–412
[50] Kolmogorov AN (1965) Three approaches to the definition of the concept "quantity of information". Problemy Peredachi Informatsii 1:3–11
[51] Bennett CH, Gacs P, Li M, Vitanyi PMB, Zurek WH (1998) Information Distance, IEEE Transacations on Information Theory 44(4):1407–1423
[52] Li M and Vitanyi PMB (1997) An Introduction to Kolmogorov Complexity and its Applications. Springer-Verlag, 2nd Edition
[53] Apostolico A and Lonardi S (2000) Compression of biological sequences by greedy off-line textual substitution. In: Data Compression Conference. IEEE Computer Society Press
[54] Chen X, Kwong S and Li M (2001) A compression algorithm for DNA sequences. IEEE-EMB Special Issue on Bioinformatics 20(4):61–66
[55] Chen X, Li M, Ma B, and Tromp J (2002) DNACompress: Fast and effective DNA sequence compression. Bioinformatics 18:1696-1698
[56] Grumbach S and Tahi F (1993) Compression of DNA sequences. In: Data Compression Conference. IEEE Computer Society Press
[57] Korodi G and Tabus I (2005) An efficient normalized maximum likelihood algorithm for DNA sequence compression. ACM Transactions on Information Systems 23(1):3–34
[58] Tabus I, Korodi G and Rissanen J (2003) DNA Sequence Compression Using the Normalized Maximum Likelihood Model for Discrete Regression. In: Data Compression Conference. IEEE Computer Socicty Press
[59] Nevill-Manning CG and Witten IH (1999) Protein is incompressible. In: Data Compression Conference. IEEE Computer Society Press
[60] Wang S, Schuurmans D, Peng F, Zhao F (2005) Combining Statistical Language Models via the Latent Maximum Entropy Principle. Machine Learning, Springer Netherlands 60(1-3):229–250
[61] Kang S, Wang S, Greiner R, Schuurmans D, Cheng L (2004) Exploiting syntactic, semantic and lexical regularities in language modeling via directed Markov random fields. International Symposium on Chinese Spoken Language Processing : 305–308

[62] Wang S, Schuurmans D, Pengun F and Zhao Y (2003) Semantic N-gram Language Modeling With The Latent Maximum Entropy Principle. In IEEE International Conference on Acoustics, Speech, and Signal Processing (ICASSP-03)
[63] Ganapathiraju M, Weisser D, Rosenfeld R, Carbonell J, Reddy R, Klein-Seetharaman J (2002) Comparative n-gram analysis of whole-genome protein sequences. Proc. HLT, San Diego 2002
[64] Liu Y, Carbonell J, et al. (2004) Context Sensitive Vocabulary And its Application in Protein Secondary Structure Prediction. ACM SIGIR Conference.
[65] Cheng, B., J. Carbonell, et al. (2004). A Machine Text-Inspired Machine Learning Approach for Identification of Transmembrane Helix Boundaries. 15th International Symposium on Methodologies for Intelligent Systems, Saratoga Springs, New York, USA
[66] Cheng, B., J. Carbonell, et al. (2005) Protein Classification based on Text Document Classification Techniques. Proteins - Structure, Function and Bioinformatics 58(4): 955-70
[67] Burkhardt S, Crauser A, Ferragina P, Lenhof HP, Rivals E, Vingron M (1999). q-gram Based Database Searching Using a Suffix Array (QUASAR). Third Annual International Conference on Computational Molecular Biology, RECOMB'99, Lyon, France.
[68] Van Compernolle D (2003) Spoken Language Science and Technology, course material
[69] Manning CD and Schütze H (2000) Foundations of statistical natural language processing. Massachusetts Institute of Technology Press, Cambridge, Massachusetts London, England 554–588
[70] Brown PF, Della Pietra AS, Della Pietra VJ, Mercer Robert LR and Jennifer CL (1992) An estimation of an upper bound for the entropy of English. In Association for Computational Linguistics, Yorktown Heights, NY 10598
[71] Jurafsky D and Martin J (2000) Speech and Language Processing. Prentice Hall(EDS)
[72] Bogan-Marta A, Gavrielides M, Pitas I and Lyroudia K (2005) A New Statistical Measure of Protein Similarity based on Language Modeling. In: IEEE International Workshop on Genomic Signal Processing and Statistics
[73] Bogan-Marta A, Pitas I, Lyroudia K (2006) Statistical Method of Context Evaluation for Biological Sequence Similarity. In: IEEE Conference on 'Artificial Intelligence in Theory and Practice', IFIP World Computer Congress 11:1–10
[74] Liao L and Noble W S (2003) Combining pairwise sequence similarity and support vector machines for detecting remoteprotein evolutionary and structural relationships. Journal of Computational Biology 10:857–868
[75] Schäffer A, Aravind L, Madden L, Shavirin S, Spouge J, Wolf Y, Koonin E, Altschul S (2001). Improving the accuracy of PSI-BLAST protein database searches with composition-based statistics and other refinements. Nucleic Acids Res 29(14):2994–3005
[76] Cover TM and Thomas AJ (1991) Elements of information theory, New York
[77] Huffman DA (1952) A method for the construction of minimum redundancy codes. Proceedings of the IRE 40:1098–1101

[78] Rissanen J (1976) Generalized Kraft inequality and arithmetic coding. IBM Journal of Research and Development 20:198–203
[79] Ross SM (1996) Stochastic processes, 2nd Edition, New York
[80] Hategan A and Tabus I (2005) Detecting local similarity based on lossless compression of protein sequences. In: International Workshop on Genomic Signal Processing 95–99
[81] Yu YK, Wootton JC and Altschul SF (2003) The compositional adjustment of amino acid subtitution matrices. PNAS 100(26):15688–15693
[82] Cao MD, Dix TI, Allison L, Mears C (2007) A simple statistical algorithm for biological sequence compression. In: DCC'07, 43–52

9

Gene Expression Imputation Techniques for Robust Post Genomic Knowledge Discovery

Muhammad Shoaib Sehgal[1], Iqbal Gondal[2] and Laurence Dooley[3]

[1] Faculty of IT, Monash University, Churchill VIC 3842, Australia and Victorian Bioinformatics Consortium, Clayton VIC 3800, Australia
Shoaib.Sehgal@infotech.monash.edu.au
[2] Faculty of IT, Monash University, Churchill VIC 3842, Australia and Victorian Bioinformatics Consortium, Clayton VIC 3800, Australia
Iqbal.Gondal@infotech.monash.edu.au
[3] Faculty of IT, Monash University, Churchill VIC 3842, Australia
Laurence.Dooley@infotech.monash.edu.au

Summary: Microarrays measure expression patterns of thousands of genes at a time, under same or diverse conditions, to facilitate faster analysis of biological processes. This gene expression data is being widely used for diagnosis, prognosis and tailored drug discovery. Microarray data, however, commonly contains missing values, which can have high impact on subsequent biological knowledge discovery methods. This has been catalyst for the manifest of different imputation algorithms, including *Collateral Missing Value Estimation* (CMVE), *Bayesian Principal Component Analysis* (BPCA), *Least Square Impute* (LSImpute), *Local Least Square Impute* (LLSImpute) and *K-Nearest Neighbour* (KNN). This Chapter investigates the impact of missing values on post genomic knowledge discovery methods like, Gene Selection and *Gene Regulatory Network* (GRN) reconstruction. A framework for robust subsequent biological knowledge inference has been proposed which has shown significant improvements in the outcomes of Gene Selection and GRN reconstruction methods.

Key words: Microarray Gene Expression Data, Missing Values Estimaiton and Post Genomic Knowledge Discovery

9.1 Introduction

Microarray gene expression data is widely used in post genomic knowledge discovery for instance, disease analysis [1], drug progression [2], evolutionary study [3] and comparative genomics [4]. This data generation however, is a complicated process and therefore, has high probability of errors [5]. These errors can occur due to various reasons, such as spotting problems, slide scratches, blemishes on the chip, hybridization error, image corruption or simply dust on the slide [6]. It is highly unlikely that the expression values extracted from these erroneous array spots contain reliable information therefore, these values are marked as erroneous and normally removed to create missing values [7]. Microarray gene expression data contains at least 5% erroneous spots and in many data sets at least 60% of the genes have one or more missing values [8]. These missing values considerably impact upon subsequent biological knowledge discovery and analysis methods as most of the methods are not easily extendible to deal with missing values [7] for example, Significant Gene Selection, Class Prediction, Gene Regulatory Network *GRN* reconstruction and Clustering algorithms [9, 10]. There are, however, few exceptions reported in the literature Rubust Singular Value Decomposition (rSVD) [33]. The simplest solution is either to repeat the experiment, though it is often infeasible for financial reasons or to ignore the samples containing missing values, which again is not a viable solution because of the limited number of samples. Other alternative simple strategies include replacing missing values by zero (ZeroImpute) and row average/median imputation (substitution by the corresponding row average/median value). Both of these strategies are high-variance approaches as, replacing missing value by zero can result in change of variance if the data is not normalized to mean = 0 and $\sigma^2 = 1$. Similarly, mean/median methods are sensitive to outliers and can disturb the variance of the data. In addition to this, these methods may cause higher accumulated errors in subsequent biological analysis [11, 12], as neither takes data correlations in consideration. A better strategy is to accurately estimate missing values by exploiting the underlying correlation structure of the data [10, 13]. This provided the rational for the manifest of various microarray gene expression imputation techniques, including *Collateral Missing Value Imputation* (CMVE) [14], Singular Value Decomposition Impute (*SVDImpute*) [12], *K-Nearest Neighbour* (KNN) [12], Least Square Impute (*LSImpute*) [13], Local LSImpute *LLSImpute* [10] and *Bayesian Principal Component Analysis* (BPCA) [6]. More importantly, despite the merits offered by the above mentioned imputation methods, the research community still prefers simple approaches like ZeroImpute to address this problem. One possible reason is due to the implicit assumption that the missing values do not affect the performance of new biological analysis methods [7], despite the outcome of various studies [15] which show that missing values highly affect the accuracy of post genomic knowledge inference methods such as, Class Prediction [11], Clustering [13], Gene Selection [16, 17]. This was a motivation behind the study to test the impact of missing values different post genomic knowledge inference methods, in particular GRN reconstruction as no study has been undertaken, to date to test the impact of missing values on GRN reconstruction. This chapter will present different imputation methods with their relative merits and demerits, in addition to a case study investigating above mentioned pervading assumption by empirically testing different post genomic knowledge discovery methods. The test methods include GRN, Gene Selection methods and the Statistical Significance Analysis [18] on three different Breast cancer datasets [19] under akin experimental conditions. The reason of choosing GRN modelling performance as a test metric is because of its significance in post genomic knowledge inference hierarchy. Since GRN facilitate to elucidate cellular functions at a molecular level where its applications are ranging from cancer research, toxicology, to drug discovery and disease prevention [20].

Similarly, gene selection using genetic expression patterns is an important problem in microarray data analysis as it helps to identify the causal genes for different biological behaviours for example, analysis of genes responsible for certain diseases or tumors [21]. The analysis has shown that the accuracy of GRN reconstruction and Gene Selection significantly increases if missing values are estimated by exploiting correlation structure of the data prior to applying knowledge inference methods (Section 9.4). Results demonstrate that several important co-regulation links are missed out when the values are simply ignored or imputed with simple methods like ZeroImpute but again are restored when missing values are estimated using more robust methods like CMVE, because of their ability to exploit the correlation structure of the data. Similarly, many important genes are missed out when missing values are simply ignored but are re-selected when gene selection is preceded after accurate imputation. Based on these results and earlier scientific studies [13, 16, 17] we recommend that missing values should be imputed by robust imputation methods prior to applying any post genomic knowledge inference method.

Our proposed knowledge discovery framework is shown in Fig 9.1. Microarray glass slide (STEP 1) is firstly converted to expression matrix after hybridization (STEP 2). Secondly, Missing values are, then, estimated using imputation methods (STEP 3). Finally, post genomic knowledge inference methods, like Class Prediction, Gene Selection, GRN reconstruction and Clustering, are then applied for subsequent biological analysis (STEP 4). The remainder of this treatise will present different imputation methods, examination of their performance in managing microarray missing values in order to improve post genomic knowledge discovery and an analysis to highlight how as a consequence, the need to repeat costly experiments can be eliminated. The chapter is organized as follows. Section 9.2, will discuss different imputation methods with their merits and demerits followed by a Section describing different post genomic inference methods used in this chapter. Section 9.4, will present analysis of empirical results of the case study on Breast cancer data supporting the validity of framework proposed in Fig. 9.1, while list of software resources is provided in Section 9.5. Finally, Section 9.6 concludes the chapter.

9.2 Missing Values Estimation Methods

9.2.1 Imputation Nomenclature

In detailing the various imputation strategies, a gene expression matrix Y is assumed to have m rows and n columns where the columns represent genes and rows represent samples as in Eq. 9.1.

$$Y = \begin{bmatrix} g_{11} & g_{12} & g_{13} & \cdots & g_{1n} \\ g_{21} & g_{22} & g_{23} & \cdots & g_{2n} \\ \cdot & \cdot & \cdot & \cdots & \cdot \\ \cdot & \cdot & \cdot & \cdots & \cdot \\ g_{m1} & g_{m2} & g_{m3} & \cdots & g_{mm} \end{bmatrix} \in \mathbb{R}^{m \times n} \quad (9.1)$$

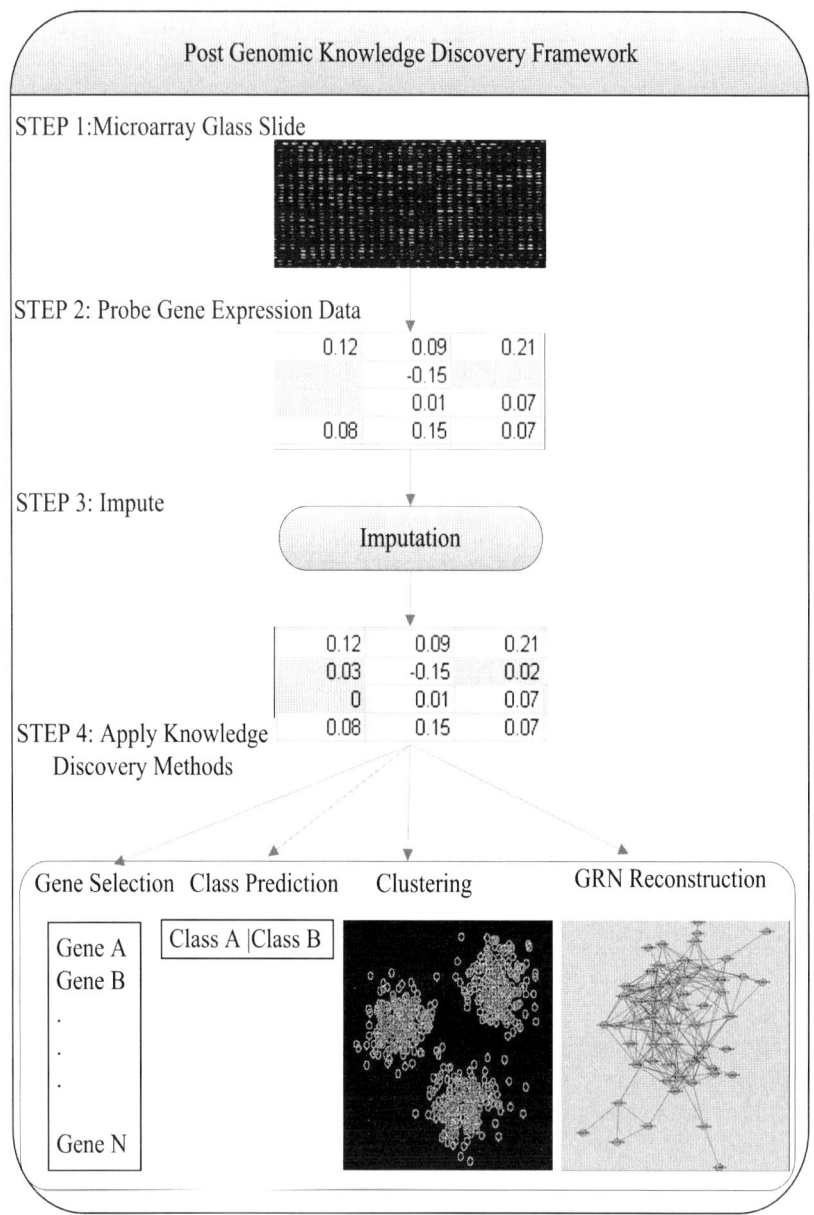

Fig. 9.1. A Robust Post Genomic Knowledge Discovery Framework

A missing value in gene expression data Y (See [1] for gene i and sample j is expressed as $Y(i,j) = g_i(j) = \Xi$. Now each imputation method will be presented in detail with their respective advantages and disadvantages.

9.2.2 Zero and Average Based Imputation [17]

The common practise to manage missing values is to replace them with Zero value as zero value is usually considered as a neutral value or by using gene average/sample average. This approach has advantage of computational efficiency and simplicity. Since, none of these methods take underlying correlation structure of the data in consideration. Therefore they disturb the variance of the data resulting in high impact on subsequent biological analysis for post genomic knowledge inference, in particular for un-normalized data and the data having very high number of missing values. The impact of missing values however, can be greatly reduced by adapting to the correlation structure of the data. Next Section discusses such techniques with their possible advantages and disadvantages.

9.2.3 Singular Value Decomposition Based Imputation (SVDImpute) [12]

The SVDImpute method uses SVD and Expectation Maximization to estimate missing values. To impute the missing value Y_{ij} of gene i in sample j, SVDImpute computes mutually orthogonal expression patterns using SVD, also can be referred as Eigen genes and can be computed as:

$$Y_{m \times n} = U_{m \times n} \sum_{m \times n} V^T_{n \times n} \qquad (9.2)$$

Matrix V^T contains Eigen genes where $\sum$ are corresponding Eigen values of the expression matrix. Since, the computation of SVD requires complete matrix therefore, the missing values are replaced by their row mean prior to the calculation of SVD. The k most effective Eigen genes are then calculated by sorting Eigen genes V^T based on their corresponding Eigen value $\sum$. Finally, missing value of Y_{ij} is computed by regressing g_i against k most effective Eigen genes. The expression values of sample j containing missing value are however, not used in this computation. The method then reduces the estimation error by recursively estimating missing values using Expectation Maximization algorithm until, the change between the newly and previously estimated matrices is less than empirically determined threshold of 0.01 [12]. Troyanskaya et al. [12] observed empirically that the method performs best when 20% of the Eigen genes are used for estimation though, there is no mathematical foundation behind the selection of these k most effective Eigen genes. Even though the method works better than above described traditional approaches, as it has odd disadvantage of being sensitive to high noise. Also, the method only considers global correlation structure of the data and has higher estimation rate when the data posses local correlations.

9.2.4 K-Nearest Neighbour (KNN) Estimation [12]

KNN estimates missing values by searching for the k nearest genes normally using a Euclidean distance function, and then taking the weighted average of the k nearest genes. In order to estimate the missing value Y_{ij} of gene i in sample j, k genes are selected whose expression vectors are similar to genetic expression of i in samples other than j. The similarity measure between gene g_i and other gene g_j is determined by the Euclidian distance Ψ over the observed components in sample j.

$$\Psi = \| g_i - g_j \| \qquad (9.3)$$

The missing value is then estimated as a weighted average of the corresponding entries in the selected k expression vectors:

$$Y_{ij} = \sum_{i=1}^{k} W_i . Y_i \qquad (9.4)$$

$$W_i = \frac{1}{\Psi \times \Delta} \qquad (9.5)$$

where $\Delta = \sum_{i=1}^{k} \Psi_i$ and Y is the input matrix containing gene expressions. Equations 9.4 and 9.5 show that contribution of each gene towards estimation is weighted by the similarity of its expression to g_i. The KNN method is flexible in terms of the choice of similarity measure where the performance of particular similarity measure is data dependent. Troyanskaya et al. [12] demonstrated that Euclidean distance performs better for microarray data than other similarity measure. The Euclidean distance measure, however, is sensitive to outliers which may be present in microarray data; although log-transforming the data significantly reduces their effects on gene similarity determination. The choice of suitable value of k also affects the imputation performance. A small k degrades the performance of the downstream analysis as the imputation process overemphasizes a few dominant genes in estimating the missing values. Conversely, a large neighborhood may include genes that are significantly different from those containing missing values, so degrading the estimation process and commensurately the analysis performance. Empirical results have demonstrated that for small data sets $k = 10$ is the best choice [9], while Troyanskaya et al. [12] observed that KNN is insensitive to values of k in the range 10 to 20.

9.2.5 Least Square Impute (LSImpute) [13]

LSImpute is a regression based estimation method that exploits the correlation between genes. The LSImpute method has three different variants namely, LSImpute-Gene, LSImpute-Array and LSImpute-Adaptive. The LSImpute-Gene estimates missing values by using the correlation between the genes while LSImpute-Array imputes missing values by exploiting correlation between the samples and LSImpute-Adaptive combines both methods for the estimation using bootstrapping approach. We'll now discuss each variant of LSImpute in detail with the relative strengths and weaknesses of each method. To estimate the missing value Y_{ij} of gene i from gene expression matrix Y containing non-missing values for gene i in sample j, the k-most correlated genes are firstly selected whose expression vectors are similar to gene i from Y in all samples except j where all the correlated genes don't have any missing value. This because LSImpute-Gene method is based on regression which requires number of parameters in the model to be much lesser than the number of observation, while microarray data suffers from the curse of dimensionality i.e. the number of parameters (number of genes) are far more than number of samples. The method then computes regression estimates for each selected gene. Finally, the missing value Y_{ij} is estimated by using weighted average of each regressed estimate. Even though the LSImpute-Gene method is more accurate than KNN, SVDImpute and other traditional methods but it suffers from the same problem of preset value of k. For example, Bø et al. [13] empirically determined the suitable value of $k = 10$ for their dataset but it may vary for other datasets [10]. One possible solution to solve the problem of curse of dimensionality for LSImpute is by regressing the mean expressions of samples. Since, array mean expressions computation requires complete values therefore missing values should be replaced by row/column mean values or any other estimation method. Bø et al [13], showed that the method works better if the values are computed first by LSImpute-Gene and then refined using LSImpute-Array. This approach has increased the estimation accuracy with added computation cost. Since, it uses LSImpute-Gene prior to any estimation therefore, it inherits above mentioned drawbacks of LSImpute-Gene e.g. use of preset value of k. LSImpute-Adaptive combines the strengths of both LSImpute-Gene and LSImpute-Array by fusing the imputation results by both methods. It adjusts the weights given to each imputation using bootstrapping technique. Empirical results by Bø et al [13] show that the method performs better than both above mentioned LSImpute variants. However, with the flexibility to adjust k (the number of predictor genes) in the regression, LSImpute performs best when data has a strong local correlation structure. This offset however, has reduced prediction accuracy compared to the new flexible imputation algorithms like LLSImpute.

9.2.6 Local Least Square Impute (LLSImpute) [10]

This algorithm estimates missing values by constructing a linear combination of correlated genes using LS regression techniques. The crucial difference between

LSImpute-Gene and LLSImpute is that in estimating Y_{ij}, the number of predictor genes k is heuristically determined directly from the dataset. To resolve the optimum value of k, LLSImpute artificially removes a known value from the most correlated gene g_i before iteratively estimating the value over a range of k values, with the k that produces the minimum estimation error is then used for the imputation of Y_{ij}. Kim et al. [10] attempted to employ the L_2 norm in addition to Pearson correlation to find the correlated genes though the difference in prediction accuracy between the two approaches is statistically insignificant while L2-norm method is reported to perform slightly better than Pearson correlation based method for their chosen data. Compared with all the aforementioned approaches, LLSImpute has the distinct advantage of adapting to the correlated data structure with an increased computational complexity, though from a microarray imputation perspective, estimation accuracy has much higher priority than computational cost.

9.2.7 Bayesian Principal Component Analysis based Estimation (BPCA) [6]

This approach estimates missing values Ξ in data matrix Y by using Y_{obs}, which have genes with no missing values. The Bayesian estimation algorithm is executed for both model parameters computed using Bayes estimates θ and Y_{miss} (similar to the Expectation Maximization repetitive algorithm) and calculates the posterior distributions for θ and Y_{miss}, $q(\theta)$ and $q(\Xi)$ [6], before the missing values in Y are imputed using:

$$\hat{Y} = \int \Xi_q(\Xi) d\Xi \qquad (9.6)$$

$$q(\xi) = p(\Xi) \mid Y^{obs}, \Theta_{true}) \qquad (9.7)$$

where Θ_{true} is the posterior distribution of the missing value. By exploiting only the global correlation in the datasets, BPCA has the advantage of prediction speed incurring a computational complexity $O(mn)$, which is one degree less than KNN, LSImpute and CMVE. Since the method only exploits the global correlation structure of the data it has high imputation errors for locally correlated data. For imputation increased estimation accuracy is a higher priority than speed.

9.2.8 Collateral Missing Value Estimation (CMVE) [14]

The CVME algorithm, which is formally presented in Fig. 9.2, imputes missing values in three stages. Firstly, the k most correlated genes with gene g_i that contains the missing value are selected for a given dataset. Secondly, it generates multiple estimation matrices using *Non-Negative Least Squares* (NNLS), *Linear Programming* (LP) and LS regression techniques to approximate missing values. Thirdly, these various estimations are weighted and fused together to form the final missing vales estimate.

Pre Condition: Gene expression matrix Y where m and n are the number of genes and samples respectively, number of predictor genes k, missing value location matrix τ and number of missing values nm.

Post Condition: Y with no missing values.

FOR l ← **1 to nm**
    STEP 1 $[i,j] \leftarrow \tau[l]$
    STEP 2 Compute absolute covariance C of a gene vector g_i of gene i using Eq. 9.8
    STEP 3 Rank genes (rows) based on C
    STEP 4 Select the k most correlated rows R_k
    STEP 5 Use the values of R_k to estimate Φ_1 using Eq. 9.9
    STEP 6 Calculate Φ_2 and Φ_3 using Eqns. 9.10 and 9.11
    STEP 7 Estimate missing value Y_{ij} using Eq. 9.15 as χ and reuse in all future predictions for other genes.
END

Fig. 9.2. The *Collateral Missing Value Imputation* (CMVE) Algorithm

To estimate the missing value $g_i(j)$, for any given data set, the absolute diagonal covariance C is computed using Eq. 9.8 for a gene vector g_i, where every gene except i is iteratively considered as a predictor gene (ω) (Step 2). The covariance function C can be formally defined as:

$$C(g_i, \omega) = \frac{1}{n-1} \sum_{l=1}^{n} (g_i(l) - \bar{g}_i)(\omega_l - \bar{\omega}) \quad (9.8)$$

An alternative strategy would be to use Pearson Correlation, though the overall effect is exactly the same for normally distributed data [22], so the covariance function is used because of its lower computation complexity. The genes are then ordered with respect to their covariance values and the first *k-ranked covariate* genes R_k are selected, whose expression vectors have the closest similarity to gene i from Y in all samples except j (Step 4). The LS regression [23] is then applied to estimate value Φ_1 for Y_{ij} (Step 5) as:

$$\Phi_1 = \alpha + \beta R_k + \zeta \quad (9.9)$$

where ζ is the error term that minimizes the variance in the LS model (parameters α and β). For a single regression, the estimate of α and β are respectively $\alpha = \bar{g}_i - \beta \bar{R}_k$ and $\beta = \frac{\Im_{xy}}{\Im_{xx}}$ where $\Im_{xy}$ is the covariance between R_k and g_i computed using Eq. 9.8

and $\mathfrak{I}_{xx} = \frac{1}{n-1}\sum_{j=1}^{n}(R_{k(j)} - \bar{R}_k)^2$ is the variance of Rk with $\bar{R}_k$; where $\bar{g}_i$ being the respective means of R_k and g_i. The two other missing value estimates Φ_2 and Φ_3 (Step 6) are respectively given by:

$$\Phi = \sum_{i=1}^{k}\phi + \eta - \sum_{i=1}^{k}\xi^2 \qquad (9.10)$$

$$\Phi_3 = \frac{\sum_{i=1}^{k}(\phi^T \times I)}{k} + \eta \qquad (9.11)$$

where ϕ is the vector that minimizes ξ_0 in Eq. 9.12, η is the normal residual and η is the actual residual. These three parameters are obtained from the *Non-Negative Least Square* (NNLS) algorithm [23]. The objective is to find a linear combination of models that best fit R_k and g_i. The objective function in NNLS minimizes the prediction error ξ_0 using Linear Programming (LP) techniques, such that:

$$\xi, \phi, \eta = min(\xi_o) \qquad (9.12)$$

$min(\xi_0)$ is a function that searches the normal vector ϕ with minimum prediction error ξ_0 and residual η. The value of ξ_0 in Eq. 9.12 is obtained from:

$$\xi_0 = max(SV(R_k \cdot \phi - g_i)) \qquad (9.13)$$

where SV are the singular values of the difference vector between the dot product of R_k and prediction coefficients ϕ with the g_i. The tolerance threshold used in the LP to compute vector ϕ is computed by:

$$Tol = k \times n \times max(SV(R_k)) \times C_n \qquad (9.14)$$

where k is the number of predictor genes, n the number of samples and C_n is a normalization factor. The final estimate χ for Y_{ij} is formed by:-

$$\chi = \rho.\Phi_1 + \Delta.\Phi_2 + \Lambda.\Phi_3 \qquad (9.15)$$

where ρ, Δ and Λ, are the weights applied to each estimate. Next Section presents different post genomic knowledge inference and statistical significance test, used to evaluate the affect of missing values on various post genomic knowledge discovery methods.

9.3 Post Genomic Knowledge Discovery Methods

The impact of missing values on Gene Selection method is tested by applying BSS/WSS gene selection method. The rationale behind choosing this method is that this method identifies those genes which have large inter-class variations while concomitantly having small intra-class variations. Next Sub-Section explains this method in detail [24].

9.3.1 Gene Selection

For any gene i in $Y \in R^{m \times n}$ BSS/WSS is calculated as follows:

$$BSS(i)/WSS(i) = \frac{\sum_{t=1}^{T} \sum_{q=1}^{Q} = 1 F(L_t = q)(\bar{Y}_q i - \bar{Y}_i)^2}{\sum_{t=1}^{T} \sum_{q=1}^{Q} F(L_t = q)(Y_{it} = \bar{Y}_{qi})^2} \qquad (9.16)$$

where T is the size of a training sample, Q is the number of classes and $F(\cdot)$ is a Boolean function which results in one if the condition is true, and zero otherwise, $\bar{Y}_i$ denotes the average expression level of gene i across all samples and $\bar{Y}_{qi}$ is the average expression level of gene i across all samples belonging to class q. The genes G are ranked from highest to lowest BSS/WSS ratios to form significant gene expression matrix, ϑ. The first p significant genes are then selected from ϑ. To evaluate the affect of missing values on GRN the *Algorithm for the Reconstruction of Accurate Cellular Networks* (ARACNe) [24] is used because it offers higher accuracy other commonly used algorithms such as, Bayesian Networks [25]. Also, the method has also been tested for mammalian gene network reconstruction compared to the other methods, which are normally tested on simple eukaryotes e.g. *Saccharomyces Cerevisiae* [26]. Following Sub-Section describes the method in greater detail.

9.3.2 Gene Regulatory Network Reconstruction

ARACNe first computes pair wise mutual information between all the genes to construct gene networks using:

$$I(g_1, g_2) = \frac{1}{m} \sum_{i=1}^{m} log[\frac{p(g_{1i}, g_{2i})}{p(g_{1i})p(g_{2i})}] \qquad (9.17)$$

where genes g_1 and g_2 are gene expression vectors,

$$p(g_1 i) = \frac{1}{\sqrt{2\pi N \alpha_1}} \sum_j e^{\frac{(g_{1i} - g_{1j})}{2\alpha_1^2}}, \qquad (9.18)$$

$$p(g_2 i) = \frac{1}{\sqrt{2\pi N \alpha_1}} \sum_j e^{\frac{(g_{2i} - g_{2j})}{2\alpha_1^2}} \qquad (9.19)$$

and

$$p(g_{1i}, g_{2i}) = \frac{1}{\sqrt{2\pi N \alpha_2}} \sum_j e^{\frac{(g_{1i} - g_{1j}) + (g_{2i} - g_{2j})}{2\alpha_2^2}} \qquad (9.20)$$

Adjustable parameters α_1 and α_2 in the above equations are computed by Monte Carlo Simulations [27] using bivariate normal probability densities [24]. The network is then pruned using *Data Processing Inequality* (DPI) which can be defined as: when two genes g_1 and g_2 are interacting through an intermediate gene g_3 and

$I(g_1,g_2|g_3)$ is zero then these genes are directly interacting if and only if: Adjustable parameters α_1 and α_2 in the above equations are computed by Monte Carlo Simulations [27] using bivariate normal probability densities [24]. The network is then pruned using *Data Processing Inequality* (DPI) which can be defined as: when two genes g_1 and g_2 are interacting through an intermediate gene g_3 and $I(g_1,g_2|g_3)$ is zero then these genes are directly interacting if and only if:

$$I(g_1,g_3) \leq I(g_1,g_2) and I(g_1,g_3) \leq I(g_2,g_3). \tag{9.21}$$

The asymmetric property of DPI however, can cause the rejection of some of the loops or interactions between three genes whose information may not be fully modelled by pair wise mutual information. Therefore, ARACNe introduces tolerance threshold which prevents the rejection of some of the triangular links and loops [24]. To further augment the fact that missing values change the data distribution and thus affect the performance of different subsequent biological analysis methods, we applied *two-sided Wilcoxon Rank sum statistical significance* test. The motivation for using this particular test is that compared to some other parametric significance tests [18], it does not mandate data to be of equal variance, which is vital given that the variance of data can be disturbed due to erroneous estimations, especially for simple imputation methods like row average.

9.3.3 Statistical Significance Test

The method calculates P-value of the hypothesis tests $H_0, Y \neq Y_{est}$ where Y and Y_{est} are the actual and estimated matrices respectively, using:

$$H_0, P - Value = 2P_r(R \leq y_r) \tag{9.22}$$

where y_r is the sum of the ranks of observations for Y and R is the corresponding random variable. Next section will provide the analysis of imputation results for gene selection, GRN reconstruction and statistical significance test.

9.4 Analysis and Discussion of Results

To quantitatively evaluate the performance of the different imputation methodologies and to improve gene selection and GRN reconstruction, the established breast cancer microarray dataset [19] was used in all the experiments. The rationale behind selecting this particular datasets is that in general, cancer data lacks molecular homogeneity in tumour tissues so missing values are hard to predict in cancerous data [28]. The dataset contains 7, 7 and 8 samples of BRCA1, BRCA2 and Sporadic mutations (neither BRCA1 nor BRCA2) respectively, with each data sample containing logarithmic microarray data of 3226 genes. The data was log transformed to minimize the effect of outliers. To rigorously evaluate the impact of missing values on GRN both gene networks before and after imputation the number of *Conserved Links* were computed which can be defined as: a co-regulation link present in both GRN_{org} and $GRN_{imputed}$. Where the GRN_{org} is a gene network constructed from the original data Y, with no missing values and $GRN_{imputed}$ is GRN constructed after imputation of randomly introduced missing values. To model $GRN_{imputed}$ iteratively, up to 20% missing values were randomly introduced in the data. These missing values were then later on imputed using CMVE, LLSImpute, BPCA, KNN and ZeroImpute methods to form Y_{est}. The gene networks, $GRN_{imputed}$ were then constructed from this imputed data Y_{est}. GRN_{org} and $GRN_{imputed}$ were then finally compared to compute the number of *Conserved Links* to test the impact of missing values on GRN reconstruction.

Figs. 9.3-9.5, show that the ARACNe method, which is reported to be robust [29] for GRN construction, could not maintain its performance in the presence of missing values, chiefly when values were imputation by commonly used ZeroImpute. In contrast when robust methods like CMVE were used, ARACNe was able to conserve the links even for higher number of missing values. Fig. 9.3, shows that for BRCA1 data ARACNe could reconstruct at least 70% of the links for the whole range of missing values (1-20%) when GRN was constructed proceeded by CMVE imputation. It missed however, most of the co-regulation links when GRN was constructed after imputation by other contemporary methods like KNN, BPCA, LLSImpute and most commonly used strategy i.e. ZeroImpute. Importantly, the GRN reconstruction performance badly suffered for higher number of missing values while CMVE held its performance even for higher percentage of missing values (Fig. 9.3). Similarly Fig. 9.4, shows that for BRCA2 data again CMVE had higher accuracy than the above mentioned strategies. For Sporadic data, after imputation by CMVE, ARACNe was able to reconstruct the GRN links while other imputation methods again feebly performed, in particular for higher number of missing values. This corroborates that GRN reconstruction is highly affected by missing values and suitable strategy for estimation like CMVE should be used prior to GRN modelling (Fig. 9.1, STEP 3). To assess the effect of missing values on gene selection, a set of significant genes ϑ was selected using the BSS/WSS from the original data with no missing values, to serve as a bench mark. Then, between 1% and 20% of expression values were randomly removed from the actual dataset. This was followed by imputation using ZeroImpute, BPCA, LLSImpute, KNN and CMVE respectively. Significant genes were selected from these imputed matrices iteratively and compared with the Γ to compute % Accuracy. Figs. 9.6-9.7, show the impact of missing values on Gene Selection accuracy when missing values were imputed by above mentioned techniques. Fig. 9.6, shows the gene selection accuracy of first 50 significant genes where it was observed that CMVE proved to be a better estimator of missing values compared to other imputation strategies especially for higher number of missing values while other methods couldn't hold their performances. For example, LLSimpute method had relatively better performance accuracy for 1% missing values but couldn't maintain its performance for higher number of missing values (Fig. 9.6). Similarly for the first 1000 significant genes again CMVE demonstrated to be a robust estimator where other algorithms couldn't keep their performances (Fig. 9.7).

Figs. 9.8-9.10, plot the P value of H_0 for the range of estimations for between 1% and 20% missing values for each of the aforementioned imputation techniques. The results show CMVE provides the best performance, as a high P value of H_0 accepts the hypothesis [18] while not surprisingly ZeroImpute exhibits the largest disparity with the original data because it does not consider any underlying correlation structure latent in the data. The performance of imputation and knowledge discovery can be data dependent. Therefore, the experiments are performed on a broader range of data sets. The results corroborate to the same observation that missing values should be imputed correctly prior to using subsequent biological analysis methods. We refer interested reader to go through [30–32], for the detailed experimental description and the analysis of results.

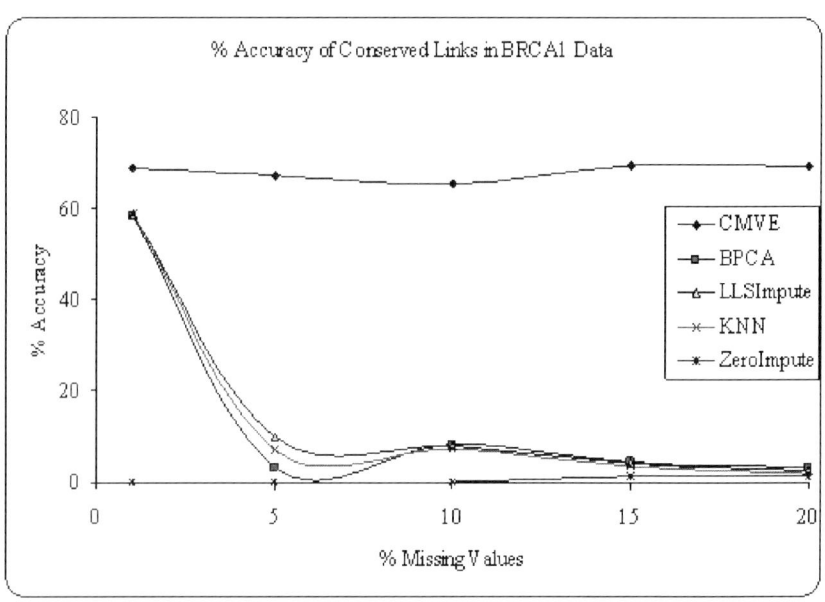

Fig. 9.3. Accuracy of Conserved Links in BRCA1 Breast Cancer Data

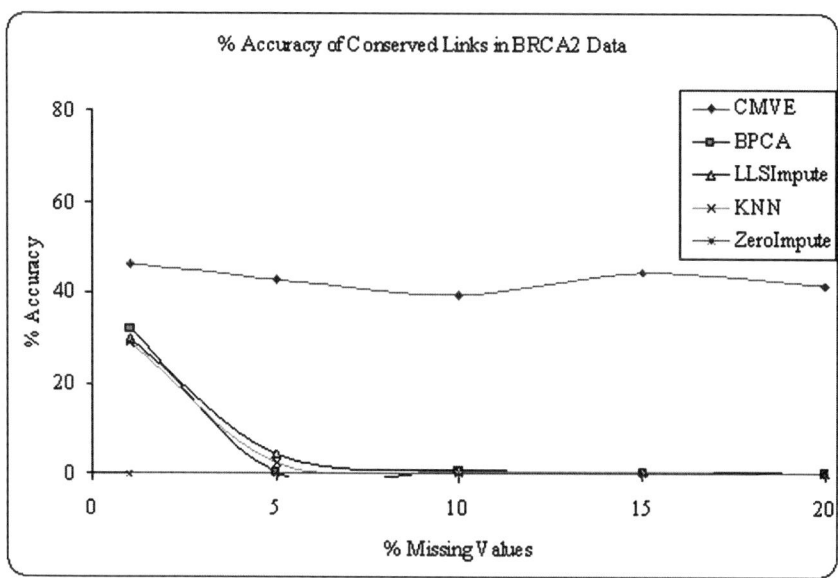

Fig. 9.4. Accuracy of Conserved Links in BRCA2 Breast Cancer Data

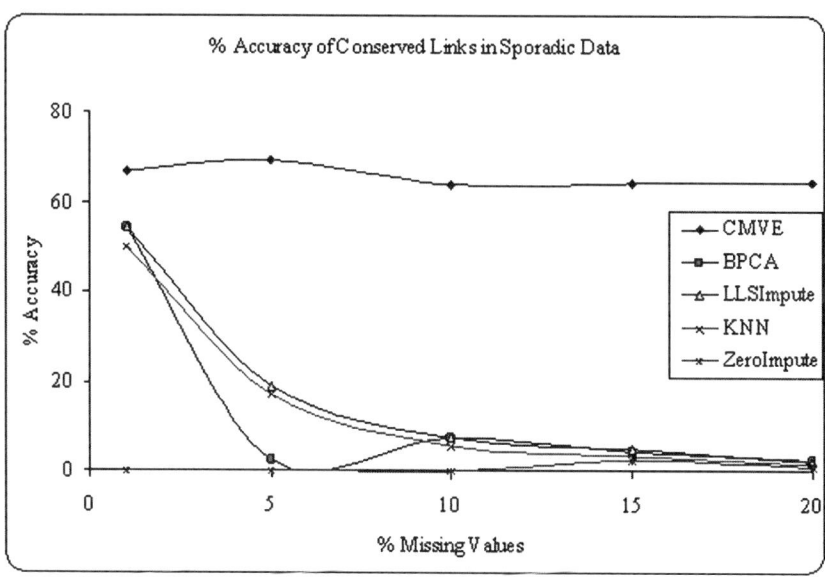

Fig. 9.5. Accuracy of Conserved Links in Sporadic Breast Cancer Data

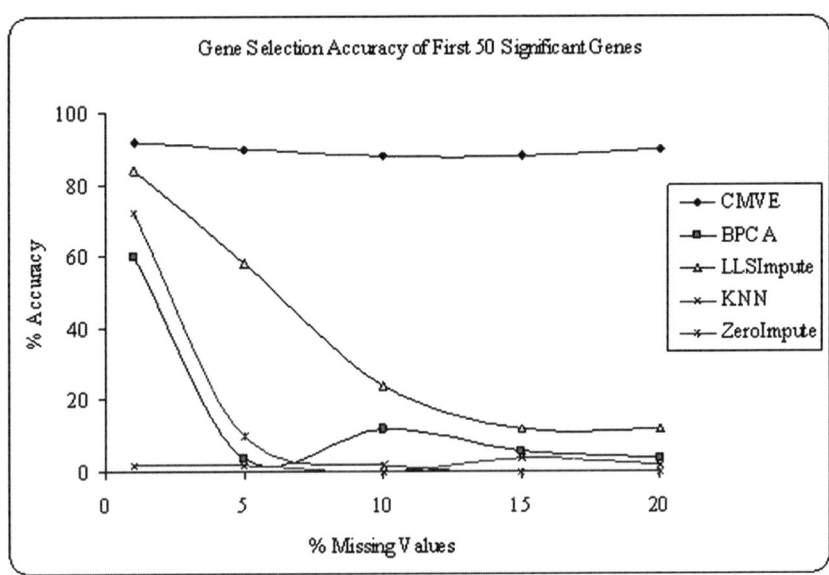

Fig. 9.6. Gene Selection Accuracy of First 50 Genes

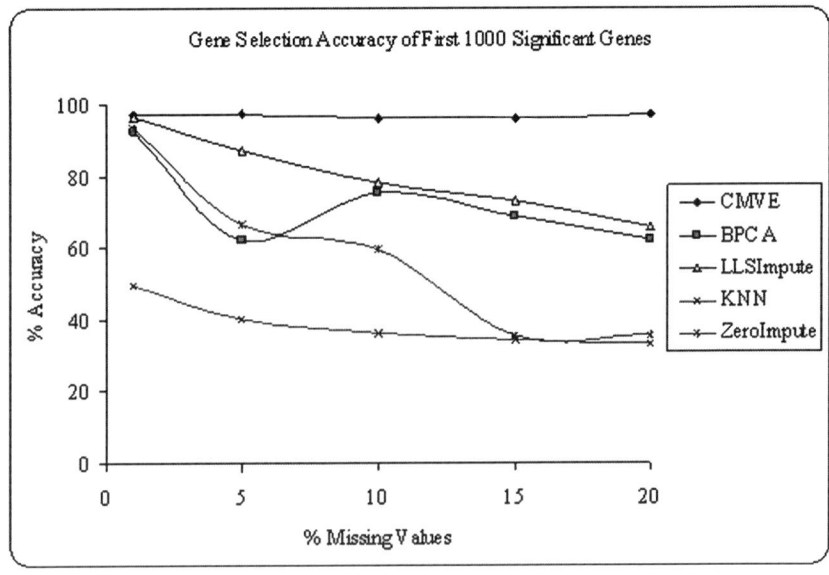

Fig. 9.7. Gene Selection Accuracy of First 1000 Genes

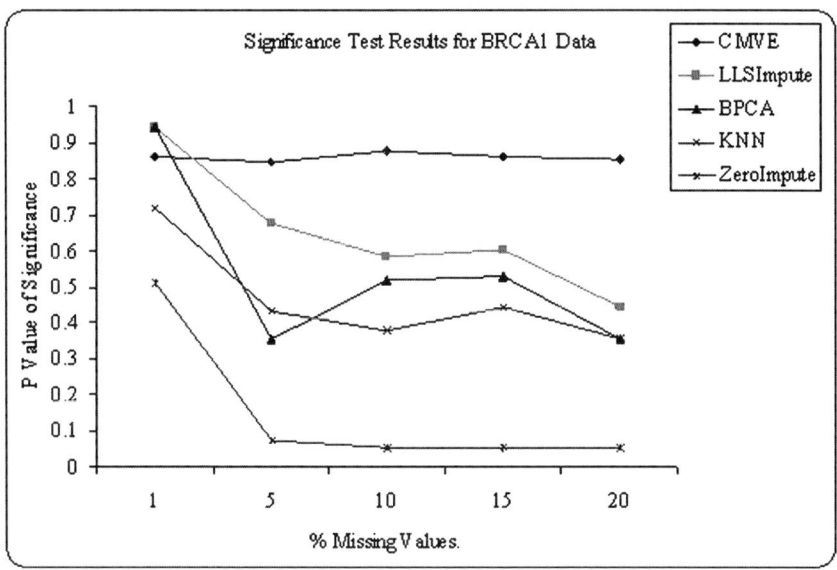

Fig. 9.8. Two-Sided Wilcoxon Rank Sum Significance Test Results for BRCA1 Data

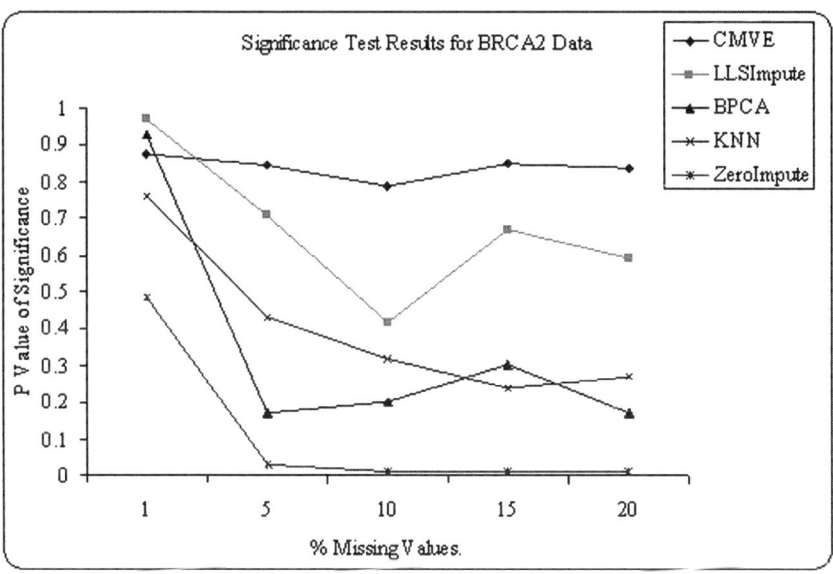

Fig. 9.9. Two-Sided Wilcoxon Rank Sum Significance Test Results for BRCA2 Data

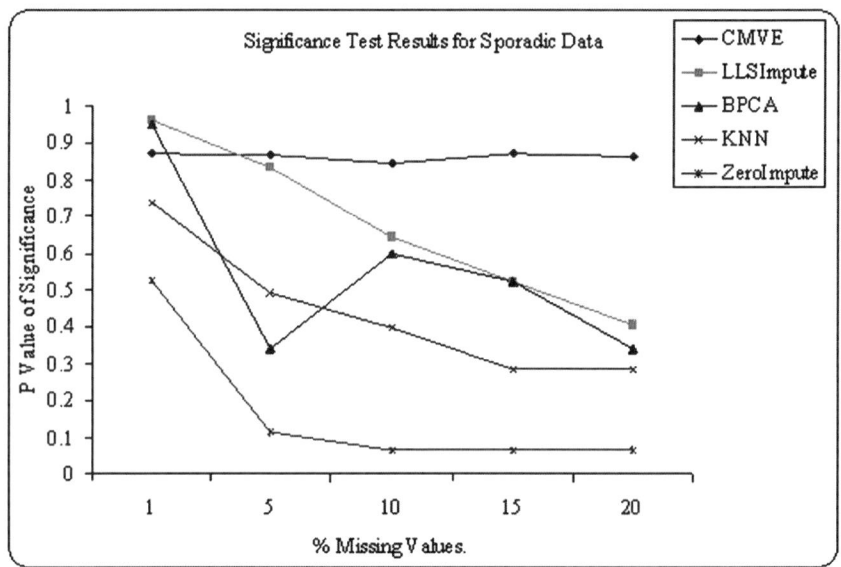

Fig. 9.10. Two-Sided Wilcoxon Rank Sum Significance Test Results for Sporadic Data

9.5 Software Availability

Imputation Method	Software Availability
CMVE	www.gscit.monash.edu.au/~shoaib
	Shoaib.Sehgal@gmail.com
BPCA	http://hawaii.aist-nara.ac.jp/~shige-o/tools/BPCAFill.html
	shige-o@is.aist-nara.ac.jp
LLSImpute	http://www-users.cs.umn.edu/~hskim/tools.html
	hskim@cs.umn.edu
LSimpute	http://www.ii.uib.no/~trondb/imputation
	trondb@ii.uib.no
KNN	http://bioinfo.cnio.es/~jherrero/downloads/KNNimpute
ARACNe	http://amdec-bioinfo.cu-genome.org/html/ARACNE.htm

Table 9.1. Downloadable imputation softwares resources

9.6 Conclusions

This chapter has provided a comprehensive study on how missing values in microarray data can affect on post genomic knowledge inference methods for instance, significant gene selection and GRN reconstruction. We have proposed a framework which minimizes the impact of these missing values upon post genomic knowledge discovery. GRN reconstruction and Gene Selection results demonstrate that missing values should be imputed by using the latent correlation structure of the data. The *Collateral Missing Value Estimation* (CMVE) algorithm, which estimates missing values using correlation structure of the data, has consistently proven to be improving GRN and Gene Selection accuracy compared to other contemporary estimation methods such as, *K Nearest Neighbour, Bayesian Principal Component Analysis, Local Least Square Impute* and commonly used *ZeroImpute* which substantiates the verity that missing values should be imputed by CMVE or any robust imputation method, prior to post genomic knowledge discovery.

Acknowledgements

The authors would like to formally acknowledge Ms. Megan Woods, Faculty of IT, Monash University, Australia for her help with the camera ready version of the Chapter.

References

[1] P. D. Sutphin, S. Raychaudhuri, N. C. Denko, R. B. Altman, and A. J. Giaccia1, "Application of supervised machine learning to identify genes associated with the hypoxia response," Nature Genetics, vol. 27, pp. 90, 2001.

[2] D. Schmatz and S. Friend, "A simple recipe for drug interaction networks earns its stars," Nature Genetics, vol. 38, pp. 405-406, 2006.

[3] M. Joron, C. D. Jiggins, A. Papanicolaou, and W. O. McMillan, "Heliconius wing patterns: an evo-devo model for understanding phenotypic diversity," Heredity, vol. 97, pp. 157-167, 2006.

[4] I. P. Ioshikhes, I. Albert, S. J. Zanton, and B. F. Pugh, "Nucleosome positions predicted through comparative genomics," Nature Genetics, vol. doi:10.1038/ng1878, 2006.

[5] A. Brazma, P. Hingamp, J. Quackenbush, G. Sherlock, P. Spellman, C. Stoeckert, J. Aach, W. Ansorge, C. A, and et al, "Minimum information about a microarray experiment (MIAME)-toward standards for microarray data," Nature Genetics, vol. 29, pp. 365-371, 2001.

[6] S. Oba, M. A. Sato, I. Takemasa, M. Monden, K. Matsubara, and S. Ishii, "A Bayesian Missing Value Estimation Method for Gene Expression Profile Data," Bioinformatics, vol. 19, pp. 2088-2096, 2003.

[7] E. Wit and J. McClure, Statistics for Microarrays: Design, Analysis and Inference: John Wiley & Sons, 2004.

[8] J. Tuikkala, L. Elo, O. S. Nevalainen, and T. Aittokallio, "Improving missing value estimation in microarray data with gene ontology 10.1093/bioinformatics/btk019," Bioinformatics, pp. btk019, 2005.

[9] E. Acuna and C. Rodriguez, "The treatment of missing values and its effect in the classifier accuracy," Classification, Clustering and Data Mining Applications, pp. 639-648, 2004.

[10] H. Kim, G. H. Golub, and H. Park, "Missing value estimation for DNA microarray gene expression data: local least squares imputation 10.1093/bioinformatics/bth499," Bioinformatics, vol. 21, pp. 187-198, 2005.

[11] M. S. B. Sehgal, I. Gondal, and L. Dooley, "Collateral Missing Value Estimation: Robust missing value estimation for consequent microarray data processing," Lecture Notes in Artificial Intelligence *LNAI*, Springer-Verlag, pp. 274-283, 2005.

[12] O. Troyanskaya, M. Cantor, G. Sherlock, P. Brown, T. Hastie, R. Tibshirani, D. Botstein, and R. Altman, "Missing Value Estimation Methods for DNA Microarrays," Bioinformatics, vol. 17, pp. 520-525, 2001.

[13] T. H. Bø, B. Dysvik, and I. Jonassen, "LSimpute: Accurate estimation of missing values in microarray data with least squares methods," Nucleic Acids Res., pp. 32(3):e34, 2004.

[14] M. S. B. Sehgal, I. Gondal, and L. Dooley, "Collateral Missing Value Imputation: a new robust missing value estimation algorithm for microarray data," Bioinformatics, vol. 21(10), pp. 2417-2423, 2005.

[15] M. S. B. Sehgal, I. Gondal, and L. Dooley, "Missing Values Imputation for DNA Microarray Data using Ranked Covariance Vectors," The International Journal of Hybrid Intelligent Systems *IJHIS*, vol. ISSN 1448-5869, 2005.

[16] R. Jornsten, H.-Y. Wang, W. J. Welsh, and M. Ouyang, "DNA microarray data imputation and significance analysis of differential expression 10.1093/bioinformatics/bti638," Bioinformatics, vol. 21, pp. 4155-4161, 2005.

[17] M. S. B. Sehgal, I. Gondal, and L. Dooley, "Missing Value Imputation Framework for Microarray Significant Gene Selection and Class Prediction," Lecture Notes in Bioinformatics (LNBI), Springer-Verlag, vol. 3916/2006, pp. 131-142, 2006.
[18] Z. Sidak, P. K. Sen, and J. Hajek, Theory of Rank Tests *Probability and Mathematical Statistics*: Academic Press, 1999.
[19] I. Hedenfalk, D. Duggan, Y. Chen, M. Radmacher, M. Bittner, R. Simon, P. Meltzer, B. Gusterson, M. Esteller, O. P. Kallioniemi, B. Wilfond, A. Borg, and J. Trent, "Gene-expression profiles in hereditary breast cancer," N. Engl. J. Med, pp. 22; 3448:539-548, 2001.
[20] X.-w. Chen, G. Anantha, and X. Wang, "An effective structure learning method for constructing gene networks 10.1093/bioinformatics/btl090," Bioinformatics, vol. 22, pp. 1367-1374, 2006.
[21] K. E. Lee, N. Sha, E. R. Dougherty, M. Vannucci, and B. K. Mallick, "Gene selection: a Bayesian variable selection approach 10.1093/bioinformatics/19.1.90," Bioinformatics, vol. 19, pp. 90-97, 2003.
[22] P. Y. Chen and P. M. Popovich, Correlation: Parametric and Nonparametric Measures, 1st edition ed: SAGE Publications, 2002.
[23] M. Harvey and C. Arthur, "Fitting models to biological Data using linear and nonlinear regression," Oxford University Press, 2004.
[24] K. Basso, A. A. Margolin, G. Stolovitzky, U. Klein, R. Dalla-Favera, and A. Califano, "Reverse engineering of regulatory networks in human B cells," Nature Genetics, vol. 37, pp. 382-390, 2005.
[25] F. V. Jensen, Bayesian Networks and Decision Graphs, 2 ed: Springer, 2002.
[26] J. Ihmels, R. Levy, and N. Barkai, "Principles of transcriptional control in the metabolic network of Saccharomyces cerevisiae," Nature Biotechnology, vol. 22, pp. 86-92, 2003.
[27] G. Casella and C. P. Robert, Monte Carlo Statistical Methods: Springer, 2005.
[28] E. Jansen, J. S. E. Laven, H. B. R. Dommerholt, J. Polman, C. van Rijt, C. van den Hurk, J. Westland, S. Mosselman, and B. C. J. M. Fauser, "Abnormal Gene Expression Profiles in Human Ovaries from Polycystic Ovary Syndrome Patients 10.1210/me.2004-0074," Mol Endocrinol, vol. 18, pp. 3050-3063, 2004.
[29] A. A. Margolin, I. Nemenman, K. Basso, C. Wiggins, G. Stolovitzky, R. D. Favera, and A. Califano, "ARACNE: An Algorithm for the Reconstruction of Gene Regulatory Networks in a Mammalian Cellular Context," BMC Bioinformatics, vol. 7, 2006.
[30] M. S. B. Sehgal, I. Gondal, and L. Dooley, "CF-GeNe: Fuzzy Framework for Robust Gene Regulatory Network Inference," Journal of Computers, Academy Press, vol. 7, pp. 1-8, 2006.
[31] M. S. B. Sehgal, I. Gondal, and L. Dooley, "Missing Value Imputation Framework for Microarray Significant Gene Selection and Class Prediction," Lecture Notes in Bioinformatics (LNBI), Springer-Verlag, vol. 3916, pp. 131-142, 2006.

[32] M. S. B. Sehgal, I. Gondal, and L. Dooley, "Missing Values Imputation for DNA Microarray Data using Ranked Covariance Vectors," The International Journal of Hybrid Intelligent Systems (IJHIS), vol. ISSN 1448-5869, 2005.

[33] L. Liu, D. M. Hawkins, S. Ghosh, and S. S. Young, "Robust singular value decomposition analysis of microarray data." vol. 100, 2003, pp. 13167-13172.

10

Computational Modelling Strategies for Gene Regulatory Network Reconstruction

Muhammad Shoaib Sehgal[1], Iqbal Gondal[2] and Laurence Dooley[3]

[1] Faculty of IT, Monash University, VIC 3842 Churchill Australia and Victorian Bioinformatics Consortium, Clayton VIC 3800 Australia
Shoaib.Sehgal@infotech.monash.edu.au

[2] Faculty of IT, Monash University, VIC 3842 Churchill Australia and Victorian Bioinformatics Consortium, Clayton VIC 3800 Australia
Iqbal.Gondal@infotech.monash.edu.au

[3] Faculty of IT, Monash University, VIC 3842 Churchill Australia
Laurence.Dooley@infotech.monash.edu.au

Summary: Gene Regulatory Network (GRN) modelling infers genetic interactions between different genes and other cellular components to elucidate the cellular functionality. This GRN modelling has overwhelming applications in biology starting from diagnosis through to drug target identification. Several GRN modelling methods have been proposed in the literature, and it is important to study the relative merits and demerits of each method. This chapter provides a comprehensive comparative study on GRN reconstruction algorithms. The methods discussed in this chapter are diverse and vary from simple similarity based methods to state of the art hybrid and probabilistic methods. In addition, the chapter also underpins the need of strategies which should be able to model the stochastic behavior of gene regulation in the presence of limited number of samples, noisy data, multi-collinearity for high number of genes.

Key words: Gene Regulatory Networks, Deterministic Modelling, Stochastic Modelling and Computational Intelligence Methods for GRN Modelling

10.1 Introduction

Basic cellular functionality is highly dependent on the transcriptional process of DNA to form proteins. For production of proteins, a DNA is first converted to mRNA (Transcription, Fig. 10.1) which then leads to the production of proteins (Translation, Fig. 10.1) where the basic production codes are provided by the genes for the synthesis of proteins. Several statistical and computational intelligence techniques have been used for class prediction [1–3], differentially expressed gene selection [4, 5] and to cluster functionally related genes under variety of conditions. Even though, these techniques give biologists valuable insights of different biological systems but still there is a need of methods which can model uncertainty, can cope with thousands of genes at a time and help to understand complex genetic interactions. In addition to that, since most of the analysis are based on over/under expressed genes studies despite the fact that differential expression analysis doesn't harness full potential of microarray gene expression data because genes are treated independent of each other and interactions among them are not considered [6]. *Gene Regulatory Network* (GRN) can model how genes interact with each other to regulate different metabolism to carry out the cellular functionality [7]. This GRN modelling has overwhelming applications in biology starting from diagnosis through to drug target identification.

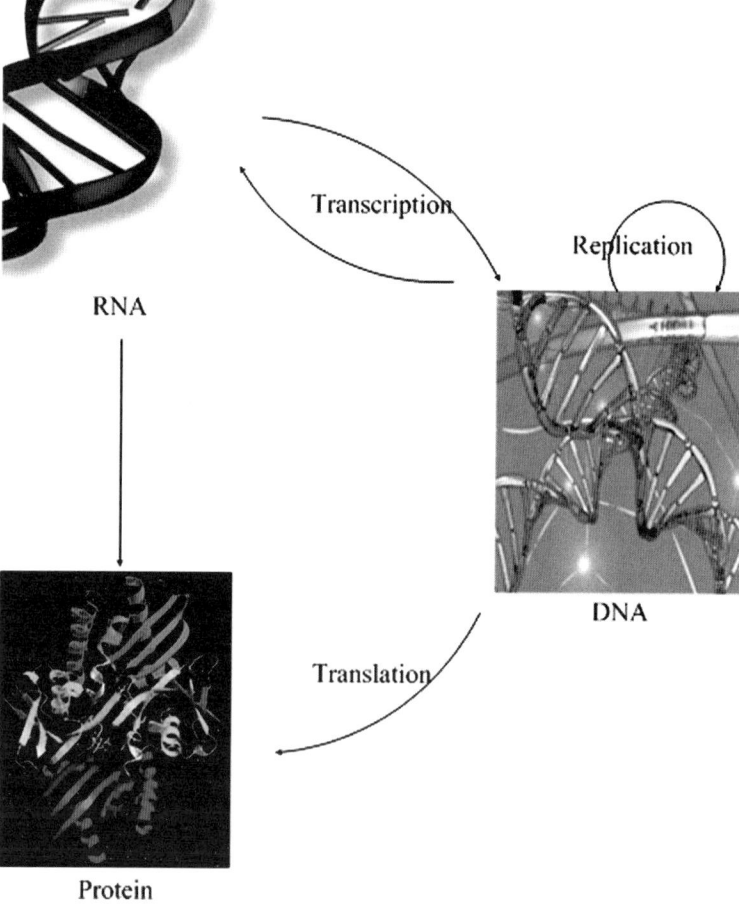

Fig. 10.1. Central Dogma [35–37]

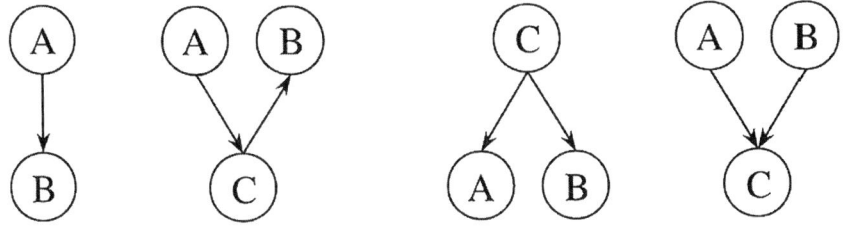

Fig. 10.2. Interaction Patterns [9]

A link between two genes g_i and g_j shows that the product of a gene g_i can inhibit or activate gene g_j which means that the protein product of gene g_i is a transcriptional factor that binds to the operator site in the promoter region of gene g_j and regulates its expression levels. Normally the links are analyzed by number of regulating *Transcriptional Factors* (TF) (incoming links to a gene) and the number of regulated genes per TF i.e. number of out coming links due to the inherent directionality property [8], to determine their distribution is followed by power law or exponent like models and to find hub genes (Hubs: The genes with max number of links). For example yeast network belongs to mix class of networks i.e. power and exponent. There are various possibilities by which genes interact with each other which are outlined in Fig. 10.1. A gene can directly trigger the other gene (Direct Link), a gene can indirectly trigger the other gene (Indirect Interaction), a gene can activate or repress two or more genes (Divergence) or two or more genes activate/repress a gene (Convergence).

Gene network construction, however, is a difficult task due to noisy nature of microarray data, curse of dimensionality (number of features are much higher than number of samples) and multi-collinearity [10]. Several techniques have been developed to model these Gene Regulatory Networks but in general GRN reconstruction consists of following series of steps (Fig. 10.1): Firstly, a sample is prepared under experimental conditions for example yeast for heat shock etc. Then microarray gene expression data is generated from the prepared sample. This is followed by a normalization step and then GRN is constructed using GRN modelling methods. The GRN modelling methods are diverse and it is important to have their in depth understanding and to know their relative strengths and weakness [9]. This chapter will provide details of commonly used Computational Intelligence methods such as: Similarity Based Methods, Probabilistic, Deterministic, Boolean and hybrid modelling techniques with their respective pros and cons.

In detailing the various GRN modelling strategies, a gene expression matrix Y is assumed to have m rows and n columns where the columns represent genes and rows represent samples as in Eq. 10.1. A gene expression vector in sample i can be referred as g_i

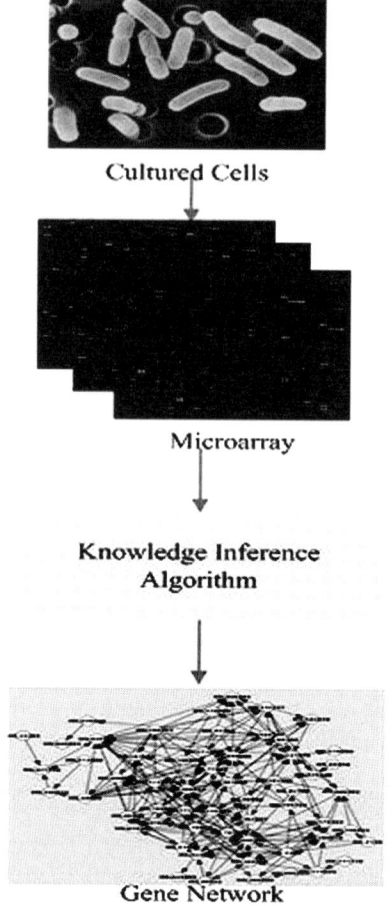

Fig. 10.3. GRN Reconstruction Framework [38, 39]

$$Y = \begin{bmatrix} g_{11} & g_{12} & g_{13} & \cdots & g_{1n} \\ g_{21} & g_{22} & g_{23} & \cdots & g_{1n} \\ \cdot & \cdot & \cdot & \cdots & \cdot \\ \cdot & \cdot & \cdot & \cdots & \cdot \\ g_{m1} & g_{m2} & g_{m3} & \cdots & g_{mn} \end{bmatrix} \in \mathbb{R}^{m \times n} \qquad (10.1)$$

10.2 Pair Wise GRN Reconstruction Methods

The regulatory interactions can be modelled by pair wise genetic interactions in which both the regulators and targets can be modelled by similarity measures. The algorithm consists of three major steps [11]:

1. Compute pair wise similarity/dissimilarity measure between each pair of genes in Y.

2. Rank all the genes based on their relative similarity/dissimilarity values.

3. Use a cut off threshold value δ to select co-regulated genes.

Following sub sections will outline some of the commonly used similarity measures and their respective merits and demerits.

Correlation and Distance Functions

Pearson correlation is the most commonly used similarity measure [12], to find the co-regulated links [13] due to its simplicity and relatively better performance for microarray data [14]. Pearson correlation r between two genes g_i and g_j can be computed as:

$$r = \frac{\sum g_i g_j - \frac{\sum g_i g_j}{n}}{\sqrt{\left(g_i^2 - \frac{(\sum g_i)^2}{n}\right)\left(g_j^2 - \frac{(\sum g_j)^2}{n}\right)}} \qquad (10.2)$$

However, Pearson correlation can lead to spurious correlate genes as it uses absolute gene expression values to compute the similarity. Also, the method is highly sensitive to outliers [15] between the genes so an alternative solution is to use rank statistics like Spearman ranked correlation, as proposed in [16] or Jackknife correlation [17], though the former is computationally intensive. Spearman correlation between two genes g_i and g_j can be computed as:

$$\rho = \frac{6 \sum D_g^2}{N_g (N_g^2 - 1)} \qquad (10.3)$$

where D_g is the distance between ordered pairs of genes g_i and g_j and N_g is the number of pairs. Several dissimilarity measures like Euclidean Distance, Manhattan metric, percent remoteness, chord distance and geodesic distance [15] can also be applied to find gene co-regulation. While the most common one being Euclidean distance, as proposed in [18]. The Euclidean distance is simple to compute and is less computational intensive though, it is sensitive to outliers [19] and can ignore the negative correlations [3] so it can ignore the co-regulation involving repression of a gene by the other gene.

Mutual Information

The mutual information $I(g_i, g_j)$, between two discrete gene expression vectors g_i and g_j can be computed as:

$$I(g_i, G_j) = \frac{1}{m} \sum_{k=1}^{m} \log \left[\frac{p(g_{ik}, g_{jk})}{p(g_{ik}) p(g_{jk})} \right] \qquad (10.4)$$

where $P(g_i, g_j)$ is a joint probability, $P(g_i)$ and $P(g_j)$ are respective marginal probabilities of expression vectors and m is number of samples. Since, the gene expression values are continuous values so they are discredited prior using above definition. This process however, can lose the information [20] therefore, various methods are proposed to compute the mutual information from continuous variables with the famous one being *Gaussian Kernel Estimator* to compute the probabilities and can be expressed as:

$$p(g_{ik}) = \frac{1}{\sqrt{2\pi N \alpha_1}} \sum_{l} e^{\frac{(g_{ik}-g_{il})}{2\alpha_1^2}} \qquad (10.5)$$

$$p(g_{jk}) = \frac{1}{\sqrt{2\pi N \alpha_1}} \sum_{l} e^{\frac{(g_{jk}-g_{jl})}{2\alpha_1^2}} \qquad (10.6)$$

$$p(g_{ik}, g_{ik}) = \frac{1}{\sqrt{2\pi N \alpha_2}} \sum_{l} e^{\frac{(g_{ik}-g_{il})+(g_{jk}-g_{jl})}{2\alpha_2^2}} \qquad (10.7)$$

where α_1 and α_2 are tunable parameter and can be computed by Monte Carlo Simulations [21] using bi-variate normal probability densities [22].

The mutual information between two variables is always ≥ 0, where mutual information zero means two genes are functionally independent of each other. Mutual information is considered to be providing a more general framework than correlation and dissimilarity measures like Pearson correlation to measure the dependency between the variables [12] due to its theoretical and probabilistic basis.

The above mentioned similarity measures use the complete expression profiles of the data to compute the degree of similarity and normalized the data to remove the expression profiles which have insignificant changes. The transcriptional regulators which act as switches in a transcriptional network however, may be expressed at very low levels so normalization can miss such key regulations. Also, above mentioned similarity measures are normally sensitive to noise and outliers like Pearson correlation. Moreover, the relationship between the genes is often expressed local similar patterns rather than global patterns which can be missed if the complete expression profiles are considered for similarity measure [23]. Above mentioned problems can be addressed by using local shape based similarity measures which will be explained in greater detail in forthcoming Sub Section.

Local Shape Based Similarity

Local shape based similarity method introduced by Balasubramaniyan *et al.* [23] searches for local relationships between genetic expressions. The similarity between genes g_i and g_j is computed by:

$$Sim(g_i, g_j) = \max_{k_m \leq k \leq n} Sim_k(g_i, g_j) \qquad (10.8)$$

where $Sim_k(g_i, g_j) = \max_{1 \leq l, o \leq n-k+1} S(g_i[l, l+k-1], g_j[o, o+k-1])$, S is a similarity measure, k is the lower bound of length of alignment and k is the best alignment length. The Sim is computed like sequence alignment algorithm such as, BLAST, Needleman-Wunsch [24], Smith-Waterman algorithm [25] or simple sliding window algorithm. Since Spearman correlation uses ranks to compute the similarity therefore Balasubramaniyan et al, suggested the use of Spearman correlation for their proposed local shape based similarity measure. Local shape based similarity algorithm though, claimed to be extracting locally similar patterns lacks evidence that the method can extract non linear relationships between the genes especially, when it is using Spearman correlation as a similarity metric.

10.3 Deterministic Methods for GRN Inference

Differential Equations

Different types of differential equations have been widely used to model GRN systems for example, Nonlinear Ordinary Differential Equations, Piecewise Linear Differential Equations and Qualitative Differential Equations. The ordinary differential equations model the rate of the regulation of a gene as a function of expression values of other genes by:

$$\frac{dg_{ik}}{dt} = f_k(g_i), l \leq k \leq n \qquad (10.9)$$

where $g = [g_1, \cdots, g_n] \geq 0$ contains concentrations of different interacting genes, proteins or small molecules [26] where discrete time delays to model transcription, translation and diffusion can be represented as:

$$\frac{dg_{ik}}{dt} = f_k(g_1(t - \tau_{k1}), \cdots, g_n(t - \tau_{kn})) 1 \leq k \leq n \qquad (10.10)$$

where $\tau_{k1}, \cdots, \tau_{kn} > 0$ represents discrete time delay. The differential equations has the ability to scale up to genomic level and can incorporate the delay between transcription and translation [27]. However, due to their deterministic change assumption i.e. d/dt is not always valid due to cellular fluctuations. Also, differential equations implicitly assume that the GRN system is spatially homogeneous which is not always true [26] which can lead to erroneous inference.

Boolean GRN Modelling Methods

The level of gene expression can depend on multiple transcriptional factors and thus on many genes. So the working principal of gene co-regulation can be modelled by using Boolean network model which functionally relate expression states of genes with the other genes using Boolean logic rules. For example, some genes are activated by different possible transcriptional factors so they can be connected using OR logic (Fig. 10.4) while other require two or more genes to be involved in a gene regulation (AND logic). Similarly inhibitory relationship between genes can be modelled by NOT logic (Fig. 10.4) and more complex rules can be modelled using combination of Boolean logics such as, if a gene is regulated only if one of its possible activator is active, while it is not repressed its one of possible inhibitors, can be modelled by OR-NOR logic (Fig. 10.4) [28].

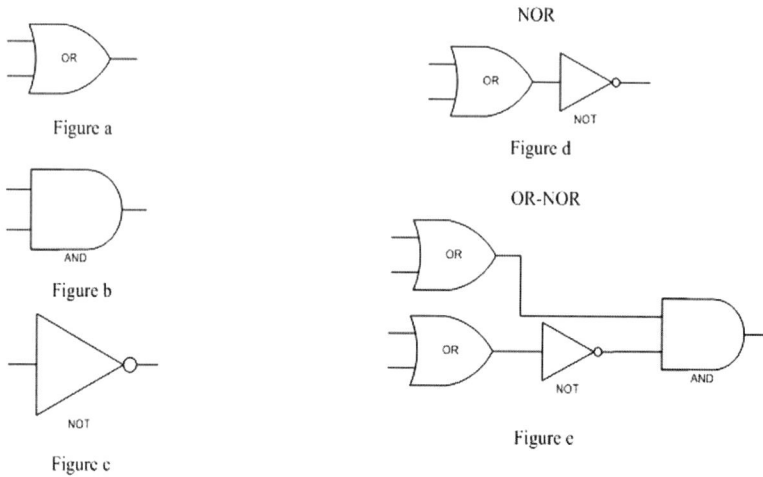

Fig. 10.4. Logical Representation of Different Gene Regulatory Relationships using Boolean Logic

10.4 Probabilistic GRN Reconstructed Strategies

Probabilistic models are one of the most commonly used GRN modelling methods due to their ability to model highly stochastic nature of gene co-regulation, as shown by most of the experimental studies [29]. The methods include: Bayesian Networks, Dynamic Bayesian Networks and various hybrid probabilistic models.

Bayesian networks model causal relationship between genes by applying probability theory [24]. A Bayesian network represents GRN by *Directed Acyclic Graph* (DAG), G(V,E) where each gene is represented by different vertex V and edge E represents the regulation pathway [20]. For instance, if gene gi is regulated by g_j it is represented by a link from g_i to g_j ($g_i \rightarrow g_j$). The dependency between a gene and its regulators is calculated by using a joint probability of a gene given its regulators.

For instance, if p_i represents the set of regulators (parents) of gene g_i then the joint probability can be computed by chain rule, such as:

$$P(g_i, g_j, \cdots, g_m) = \prod_{i=1}^{m} P(g_i|p_i) \tag{10.11}$$

Causal relationship modeling between genes using Bayesian networks can be divided into two main modules:

1. Scoring Function
2. Search Method

where scoring function computes how well the data fits to structure and search method searches for the network with the highest scores [30]. The most common scoring functions are *Bayesian Score* [31] and *Minimum Description Length* (MDL) [20, 32]. An important property of scoring functions is decomposability which can be defined as:

$$Score(S,Y) = \sum_i Score(g_i, P_i), Y(g_i, P_i) \tag{10.12}$$

where Score is a scoring function, $Y(g_i, P_i)$ is data involving g_i and P_i.

As alluded earlier, the second step in GRN reconstruction using Bayesian networks is defining a search function. The search problem is NP hard therefore heuristic methods are used to search the sub-optimal structure of the network. The search method applies three basic operations to the network with the objective to optimize the score: Addition, Deletion and Reversing the link direction as shown in Fig. 10.5. For each change the graph, search algorithm computes the score using scoring function and also, nullifies the invalid moves e.g. addition formed a cycle which is invalid in Bayesian networks (Fig. 10.5). Finally, the graph with the highest score is selected [33]. However it is worth noting that two graphs may have same score which is one of the disadvantages of using Bayesian networks. The most common heuristic search algorithms used in this context are: Hill Climbing, Simulated Annealing, Genetic Algorithms and K2.

The Bayesian networks takes the advantage of their sound probabilities semantics, ability to deal with noise & missing data which will help to cope with incomplete knowledge about biological system and flexibility to integrate prior biological knowledge into the system [30]. However, Bayesian networks have disadvantage of their high computational complexity, lack of scalability [17] and acyclic restriction [20]. The acyclic problem can be solved by using dynamic Bayesian networks [24] at additional computational cost by adding time delay [33].

Due to the relative advantages of above mentioned methods several hybrid methods have been evolved over the years to utilize the advantages [22] of each method.

10.5 Hybrid GRN Inference Methods

This section provides overview of different hybrid GRN reconstruction methods. Zhao *et al.* [20] introduced a hybrid model based on Mutual information and MDL

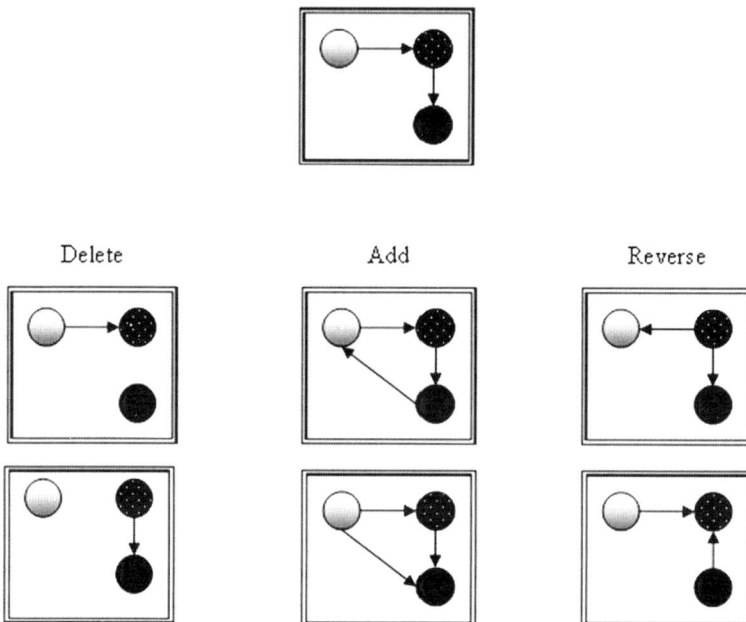

Fig. 10.5. Possible Moves of a Search Function

principal. The method computes pair wise mutual information and used MDL to automatically determine the selection threshold. It then removes the links and computes the score. Finally, the network with the highest score is selected. The method has advantage of automatically threshold selection compared to trial and error method and is scalable than simple Bayesian network. The technique however, computes discrete mutual information which can loose some valuable information.

Basso et al, introduced *Algorithm For The Reconstruction of Accurate Cellular Networks* (ARACNe) which computes the pair wise mutual information by using *Gaussian Kernel Estimator* (Section 10.2) [22]. Mutual information computation step is followed by network pruning using Data Processing Inequality which can be defined as, when two genes g_i and g_j are interacting through a third gene g_k and $I(g_i, g_j | g_k)$ is zero then these genes are directly interacting with each other if:

$$I(g_i, g_k) \leq (g_i, g_j) and I(g_i, g_k) \leq (g_j, g_k) \tag{10.13}$$

This property is asymmetric and therefore has the possibility of rejecting some of the loops or interaction between three genes whose information may not be fully modelled by pair wise mutual information. The use of tolerance threshold can solve this problem as has advantage of avoiding rejection of some of the triangular links and loops [22].

The ARACNe method is robust against noise and is proven to be showing better modelling than Bayesian networks.

Gene regulation is fuzzy in nature therefore different fuzzy GRN modelling methods have been proposed. Du *et al.* [34] introduced a method based on Fuzzy k means algorithm. The method first clusters functionally related genes using fuzzy k means algorithm and then constructs the network using following linear model:

$$g_t(i+\Gamma_i) - \sum w_{ji}g_j + b_i \qquad (10.14)$$

where g_i is the expression level of ith gene at time t, Γ is a regulation time delay of g_i, w_{ji} is the weight associated to the inference of g_j to g_i and b_i is the bias indicating default expression of g_i without regulation. The method finally evaluates the link strength using fuzzy metric based on Gene Ontology evidence strength and co-occurrence of similar gene functions. The method utilized fuzzy logic to model the fuzzy nature of gene co-regulation. However the method uses predetermined number of clusters which may loose some of the regulated links. To overcome this disadvantage Sehgal *et al.* [7] introduced a method, *Adaptive Fuzzy Evolutionary GRN Reconstruction* (AFEGRN) for modelling GRNs. The AFEGRN automatically determines model parameters such as, number of clusters for fuzzy c-means using fuzzy-PBM index and evolutionary *Estimation of Gaussian Distribution Algorithm*. Finally the network is reconstructed using Spearman correlation Eq. 10.3. The method adapts to the data distribution compared to the earlier described method by [34] which uses preset value of number of clusters. Since the method used Spearman correlation so it has the disadvantage like other correlation based matrices that it may introduce spurious co regulated links. To overcome this disadvantage Chen *et al.* [30] introduced a hybrid algorithm based on mutual information. The method first computes the mutual information between the genes and then uses K2 algorithm to finally construct the network. Since, the K2 algorithm is highly sensitive to missing values and microarray data contains at least 5% missing values and in most data sets, at least 60% of genes have one or more missing values [35], therefore the method can miss important regulation links.

10.6 Conclusions

Gene Regulatory Network (GRN) models the genetic interaction between the genes and other cellular components to elucidate the cellular functionality. This GRN modelling has overwhelming applications in biology starting from diagnosis through to drug target identification. Several GRN modelling methods have been proposed and it is important to study the relative merits and demerits of each method. This chapter has provided a comprehensive study on GRN reconstruction algorithms by highlighting their respective merits and demerits. The chapter introduced simple similarity based methods to state of the art hybrid and probabilistic methods. It is clear however, that despite the significant contribution of the proposed methods still there is a need of technique which should be able to model the stochastic behavior of gene regulation in the presence of limited number of samples, noisy data, multi-collinearity for high number of genes.

Acknowledgements

The authors would like to formally acknowledge Ms. Megan Woods, Faculty of IT, Monash University, Australia for her help with the camera ready version of the Chapter.

References

[1] T. R. Golub, D. K. Slonim, P. Tamayo, C. Huard, M. Gaasen-beek, J. P. Mesirov, H. Coller, M. L. Loh, J. R. Down-ing, M. A. Caligiuri, C. D. Bloomfield, and E. S. Lan-der, "Molecular classification of cancer: class discovery and class prediction by gene expression monitoring," Science, pp. 286(5439):531-537, 1999.

[2] M. S. B. Sehgal, I. Gondal, and L. Dooley, "Statistical Neural Networks and Support Vector Machine for the Classification of Genetic Mutations in Ovarian Cancer," IEEE Symposium on Computational Intelligence in Bioinformatics and Computational Biology (CIBCB)'04, USA., pp. 140-146, 2004.

[3] M. S. B. Sehgal, I. Gondal, and L. Dooley, "Missing Values Imputation for DNA Microarray Data using Ranked Covariance Vectors," The International Journal of Hybrid Intelligent Systems (IJHIS), vol. ISSN 1448-5869, 2005.

[4] S. Dudoit, J. Fridlyand, and T. P. Speed, "Comparison of discrimination methods for the classification of tumors using gene expression data," Journal of the American Statistical Association, pp. 77-78, 2002.

[5] M. S. B. Sehgal, I. Gondal, and L. Dooley, "Collateral Missing Value Estimation: Robust missing value estimation for consequent microarray data processing," Lecture Notes in Artificial Intelligence (LNAI), Springer-Verlag, pp. 274-283, 2005.

[6] J. K. Choi, U. Yu, O. J. Yoo, and S. Kim, "Differential coexpression analysis using microarray data and its application to human cancer," Bioinformatics, vol. 21, pp. 4348-4355, December 15, 2005 2005.

[7] M. S. B. Sehgal, I. Gondal, L. Dooley, and R. Coppel, "AFEGRN- Adaptive Fuzzy Evolutionary Gene Regulatory Network Reconstruction Framework," IEEE- World Congress on Computational Intelligence-FUZZ-IEEE, pp. 1737-1741, 2006 2006.

[8] I. Farkas, C. Wu, C. Chennubhotla, I. Bahar, and Z. Oltvai, "Topological basis of signal integration in the transcriptional-regulatory network of the yeast, Saccharomyces cerevisiae," BMC Bioinformatics, vol. 7, p. 478, 2006.

[9] A. V. Werhli, M. Grzegorczyk, and D. Husmeier, "Comparative evaluation of reverse engineering gene regulatory networks with relevance networks, graphical gaussian models and bayesian networks 10.1093/bioinformatics/btl391," Bioinformatics, vol. 22, pp. 2523-2531, October 15, 2006 2006.

[10] G. Fort and S. Lambert-Lacroix, "Classification using partial least squares with penalized logistic regression," Bioinformatics, vol. 21, pp. 1104-1111, 2005 2005.
[11] P. Y. Chen and P. M. Popovich, Correlation: Parametric and Nonparametric Measures, 1st edition ed.: SAGE Publications, 2002.
[12] R. Steuer, J. Kurths, C. O. Daub, J. Weise, and J. Selbig, "The mutual information: Detecting and evaluating dependencies between variables 10.1093/bioinformatics/18.suppl_2.S231," Bioinformatics, vol. 18, pp. S231-240, October 1, 2002 2002.
[13] J. M. Stuart, E. Segal, D. Koller, and S. K. Kim, "A Gene-Coexpression Network for Global Discovery of Conserved Genetic Modules 10.1126/science.1087447," Science, vol. 302, pp.249-255, October 10, 2003 2003.
[14] G. Yona, W. Dirks, S. Rahman, and D. M. Lin, "Effective similarity measures for expression profiles 10.1093/bioinformatics/btl127," Bioinformatics, vol. 22, pp. 1616-1622, July 1, 2006 2006.
[15] X. Xia and Z. Xie, "AMADA: analysis of microarray data," Bioinformatics Application Note, vol. 17, pp. 569-570, 2001.
[16] M. S. B. Sehgal, I. Gondal, L. Dooley, and R. Coppel, "AFEGRN: Adaptive Fuzzy Evolutionary Gene Regulatory Network Re-construction Framework," World Congress on Computational Intelligence: Fuzzy Systems., 2006.
[17] X. J. Zhou, Ming-Chih, J. Kao, H. Huang, A. Wong, J. Nunez-Iglesias, M. Primig, O. M. Aparicio, C. E. Finch, T. E. Morgan, and W. H. Wong, "Functional annotation and network reconstruction through cross-platform integration of microarray data," Nature Biotechnology, vol. 23, pp. 238-243, 2005.
[18] L. J. Heyer, S. Kruglyak, and S. Yooseph, "Exploring Expression Data: Identification and Analysis of Coexpressed Genes 10.1101/gr.9.11.1106," Genome Res., vol. 9, pp. 1106-1115, November 1, 1999 1999.
[19] O. Troyanskaya, M. Cantor, G. Sherlock, P. Brown, T. Hastie, R. Tibshirani, D. Botstein, and R. Altman, "Missing Value Estimation Methods for DNA Microarrays," Bioinformatics, vol. 17, pp. 520-525, 2001.
[20] W. Zhao, E. Serpedin, and E. R. Dougherty, "Inferring gene regulatory networks from time series data using the minimum description length principle," Bioinformatics, vol. 22(17), pp. 2129-2135, 2006.
[21] G. Casella and C. P. Robert, Monte Carlo Statistical Methods: Springer, 2005.
[22] K. Basso, A. A. Margolin, G. Stolovitzky, U. Klein, R. Dalla-Favera, and A. Califano, "Reverse engineering of regulatory networks in human B cells," Nature Genetics, vol. 37, pp. 382-390, 2005.
[23] R. Balasubramaniyan, E. Hullermeier, N. Weskamp, and J. Kamper, "Clustering of gene expression data using a local shape-based similarity measure 10.1093/bioinformatics/bti095," Bioinformatics, vol. 21, pp. 1069-1077, April 1, 2005 2005.
[24] A. T. Kwon, H. H. Hoos, and R. Ng, "Inference of transcriptional regulation relationships from gene expression data 10.1093/bioinformatics/btg106," Bioinformatics, vol. 19, pp. 905-912, May 22, 2003 2003.

[25] J. Qian, M. Dolled-Filhart, J. Lin, H. Yu, and M. Gerstein, "Beyond Synexpression Relationships: Local Clustering of Time-shifted and Inverted Gene Expression Profiles Identifies New, Biologically Relevant Interactions," J. Mol. Biol., pp. 1053-1066, 2001.

[26] H. D. Jong, "Modeling and Simulation of Genetic Regulatory Systems: A Literature Review," Journal of Computational Biology, vol. 9, pp. 67-103, 2002.

[27] T. Chen, "Modeling Gene Expression With Differential Equations," Pacific Symposium in Bioinformatics (PSB), World Scientific, vol. 4, pp. 29-40, 1999.

[28] S. Bulashevska and R. Eils, "Inferring genetic regulatory logic from expression data 10.1093/bioinformatics/bti388," Bioinformatics, p. bti388, March 22, 2005 2005.

[29] L. Mao and H. Resat, "Probabilistic representation of gene regulatory networks 10.1093/bioinformatics/bth236," Bioinformatics, vol. 20, pp. 2258-2269, September 22, 2004 2004.

[30] X.-w. Chen, G. Anantha, and X. Wang, "An effective structure learning method for constructing gene networks 10.1093/bioinformatics/btl090," Bioinformatics, vol. 22, pp. 1367-1374, June 1, 2006 2006.

[31] G. F. Cooper and E. Herskovits, "A Bayesian method for the induction of probabilistic networks from data," Machine Learning, vol. 9, pp. 309-347 1992.

[32] J. Suzuki, "A construction of Bayesian networks from databases based on an MDL scheme," Ninth Conference on Uncertainty in Artificial Intelligence, pp. 266-273, 1993.

[33] D. Husmeier, "Sensitivity and specificity of inferring genetic regulatory interactions from microarray experiments with dynamic Bayesian networks," Bioinformatics, vol. 19, pp. 2271-2282, 2003.

[34] P. Du, J. Gong, E. S. Wurtele, and J. A. Dickerson, "Modeling gene expression networks using fuzzy logic," IEEE Transactions on Systems, Man, and Cybernetics, vol. 35, pp. 1351-1359, 2005.

[35] J. Tuikkala, L. Elo, O. S. Nevalainen, and T. Aittokallio, "Improving missing value estimation in microarray data with gene ontology 10.1093/bioinformatics/btk019," Bioinformatics, p. btk019, December 23, 2005 2005.

[36] http://www.berkeley.edu/news/media/releases/2003/02/18_table.shtml

[37] http://www.union.wisc.edu/rna/newpics/bottom.jpg

[38] http://nanopedia.case.edu/image/dna.jpg

[39] http://alumni.media.mit.edu/ saul/PhD/imgs/ecoli.jpg

[40] http://www.med.monash.edu.au/assets/images/microbiology/microarray.jpg

11

Integration of Brain-Gene Ontology and Simulation Systems for Learning, Modelling and Discovery

Nik Kasabov, Vishal Jain, Lubica Benuskova, Paulo C. M. Gottgtroy and Frances Joseph

Knowledge Engineering and Discovery Research Institute, Auckland University of Technology, Auckland, New Zealand
E-mail: nkasabov@aut.ac.nz

Summary: This chapter discusses and presents some preliminary results on the Brain-Gene Ontology project that is concerned with the collection, presentation and use of knowledge in the form of ontology equipped with the Knowledge Discovery means of Computational Intelligence. Brain-Gene Ontology system thus includes various concepts, facts, data, graphs, visualizations, animations, and other information forms, related to brain functions, brain diseases, their genetic basis and the relationship between all of them, and various software simulators. The first version of the Brain-Gene Ontology has been completed as an evolving hierarchical structure in the Protégé ontology building environment endowed with plugins into the CI knowledge discovery packages like NeuCom, Weka, Siftware, and others.

Key words: Ontology, Brain, Genes, Knowledge Discovery, Computational Intelligence

11.1 Introduction

The explosion of biomedical data and the growing number of disparate data sources are exposing researchers to a new challenge – how to acquire, represent, maintain and share knowledge from large and distributed databases in the context of rapidly evolving research. In the biomedical domain, for instance, the problem of discovering knowledge from biomedical data and making biomedical knowledge and concepts sharable over applications and reusable for several purposes is both complex and crucial. It is central to support the decision in the medical practice as well as to enabling comprehensive knowledge-acquisition by medical research communities and molecular biologists involved in biomedical discovery.

The term ontology has its origin in philosophy. In philosophy, ontology is the study of being or existence. It seeks to describe or posit the basic categories and relationships of being or existence to define entities and types of entities. Ontology can be said to study conceptions of reality. In modern computer science and information science, ontology is a data model that represents a set of concepts within a domain and the relationships between those concepts. Ontology is used to reason about the objects within that domain. Ontology specifies at a higher level the classes of concepts that are relevant to the domain and the relations that exist between these classes. Ontology captures the intrinsic conceptual structure of a domain. For any given domain, its ontology forms the heart of the knowledge representation. According to Gruber, the meaning of ontology in the context of computer science is the description of concepts and relationships that can exist for an agent or a community of agents [10]. By agent(s) we mean a database, software tool, or any computational system. Thus, ontology is a description (like a formal specification of a program) of the concepts and relationships between them to support the sharing and reuse of formally represented knowledge among AI systems [5] [6]. In recent years, ontologies have been adopted in many business and scientific communities as a way to share, reuse and process domain knowledge (Fensel 2004). For experimental purposes the medical ontologies [7], Biomedical Ontology http://www.bioontology.org/) and the Gene Ontology have been created http://www.geneontology.org/) [2]. Disease Ontology is a controlled medical vocabulary designed to facilitate the mapping of diseases and associated conditions to particular medical codes such as ICD9CM, SNOMED and others (http://diseaseontology.sourceforge.net/). The goal of the Biomedical Ontology is to allow scientists to create, disseminate, and manage biomedical information and knowledge in machine-processable form for accessing and using this biomedical information in research. The Gene Ontology (GO) project provides a controlled vocabulary to describe gene and gene product attributes in any organism addressing the need for consistent descriptions of gene products in different databases.

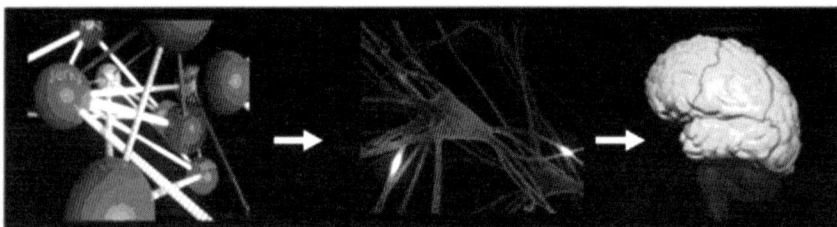

Fig. 11.1. Brain-Gene Ontology is concerned with complex relationships between genes, their influence upon neurons and the brain

Our project of Brain-Gene Ontology (BGO) development is focused on the brain and has a broader scope that GO in that it integrates information from different disciplinary domains such as neuroscience, bioinformatics, genetics, computer and information sciences [13] [14] (Fig. 11.1). It is based on growing data on influence of genes upon brain functions [1]. The BGO is an evolving system that is changing and developing with the addition of new facts and knowledge in it. The system is designed to be used for research, simulation and teaching at different levels of tertiary education. Linking selected structured bodies of physiological, genetic and computational information provides a pathway for different types of users. Designing an interface that enables users with different levels of expertise, specialization and motivation to access the project – either through a familiar or specialist approach, or through a more general introduction – is a critical issue.

In this contribution we describe the information structure of BGO (Fig. 11.2), the environment in which the BGO is implemented, and how we can use the BGO for new discoveries by means of computational intelligence and for teaching. We conclude with future directions for BGO development.

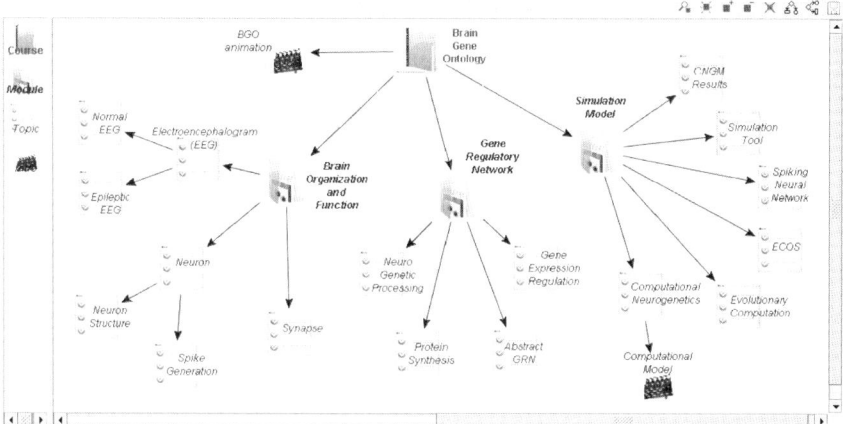

Fig. 11.2. Snapshot of the BGO information structure with three main parts and their divisions

11.2 Evolving Implementation of BGO in Protégé

BGO can be viewed as a declarative model that defines and represents the concepts existing in the domain of brain and genes, their attributes and the relationships between them. The first version has been implemented in Protégé, which is open source ontology building environment developed by the Medical Informatics Department of the Stanford University (protege.stanford.edu). BGO is based on the two most used biological data sources, named Gene Ontology, and Unified Medical Language System - UMLS, along with knowledge integrated from gene expressions databases like SwissProt, Gene Ontology, and others [8]. It also incorporates knowledge acquired from biology domain experts and from different literature databases such as PubMed. Another feature is the graphical presentation of relations by specific Protégé means (dynamic graphs, attached documents and pictures). Fig. 11.2 shows the overall information structure of the BGO. BGO is comprised of three main parts: 1. brain organization and function, 2. gene regulatory network, and 3. a simulation model. Brain organization and function contains information about neurons, about their structure and process of spike generation. It also describes processes in synapses and electroencephalogram (EEG) data for different brain states, in particular for the normal and epileptic state. Gene regulatory network (GRN) part is divided into sections on neurogenetic processing, gene expression regulation, protein synthesis and abstract GRN. The third large part, simulation model has sections on computational neurogenetic modeling (CNGM) [4], evolutionary computation, evolving connectionist systems (ECOS) [15], spiking neural network (Kasabov and Benuskova 2004), simulation tool [17] and CNGM results. The user can dive into these sections and their subsections down to the genetic level and use the information for learning and research (Fig. 11.3).

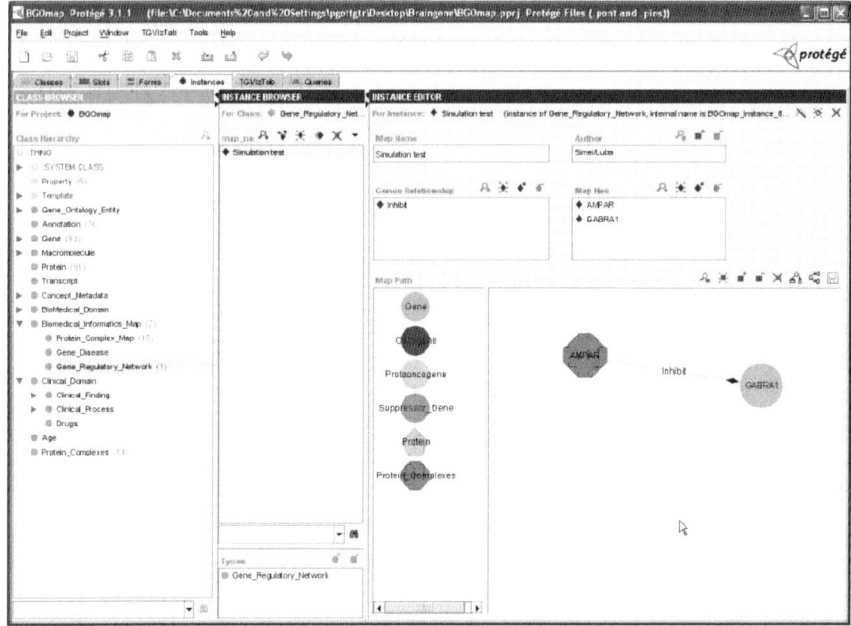

Fig. 11.3. Snapshot of the BGO showing information available in the BGO about genes, proteins, functions, annotations, molecular length, weight, expression, interactions, species, diseases, etc

As we will see below, data from the BGO can be used in simulation systems, such as computational neurogenetic simulation tool [12] [3], NeuCom (www.theneucom.com), Siftware, and Weka. NeuCom is a learning and reasoning computer environment based on connectionist (Neurocomputing) modules. It is designed to solve such problems as clustering, classification, prediction, adaptive control, data mining and pattern discovery from databases in a multidimensional, dynamic and changing data environment. Siftware is a software system for gene expression data analysis, modelling and profiling (license available from PEBL, www.peblnz.com). Weka is a collection of machine learning algorithms for data mining tasks (http://www.cs.waikato.ac.nz/ml/weka/). Weka contains tools for data preprocessing, classification, regression, clustering, association rules, and visualization. Results from these simulators can be added back to the BGO to update the BGO current knowledge base. Hence BGO evolves based on the knowledge input from outside and also based on creation of new knowledge by means of Computational Intelligence.

11.3 New Discoveries with BGO

The developed BGO system provides conceptual links between data on brain functions and diseases, their genetic basis, experimental publications, graphical illustrations and the relationships between the concepts. Each instance in BGO represents experimental research and as shown in Fig. 11.4 these instances are traceable through a query plug-in that allows us, for example, to answer questions such as – which genes are related to the occurrence of epilepsy? – by simply typing the key word epilepsy into the query window and selecting the class gene and the slot function comment. The system return the list of genes potentially related to epilepsy. By selecting any of them we can obtain detailed information about that particular gene like its GO function, chromosomal location, synonyms, brain expression profile, etc. Next we can select gene(s) of interest to visualize their relationships to other concepts in the BGO. For that we use another inbuilt Protégé mean, the TGVizTab, which enables visualization of relations between genes, proteins, molecular and neuronal functions (see Fig. 11.5). This visualization enables the user to discover previously unrevealed relationships between concepts and follow them up.

We have developed a set of plugins to enable to visualize, extract and import knowledge from/into different data sources and destinations. BGO thus allows users to select and export the specific data of their interest like chromosomal location or molecular sequence length, or expression patterns, which can then be analyzed in a software machine learning environment, such as WEKA and NeuCom to train prediction or classification models and to visualize relationship information. Such exported data on gene/protein identification numbers can also be analysed in a different manner by standard bioinformatics softwares like BLAST and FASTA for revealing homology patterns for those genes/proteins of interest, etc.

In the future, the integral part of BGO will become the module of computational neurogenetic modelling to aid discoveries of complex gene interactions underlying oscillations in neural systems (Fig. 11.6) [3]. Computational Neurogenetic Modelling (CNGM) is to model GRN within artificial neural networks using evolutionary computation methods for optimization. CNGM is the combination of two ideas: (1) using an Artificial Neural Network (ANN) to model the brain, and (2) using Gene Regulatory Networks (GRN) to influence the behaviour of the neurons in an ANN.

In CNGM, interactions of genes in neurons affect the dynamics of the whole neural network model through neuronal parameters, the values of which depend on gene

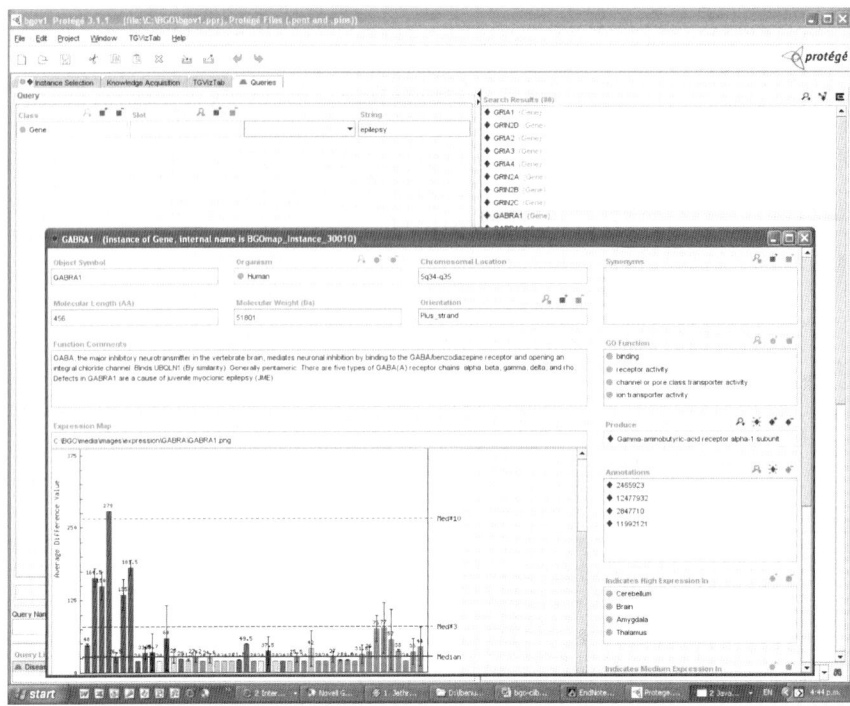

Fig. 11.4. Query search system looking for epilepsy genes and the GABRA1 gene as an example of retrieved information on its functions, annotations, molecular length, weight, expression profile in the organism, etc

expression. Through optimization of the gene interaction network, initial gene/protein expression values and neuronal parameters, particular target states of the neural network operation can be achieved, and statistics about gene interaction matrix can be extracted. In such a way it is possible to model the role of genes and their interactions in different brain states and conditions that manifest themselves as changes in local field potentials (LFP) or EEG. At present, the method and simulation tool is introduced into the BGO and described together with examples of simulation results for normal and epileptic LFP/EEG. In Fig. 11.7, there is an example of the network spiking activity that results from a complete genome and the corresponding normal filed potential. Next set of figures shows the effect of GABRA1 gene deletion upon spiking activity and the local field potential in the simulated brain cortex. Deletion of GABRA1 gene is simulated by the removal of the fast inhibition in the spiking neural network with the slow inhibition left intact. This result in spontaneous occasional global synchronizations of model neurons and peaks of high amplitude low frequency waves in the local field potential, thus simulating the epileptiform activity, which is the consequence of gene deletion or mutation leading to its impaired function.

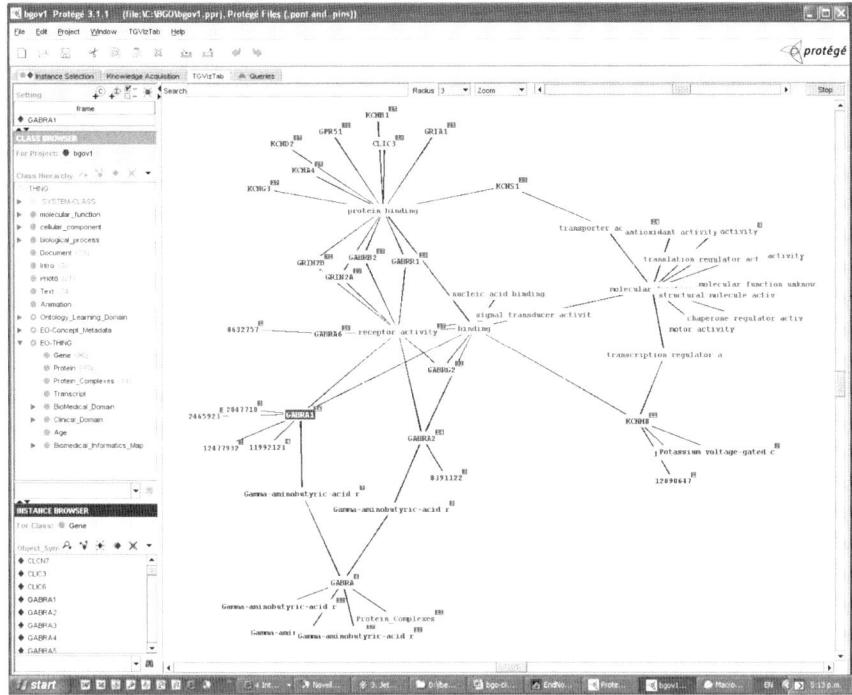

Fig. 11.5. Snapshot of the BGO detail showing relations between genes, proteins, molecular and neuronal functions for the GABRA1 gene. Each node can be expanded further so that one can identify relationships between molecular weight, chromosome location, gene product, function in neurons, mutations and related diseases, and so on

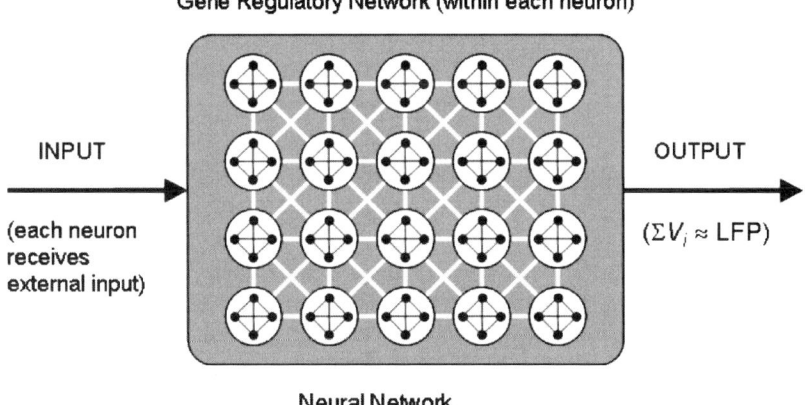

Fig. 11.6. Computational NeuroGenetic Model as a complex embedded dynamic system

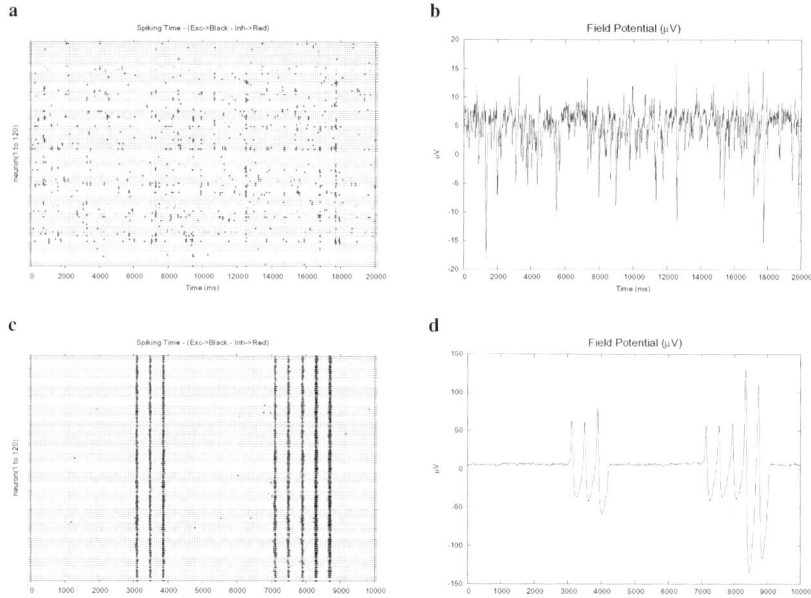

Fig. 11.7. Example of the results of computational neurogenetic model. Simulated (a) spiking activity and (b) local field potential of the spiking neural network model of a normal brain cortex. Simulation of the (c) spiking activity and (b) local field potential of the spiking neural network model of a epileptic brain cortex, the neurons of which lack fast inhibition due to the deletion of GABRA1 gene

Fig. 11.8 shows the main window of the simulation tool for neurogenetic simulations [17], which however is not available for users at the current stage of BGO. Only the theory of the computational neurogenetic modeling and presented illustrative results are included.

Another application of BGO is the integration between ontology and machine learning tools in relation to feature selection, classification and prognostic modelling with results incorporated back into the ontology. As an example, here we will take a publicly available gene expression data of 60 samples of CNS cancer (medulloblastoma) representing 39 children patients who survived the cancer after treatment, and 21 who did not respond to the treatment [16]) (Supplemental material). Fig. 11.9 illustrates the selection of the top 12 genes out of 7129 genes, as numbered in the original publication [16], using a signal to noise ratio method (SNR) in a software environment Siftwarte for which we have developed a plugin to export the data from BGO. The selected smaller number of genes, out of thousands, can be further analyzed and modeled in terms of their interaction and relation to the functioning of neurons, neural networks, the brain and the CNS. The results then can be imported back to BGO:

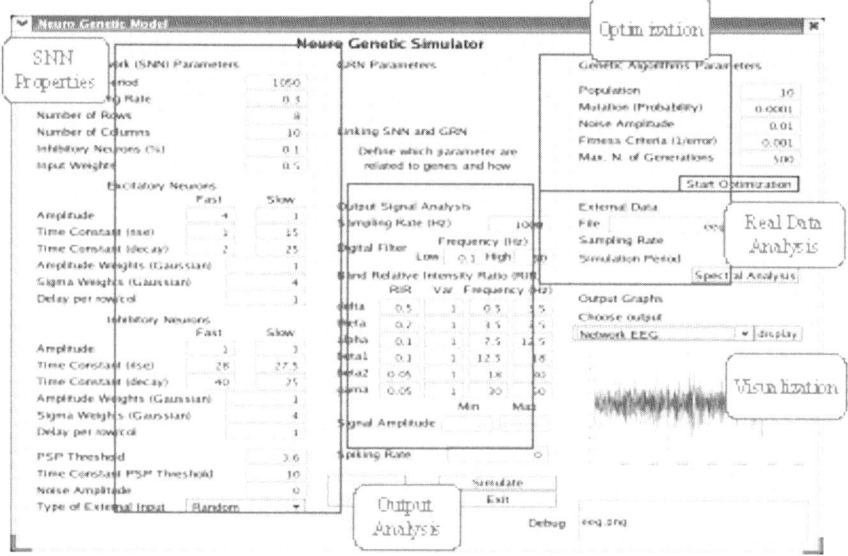

Fig. 11.8. Snapshot of the BGO neurogenetic simulation tool

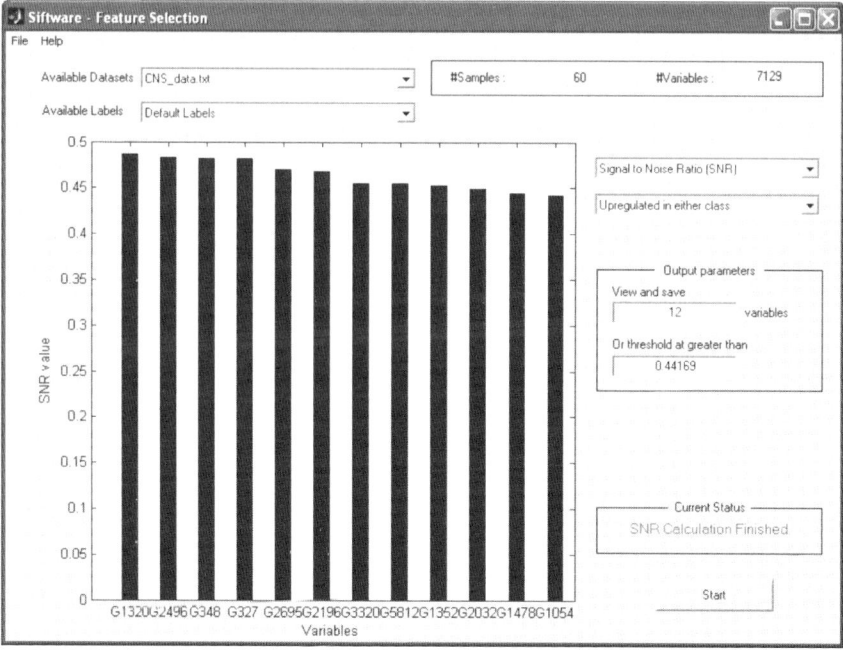

Fig. 11.9. 12 genes selected as top discriminating genes from the Central Nervous System (CNS) cancer data that discriminates two classes – survivals and not responding to treatment [16]. The Siftware system is used for the analysis and the method is called Signal-to-Noise ratio

After the features are selected, a multilayer-perceptron (MLP) classifier can be built (Fig. 11.10). An MLP that has 12 inputs (12 gene expression variables), 1 output (the class - survival or failure) and 5 hidden nodes is trained on all 60 samples of the gene expression data from the CNS cancer case study data. The error decreases with the number of iterations applied until the system reaches 100% accuracy of classification on all data. Then the trained system can be used to make prognosis on a new gene dataset from a new patient. For a full validation of the classification accuracy of the method used (here it is MLP) and the features selected (here they are 12 genes) a cross-validation experiment needs to be done, where a model is trained on part of the data and tested for generalization on the other part. Another option will be to include also the clinical information about the age of the patient, stage of the tumor, etc.

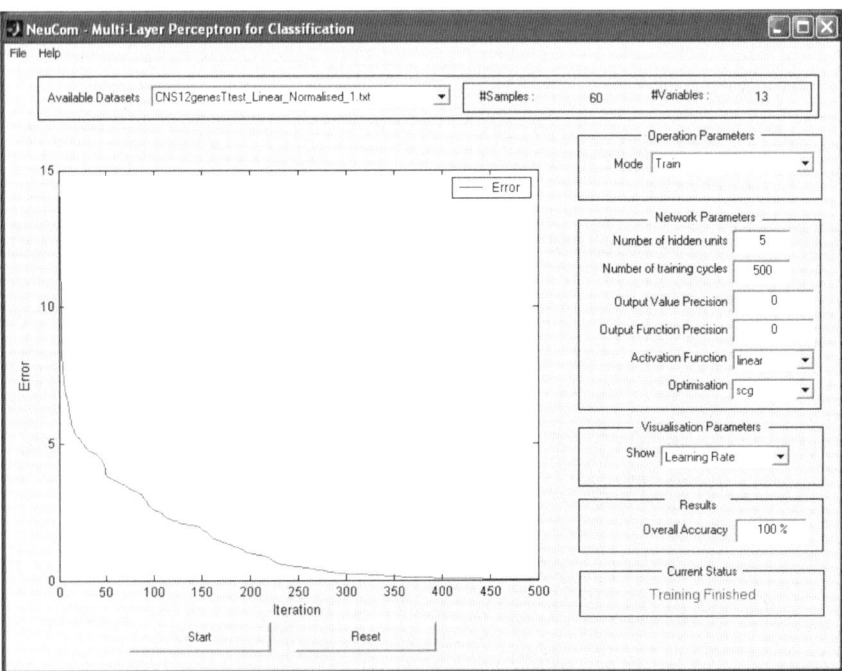

Fig. 11.10. MLP that has 12 inputs (12 gene expression variables from Fig. 9), 1 output (the class of survivals vs not responding to treatment) and 5 hidden nodes, is trained on all 60 samples of the gene expression data from the CNS cancer case study data. The error decreases with the number of iterations applied (altogether 500). The experiments are performed in a software environment NeuCom (www.theneucom.com)

The BGO is an evolving ontology that evolves its structure and content so that new information can be added in the form of molecular properties, disease related information and so on. All of this information can be re-utilized to create further models of brain functions and diseases that include models of gene interactions.

We hope that by linking and integrating simulation results from the CNGM simulations with genetic information in the BGO, we can facilitate better understanding of metabolic pathways and modelling of gene regulatory networks, and ultimately a more complete understanding of the pathogenesis of brain diseases.

11.4 BGO for Teaching

The BGO can be used as an online teaching and learning tool for undergraduate and postgraduate students as well as researchers in bioinformatics, neuroinformatics, computer and information sciences and related areas. It exemplifies the importance of use of ontologies in nowadays knowledge management and interpreting relationships between molecules and brain functions. It enables teaching the basics of molecular biology and gene regulatory networks as well as introducing the area of computational neurogenetic modeling. The BGO can be used to better understand and explain various topics related to brain, genes and their modeling, for example: the structure of the brain; main functions of the brain; the importance of gene mutation on brain functions and behavior; importance of gene regulatory networks in neurons; mental/neurological disorders and main receptor/ion channel genes/proteins involved; understanding neural signal propagation and the role of synapses; analysis of LFP/EEG data and its relevance to brain functions; neurogenetic modeling and the role of its parameters for the outcome. The interface is built using textual, graphical, audio and visual media. The inclusion of 3D animation, gives both a dynamic narrative introduction and overview to the BGO (see Fig. 11.11).

The animation navigates and provides a sophisticated visual method of integration across the different domains of the BGO. This approach, drawn from the aesthetics and immersive experience of computer games and special effects technologies is introduced as a way of engaging a younger or novice audience in this complex, emergent, cross-disciplinary field of linking genes to brain functions.

11.5 Conclusions and Future Directions

The chapter reports on a preliminary version of the world-first brain-gene ontology that includes conceptual and factual information about the brain and gene functions and their relationships. BGO can be viewed as a declarative model that defines and represents the concepts existing in the domain of brain and genes, their attributes and the relationships between them. It is represented as a knowledge base which is available to applications that need to use and/or share the knowledge of the domain. BGO is a modern tool for teaching and research across areas of bioinformatics, neuroinformatics, computer and information sciences at different levels of education and expertise.

BGO allows users to navigate through the rich information space of brain functions and brain diseases, brain related genes and their activities in certain parts of the brain and their relation to brain diseases; to run simulations; to download data

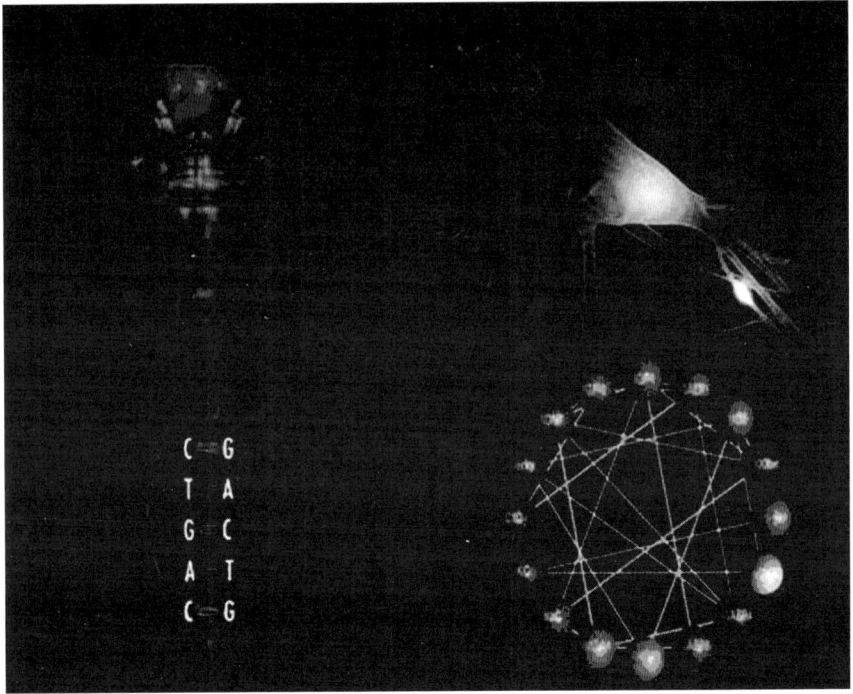

Fig. 11.11. Snapshots from animations embedded in BGO (upper left) the brain, (upper right) signal propagation in and within neurons, (lower left) gene sequence, (lower right) building an abstract GRN

that can be used in a software machine learning environment, such as WEKA and NeuCom to train prediction or classification models; to visualize relationship information; and to add new information as the BGO has an evolving structure. The BGO contains also a computational model and later a simulation tool for modeling complex relationships between genes and neural oscillations. The BGO is designed to facilitate active learning and research in the areas of bioinformatics, neuroinformatics, information engineering, and knowledge management. Different parts of it can be used by different users, from a school level to postgraduate and PhD student level. In future, more data and information will be added, that will include both, higher level information on cognitive functions and consciousness, and lower level quantum information and models.

We believe that the BGO system has the vast scope of future development. Some directions are suggested as below:

1. Further information and data integration from different sources. This phase is on its edge of its completion and we are using data sources like GO, SwissProt, Gene Expression Atlas, Pubmed, Interpro, Entrez and some datasets of interacting proteins, etc. towards evolvement of our system.

2. Inference and Knowledge Discovery. Knowledge discovery (KD) has always been a critical aspect in the ontology usage. Typical tasks for KD are the identification of classes (clustering), the prediction of new, unknown objects belonging to these classes (classification), and the discovery or inference of associations and relations between facts. Means like Query Search system, Algernon and Jess, etc. can be used in future.
3. Simulation of CNGM and Hidden Knowledge Visualization (HKV). Results obtained by simulating the neurogenetic models will become new facts to be integrated within the BGO, which will close the loop of new knowledge discovery and representation in the ontology knowledge base. Effective HKV visualization through clusters, trees, graphs, etc. using TGviz is also underway. It may reveal to some kind of valid, novel, potentially useful and understandable knowledge that varies from user to user.

11.6 Acknowledgments

This work is supported by NERF AUT0201, TAD and KEDRI. We would like to thank several colleagues who participated at different stages of the BGO development, namely Ilkka Havukkala, Rene Kroon, Laurent Antonczak, Simei G. Wysoski, William Lu, John Eyles, and Mark Howden (sound of animations). Scott Heappey is particularly acknowledged for creating all animations. For more information on BGOS, please visit the Centre of Neurocomputing and Neuroinformatics at: www.kedri.info.

References

[1] The National Center for Biotechnology Information (2007) The Nervous system. In: Genes and disease http://www.ncbi.nlm.nih.gov/books/bv.fcgi?rid=gnd.chapter.75&ref=toc
[2] Ashburner M, Ball CA, Blake JA, Botstein D, Butler H, Cherry JM, et al. (2000) Gene ontology: tool for the unification of biology. Nature Genetics 25:25–29
[3] Benuskova L, Jain V, Wysoski SG, Kasabov N (2006) Computational neurogenetic modelling: a pathway to new discoveries in genetic neuroscience. Intl. J. Neural Systems 16:215–227
[4] Benuskova L, Kasabov N (2007) Computational neurogenetic modeling. Springer, New York
[5] Chandrasekaran B, Josephson JR, Benjamins VR (1999) What are ontologies, and why do we need them? Intelligent Systems and Their Applications 14:20–26
[6] Fensel D (2004) Ontologies: a silver bullet for knowledge management and electronic commerce. Springer, Heidelberg
[7] Pisanelli DM, ed (2004) Ontologies in medicine. IOS Press, Amsterdam

[8] Gottgtroy P, Kasabov N, MacDonell S (2004) In: Zhang C, Guesgen HW, Yeap WK (eds) An ontology driven approach for knowledge discovery in Biomedicine. PRICAI 2004: Trends in Artificial Intelligence. Proc. VIII Pacific Rim Intl. Conf. AI, Lecture Notes in Artificial Intelligence, Vol. 3157. Springer-Verlag, Berlin

[9] Gottgtroy P, Kasabov N, MacDonell S (2006) Evolving ontologies for intelligent decision support. In: Sanchez E (ed) Fuzzy Logic and the Semantic Web (Capturing Intelligence). Elsevier, Amsterdam

[10] Gruber TR (1993) A translation approach to portable ontologies. Knowledge Acquisition 5:199–220

[11] Kasabov N, Benuskova L (2004) Computational neurogenetics. J. Comp. Theor. Nanoscience 1:47–61

[12] Kasabov N, Benuskova L, Wysoski SG (2005) Biologically plausible computational neurogenetic models: modeling the interaction between genes, neurons and neural networks. J. Comp. Theor. Nanoscience 2: 569–573

[13] Kasabov N, Jain V, Gottgtroy PCM, Benuskova L, Joseph F (2006) Brain gene ontology: integrating bioinformatics and neuroinformatics data, information and knowledge to enable discoveries. In: Abraham A, Kasabov N, Koeppen M, Koenig A, Song Q (eds) Proc. 6th Intl. Conf. Hybrid Intelligent Systems and 4th Conf. Neuro-Computing and Evolving Intelligence. IEEE, Auckland, New Zealand

[14] Kasabov N, Jain V, Gottgtroy PCM, Benuskova L, Wysoski SG, Joseph F (2007) Evolving Brain-Gene Ontology System (EBGOS): towards Integrating Bioinformatics and Neuroinformatics Data to Facilitate Discoveries. International Joint Conference on Neural Networks, accepted.

[15] Kasabov N (2003) Evolving connectionist systems. Methods and applications in bioinformatics, brain study and intelligent machines. Springer-Verlag, London

[16] Pomeroy, S. L., P. Tamayo, Gaasenbeek M, Sturla LM, et al (2002) Prediction of central nervous system embryonal tumour outcome based on gene expression. Nature 415:436–442

[17] Wysoski SG, Benuskova L, Kasabov N (2004) Simulation of neurogenetic models. In: Kasabov N, Chen ZSH (eds) Proc. 4th Conf. Neuro-Computing and Evolving Intelligence. AUT, Auckland, New Zealand

12

Efficiency and Scalability Issues in Metric Access Methods

Vlastislav Dohnal[1], Claudio Gennaro[2], and Pavel Zezula[1]

[1] Masaryk University
Brno, Czech Republic
{dohnal,zezula}@fi.muni.cz

[2] ISTI-CNR
Pisa, Italy
gennaro@isti.cnr.it

Summary: The metric space paradigm has recently received attention as an important model of similarity in the area of Bioinformatics. Numerous techniques have been proposed to solve similarity (range or nearest-neighbor) queries on collections of data from metric domains. Though important representatives are outlined, this chapter is not trying to substitute existing comprehensive surveys. The main objective is to explain and prove by experiments that similarity searching is typically an expensive process which does not easily scale to very large volumes of data, thus distributed architectures able to exploit parallelism must be employed.

After a review of applications using the metric space approach in the field of Bioinformatics, the chapter provides an overview of methods used for creating index structures able to speedup retrieval. In the metric space approach, only pair-wise distances between objects are quantified, so they represent the level of dissimilarity. The key idea of index structures is to partition the data into subsets so that queries are evaluated without examining entire collections – minimizing both the number of distance computations and the number of I/O accesses. These objectives are obtained by exploiting the property of metric spaces called the triangle inequality which states that if two objects are near a third object, they cannot be too distant to one another. Unfortunately, computational costs are still high and the linear scalability of single-computer implementations prevents from searching in large and ever growing data files efficiently. For these reasons, we describe very recent parallel and distributed similarity search techniques and study performance of their implementations. Specifically, Section 12.1 presents the metric space approach and its applications in the field of Bioinformatics. Section 12.2 describes some of the most popular centralized disk-based metric indexes. Consequently, Section 12.3 concentrates on parallel and distributed access methods which can deal with data collections that for practical purposes can be arbitrary large, which is typical for Bioinformatics workloads. An experimental evaluation of the presented distributed approaches on real-life data sets is presented in Section 12.4. The chapter concludes in Section 12.5.

12.1 The Metric Space Approach

Proliferation of digital contents such as video, images, text, or genome sequences imposes the use of access methods for storing and retrieving this kind of information efficiently. The concept of similarity searching based on relative distances between a query and database objects has become a solution for a number of application areas, e.g. data mining, signal processing, geographic databases, information retrieval, or computational biology.

This problem of similarity searching can be formalized by the mathematical notion of *metric space* [10, 54], so data elements are assumed to be objects from a metric space domain where only pairwise distances between the objects can be determined by a respective distance function. More formally, a metric space is defined by a domain of objects $\mathcal{D}$ (elements, points) and a distance function d – a *non-negative* and *symmetric* function which satisfies the *triangle inequality* $d(x,y) \leq d(x,z) + d(z,y)$, $\forall x, y, z \in \mathcal{D}$. In general, metric distance functions are considered as CPU demanding because a quadratic computational complexity is not exceptional. Examples of distance functions include: the *Minkowski distance* (L_p metrics), the *quadratic form distance* functions, the *edit distance*, also called the *Levenshtein distance*, the *Jaccard's coefficient*, or the *Hausdorff distance*, further details are available in [54].

Treating data items as objects of a metric space brings a great advantage in universality, because many data types and information-seeking strategies conform to the metric point of view. Accordingly, a single metric indexing technique can be applied to many specific search problems quite different in nature. In this way, the important *extensibility* property of access structures is automatically satisfied. An indexing schema that allows various forms of queries, or which can be modified to provide additional functionality, is of more value than a schema otherwise equivalent in power or even better in certain respects, but which cannot be extended.

A similarity query is defined by a query object q and a constraint on the form and extent of proximity required, typically expressed as a distance. The response to a query returns all objects that satisfy the selection conditions, presumed to be the objects close to the given query object. Probably the most common type of similarity query is the *range query*. Assuming a database X ($X \subseteq \mathcal{D}$), the range query retrieves all elements within the distance r from q, that is the set $\{x \in X, d(q,x) \leq r\}$. An alternative way to search for similar objects is to use a *k-nearest neighbors query*. The k-nearest neighbors query retrieves the k closest elements to q, that is a set $A \subseteq X$ such that $|A| = k$ and $\forall x \in A, y \in X - A, d(q,x) \leq d(q,y)$.

12.1.1 Metric Spaces in Bioinformatics

In Bioinformatics, sequence similarity is one of the most important tools for discovering relationship between genomic or protein sequences. In other words, a high degree of sequence similarity constitutes an indication for homology. The metric space represents a possible approach for addressing sequence similarity problems [22, 23, 25, 49].

The simplest form of sequence similarity is the Hamming distance. It expresses the distance between two equal-length sequences as the number of positions in which the corresponding symbols are different. However, for comparing sequences of different lengths, a more sophisticated function, e.g., the edit distance, is more appropriate. The edit distance is defined as the minimum number of insertions, deletions, or substitutions needed to transform one sequence into another.

A more natural way of formulating the similarity between sequences in computational biology is the *sequence alignment*. This method is based on identifying portions of sequences that correspond to each other. Such a correspondence can reflect evolutionary conservation, structural or functional similarity, or a random event. The sequence alignment in general introduces a more complex evaluation of sequence similarity by considering different scores for matching symbols, mismatching symbols, and for gaps. The *global sequence alignment* allows us to compare entire sequences. It can be seen as a generalization of the well-know *longest common subsequence* (LCS) problem and can be solved using the Needleman-Wunsch algorithm [29].

The sequence alignment was originally expressed in terms of similarity: Peter Sellers [27, 34] was probably the first who recognized the advantage of expressing the sequence alignment in terms of metric distances instead of similarity. In this respect, the distance measure indicates how many changes are required to change one sequence into another. In this work, Sellers proved that the triangle inequality property also makes evolutionary sense. So, we associate positive scores to substitution, instead of negative scores used by algorithms computing similarity. Subsequently, Waterman et al. [48] generalized the Sellers' distance to include gaps.

The significant step forward was the introduction of the concept of *local sequence alignment* and its corresponding metric distance function [39]. The objective is to find an optimal matching between two pairs of subsequences from two sequences. Such an alignment is locally optimal if its distance cannot be decreased either by increasing or decreasing the extent of the aligned subsequences. It must be noted that optimal methods always report the best alignment that can be achieved, even if it has no biological meaning. In fact, when searching for local alignments there may be several significant alignments. Therefore, it would be reductive to examine only the optimal one [7]. As a consequence, a further generalization of the sequence alignment problem for detecting the *n* best nonintersecting, suboptimal, local alignments were proposed. An algorithm for solving this problem (which is an extension to the Smith-Waterman algorithm) was first proposed by Sellers [35] and then deeply studied in [2, 36, 47]. In this case, the similarity function produces a set of answers. However, a metric distance function must return a single value for each pair of arguments. The solution adopted in here is to transform the problem of local alignment in several subproblems of global alignment (to which metric space approach applies) by either dividing the query or database objects into subsequences [28].

12.1.2 Software Tools

The Molecular Biological Information System (*MoBIoS*)[3] is a metric-space-based database management system developed by D. P. Miranker and his team targeting life-science data [23–26, 49]. By analogy to spatial databases which extend relational database systems with index-structures and data types that support two and three-dimensional data and form the basis of geographic information systems (GISs), MoBIoS comprises built-in biological data types and index structures to support fast object storage and retrieval based on relative distances between objects determined by metric distance functions. In MoBIoS, a modified version of M-tree is used and it differs in two aspects. First, a new initialization (bulk-loading) algorithm to build the index from a given dataset has been designed. Second, the structure is further optimized so that covering radii in index nodes are reduced, which leads to better query performance. In the contest of the MoBIoS project, three important biological data have been considered: protein k-mers with the metric PAM model, DNA k-mers with the Hamming distance, and peptide fragmentation spectra with a pseudo-metric derived from the cosine distance [22].

The Protein Fragment Motif Finder (*PFMFind*)[4] system developed by Stojmirović and his colleagues is another application of the metric space approach. PFMFind is a system that enables efficient discovery of relationships between short fragments of protein sequences by applying similarity searching. It supports queries based on score matrices and PSSMs obtained through an iterative procedure similar to PSI-BLAST. The heart of PFMFind is FSIndex, an efficient indexing scheme for similarity searching in very large datasets of short protein fragments of fixed length [31, 41]. In this approach, the authors construct a *quasi-metric* tree-like index structure. A quasi-metric is a metric which satisfies the triangle inequality but is not symmetric (i.e., $d(x,y) \neq d(y,x)$). FSIndex takes advantage of the intrinsic geometry of the dataset used, being based on amino acid alphabet reduction. The amino acid alphabet is reduced into clusters so that quasi-metric distances are, as much as possible, large between and small within clusters. Each fragment is stored in a bin indexed by its sequence in the reduced alphabet. At the search time, the bin corresponding to the query fragment is generated and then transformed, position by position, into other possible bins. Neighboring bins for which the accumulated lower bound to the distance from the query point is greater than the query range as well as their descendants are pruned.

E-Predict[5] is a system developed by Pin-Hao Chi and his collaborators [11] for protein structure classification. Through the use of structural classification, life science researchers and biologists are able to study evolutionary evidence from similar proteins that have been conserved in multiple species. E-Predict transforms relevant protein structural information into high-level features, so similar protein structures are then retrieved from a high-dimensional feature space using nearest-neighbors search in the M-tree.

---

[3] http://www.cs.utexas.edu/users/mobios/
[4] http://www.vuw.ac.nz/biodiscovery/Publications/PFMFind/index.aspx
[5] http://ProteinDBS.rnet.missouri.edu/E-Predict.php

Another software package called *MetricMap*[6] developed by J. T. L. Wang and co-workers [46] exploits the technique of embedding metric spaces (refer to Chapter 1 in [54]) for searching in both protein sequences and RNA secondary structure data.

12.2 Centralized Metric Access Methods

Many metric index structures have been designed but some of them as main memory structures only. Recent surveys [10, 19, 54] give an illustration on a variety of different index structures for metric spaces. In the following, we concentrate on two typical disk-oriented representatives that are able to manage large collections of data.

12.2.1 Metric Tree Family

The M-tree (Metric Tree) is an index structure for searching in metric spaces proposed in [13]. It is able to index dynamic datasets (i.e, when insertions and deletions of objects are frequent) modeled as generic metric spaces with reasonable costs without requiring periodical restructuring. In contrast to other structures such as VP-tree [51], GNAT [9], GH-tree [44], that are constructed in a top-down manner, the M-tree is constructed in a bottom-up fashion like B-trees by splitting its fixed-size nodes. All (internal and leaf) nodes of M-tree consist of several entries. Every internal node entry has a metric region associated with. The metric region is of a ball-like shape and is determined by a center point, called *pivot*, and a covering radius. On contrary, leaf node entries do not contain any region information, but they store data objects, usually represented as their features, directly. In Fig. 12.1a, ball metric regions around the pivots o_1, o_2, o_4, o_7 and o_{10} are shown. In particular, each internal node entry consists of a child node pointer, the pivot and the covering radius of the ball region that bounds all objects indexed below, and the distance from this pivot to its parent pivot in the parent node entry. A leaf node entry consists of a data object and its distance from the parent's pivot. An example of M-tree is presented in Fig. 12.1b. Notice that pivots can even be repeated in the M-tree several times, e.g., the objects o_1 and o_2. Obviously, since the distance to the parent pivot has no meaning for the root entries, it is expressed by '-.-' in the figure.

The search efficiency is achieved by pruning the subtrees that certainly can not contain qualifying objects. This pruning effect of search algorithms is achieved by respecting covering radii and distances from objects to their pivots in parent nodes.

Although the property of dynamicity is an important requirement in access methods like M-tree, this requisite often can have a negative impact on performance. Moreover, the insertion algorithm of M-tree is not deterministic and inserting objects in different order can result in different trees. In order to address this problem, the *bulk-loading* algorithm has been proposed in [12]. The outline of the algorithm is as follows: given a set of n objects to be inserted, the algorithm produces an initial

---

[6] http://www.cis.njit.edu/~jason/metricmap.html

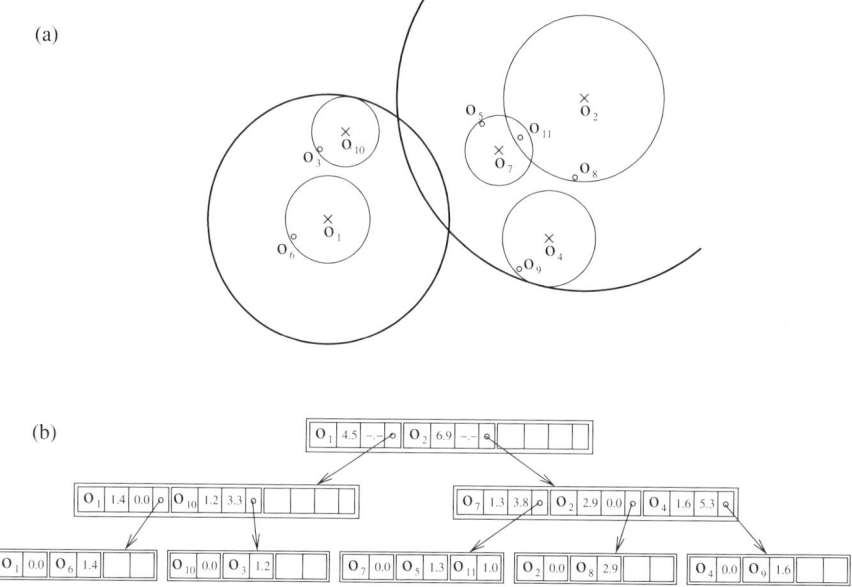

Fig. 12.1. Example of an M-tree: (a) a 2-D representation of partitioning; pivots are denoted by crosses and the circles around pivots correspond to ball metric regions; (b) a corresponding tree structure consisting of three levels.

clustering into l subsets of relatively close objects. This is accomplished by choosing l distant objects from the set and promoting them to pivots. The remaining $n-l$ objects are then assigned to their nearest pivot. Next, we proceed by invoking the bulk-loading algorithm for each of these l subsets, obtaining l subtrees. Eventually, the root node of the M-tree is created and all subtrees are connected to it. Special refinement steps are applied to make the tree balanced.

Most recently, several extensions of M-tree have been proposed in the literature (see [54] for a comprehensive survey). The Slim-tree is a metric tree structure proposed in [43] which attempts to improve performance by defining new insertion and split algorithms. Moreover, a special post-processing procedure is proposed that tries to reduce the overlap between node regions of sibling nodes. In [38], the authors provide another extension of the M-tree insertion algorithm with the objective of building more compact trees. Skopal [37] has recently introduced the Pivoting M-tree (PM-tree), a metric access method combining M-tree with the pivot-based filtering. Similar extension to this is represented by Distance Field Tree (DF-tree) [42]. A modification of M-tree able to efficiently index dense and sparse regions in data space proposed by C. Traina, Jr. and colleagues in [45].

12.2.2 Hash-based Similarity Indexing

The Similarity Hashing (SH), as proposed in [18], is built upon a completely different principle than the M-tree. This access method is inspired by hashing based approaches which organize search keys in buckets that can be directly accessed through the calculation of a hash function. In SH, the data file is arranged in a multi-tier hash structure, consisting of *separable sets* on each tier (or level). The separable sets are consequently stored in buckets. The main advantage of this approach is that for range queries up to a pre-defined value of the search radius, at most one bucket need to be accessed on each level. This property permits easy insertion and bounded search costs. Moreover, the use of pre-computed distances, obtained during insertion, significantly improves the efficiency of search operations in terms of the number of distance computations.

An efficient implementation of the similarity hashing approach has been developed in a structure called the Distance Index (D-index) [16]. In order to construct this hash organization, the D-index introduces the concept of a ρ-*split function* which exploits and extends the idea of the *excluded middle partitioning* originally proposed in [52]. In general, a ρ-split function of the first order divides a metric space domain in two non-overlapping partitions separated by a special region (the exclusion zone), which guarantees that an arbitrary object in one of the two partitions is at distance at least 2ρ from any object in the other partition. To obtain more than two sets as this partitioning does, the D-index allows combinations of several ρ-split functions. The combination of n ρ-split functions produces a new ρ-split function of order n characterized by 2^n partitions separated by one exclusion zone. An example of a combination of two functions is given in Fig. 12.2a. Notice that, the combination of more ρ-split functions still forms a single exclusion zone. This region is then recursively partitioned on the next level. This procedure creates a multilevel access structure as depicted in Fig. 12.2b. The structure in the example consists of three levels and one exclusion zone stored in the exclusion bucket of the whole structure. In contradistinction to tree-based structures, navigation along the tree branches is unnecessary, and each storage bucket is accessible directly. In order to reduce I/O costs, the D-index implements an *elastic bucket* strategy which guarantees that the I/O costs never exceed the cost of scanning a compressed sequential file. An extensive experimental study [14] conducted on real-life data sets demonstrated that the performance of SH is superior to other available tree-based structures.

The excluded middle partitioning principle is based on the ball partitioning idea; however, other types of splitting functions can be applied when implementing the similarity hashing schema. The authors of [15] define another three split functions that are able to achieve the same effect, i.e., to produce sets separable up to a pre-defined distance radius ρ. Based on well-known geometric concepts, these methods are called the *elliptic*, *hyperbolic*, and *pseudo-elliptic* ρ-split functions.

12.2.3 Performance Trials

The extensive performance evaluation published in [14] shows that, depending on the query type and the distance distribution of searched datasets, index structures can

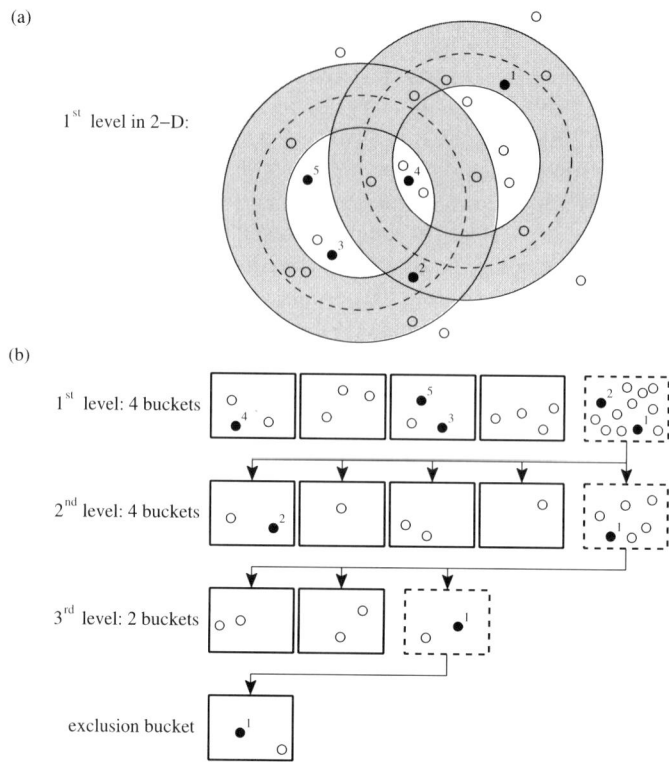

Fig. 12.2. Example of D-index structure: (a) a combination of ρ-split functions and (b) a resulting three-level structure.

speedup search time significantly. However, considering the amount of data produced and available in corporate networks, scalability of search structures with respect to data volume is probably the most important issue to investigate.

Figure 12.3 presents scalability of range and nearest neighbor queries in terms of distance computations and memory block accesses. In these experiments, the VEC dataset (45-dimensional vectors of color features extracted from images, compared by a quadratic-form distance function) is used and the amount of data grows from 100,000 up to 600,000 objects. Apart from the SEQ organization (sequential or linear scan), individual curves are labeled by a number indicating either the count of nearest neighbors or the search radius, and a letter, where 'D' stands for the D-index and 'M' for the M-tree. An interesting observation from the results is that M-tree exceeds SEQ in terms of I/O costs for queries returning larger portions of database. This is caused by low average occupation of nodes.

The basic lessons learned from these experiments are twofold:

- similarity searching is expensive;
- from the scalability point of view, the behavior of centralized indexes is practically linear.

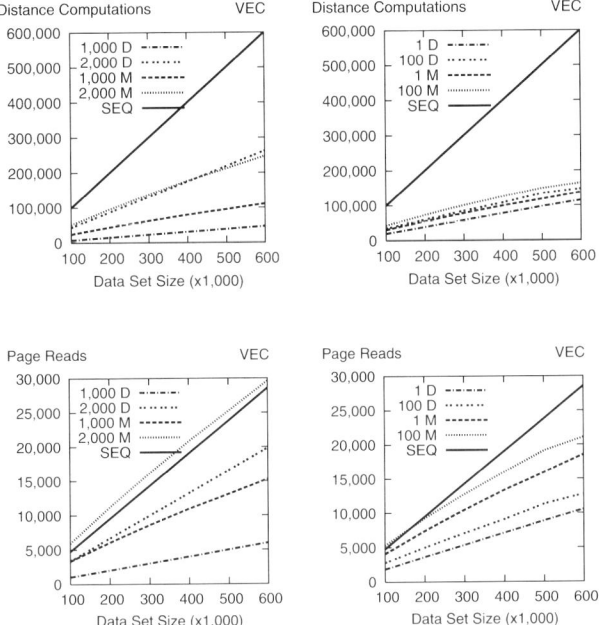

Fig. 12.3. Scalability of range (left) and nearest neighbor queries (right) for the VEC dataset.

Of course, there are differences in search costs among individual techniques, but the global outcome regardless of the type of data is that the search costs grow linearly with the dataset size. This property makes their applicability to huge data archives more difficult, because, after a certain point, centralized indexes become inefficient for users' needs, e.g., the response time becomes unacceptable.

Suitable solutions arise from two possibilities. First, increased performance may be obtained by sacrificing some precision in search results. This technique is called *approximate similarity searching* and many suitable solutions can be found in [3, 55]. Second, more storage and computational resources may be used to speed up executions of queries. The main idea here is to modify centralized solutions by considering parallel environments and to develop distributed structures. We elaborate on this issue in the following section.

12.3 Exploiting Multiple Computational Resources

The growth rate of dataset size of practically any domain of application for similarity searching now exceeds the growth rate of processor speeds. This is particularly true for Bioinformatics workloads. For instance, consider the GenBank biological database[7] (archiving nucleic acid sequences) which continues to grow at an exponential

---

[7] http://www.ncbi.nlm.nih.gov

rate, doubling every 15 months. In February 2003, the database contained over 29 billion nucleotide bases in more than 23 million sequences [8].

Though metric access methods are able to speedup retrieval considerably, the processing time is not negligible and it grows linearly with the size of the searched collection. The consequent degradation in performance of centralized access methods requires investigation of search methods that organize the database in parallel in order to speed up on-line searching. With such an infrastructure, parallel distance computations would enhance the search response time significantly. Modern computer networks have a large enough bandwidth, so it is becoming more expensive for an application to access a local disk than to access the RAM of another computer in the network.

In this section, we present current approaches to parallel and distributed similarity search processing categorized into three groups: techniques exploiting multiple resources of a single computer; index structures taking advantage of multiple computers with centralized management and distributed index structures without any centralized directory.

12.3.1 Parallel Similarity Searching

Parallelism in similarity searching can be exploited in two ways – more CPUs for computations and more disk drives for storage. In this direction, the popular M-tree has been extended and the Parallel M-tree [1, 56] has been developed. The experiments in [56] demonstrate relatively high I/O speedup and scaleup, and the effects of the sequential components of the M-tree algorithms seem not to be very restrictive. Although the experiment results show significant improvements, they are still limited considering the scalability, because the Parallel M-tree cannot dynamically increase the number of processors to preserve query response time as the file grows in size. The number of processors that can be actively used is also bounded by the maximum number of keys in a node.

12.3.2 Centralized Coordination

A much more promising solution exploits a distributed environment in which more computational units (computers, network nodes) are employed. In the following, we present a distributed access structure which is built on top of a Grid infrastructure.

Metric Grid

The idea behind the Metric Grid (M-Grid) [4] is straightforward. The D-index's partitioning schema (refer to Sec. 12.2.2) constitutes the basis of the M-Grid. In particular, we define a special Grid node named the *master node* where an addressing structure is stored. The addressing structure is formed by the hashing schema of the D-index. The difference is that bucket identifications are used instead of buckets, so the storage is distributed over all other Grid nodes. As a result, the master node is responsible for contacting Grid nodes managing buckets to be searched.

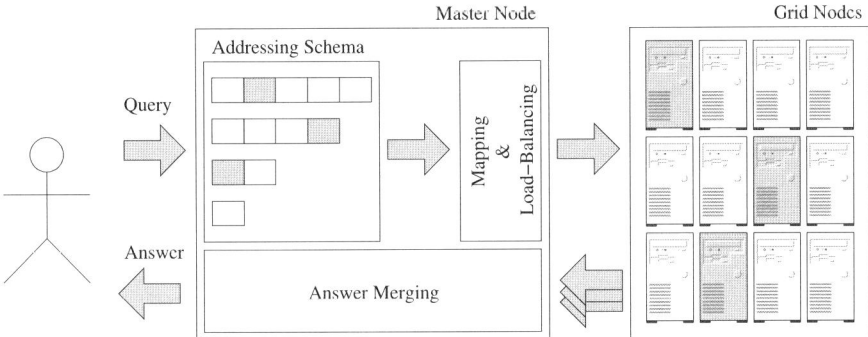

Fig. 12.4. The schema of M-Grid and the process of querying.

A schema of M-Grid and of the querying process is depicted in Fig. 12.4. When a user poses a similarity query, the master node identifies the buckets that might contain relevant data. The bucket-to-node mapping is consulted to get addresses of the corresponding Grid nodes. The master node initiates the execution phase by forwarding the query to the respective Grid nodes where the objects qualifying the query get retrieved. The individual sub-answers are then sent back to the master node which merges them to form the final answer to the query.

For performance tuning, the M-Grid allows to store more buckets on a single Grid node. Moreover, the M-Grid can also replicate some buckets which contain extensively retrieved data items. A deep performance analysis is presented in [4]. The results revealed the M-Grid's suitability for large data archives since it is scalable in our terms. The major limitation of this system is its centralized navigation directory.

More techniques suitable for distributed environments are tackled in the following section. Their main advantage lies in avoiding any centralized node or directory.

12.3.3 Scalable and Distributed Search Structures

Four scalable and distributed similarity access methods, able to execute similarity queries for any metric dataset, have been proposed recently. The main characteristics of these structures are that they exploit parallelism during the query execution and they do not have any centralized directory or master node to be accessed when searching for objects.

Two different strategies have been adopted: techniques based on partitioning principles and transformation methods. The former group comprises the VPT* which uses *ball* partitioning techniques, and the GHT* which exploits *generalized hyperplane* partitioning principles. The principle adopted by the latter group exploits a mapping from a metric space into a coordinate space of given dimensionality. This enables us to apply the well-known solution named distributed hash tables (DHT): the CAN and the Chord. The metric indexes based on them are called the MCAN and the M-Chord, respectively.

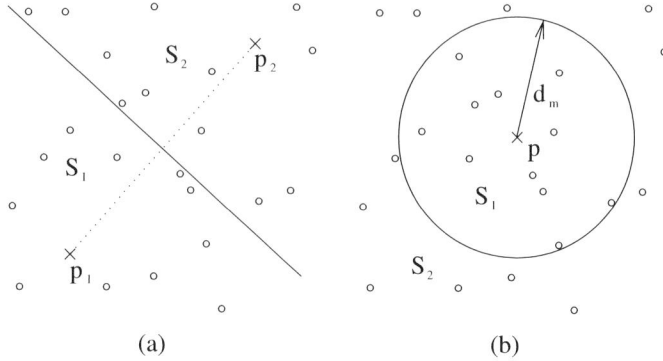

Fig. 12.5. Examples of partitioning: (a) the generalized hyperplane partitioning and (b) the ball partitioning.

Native Metric Search Structures

The Distributed Generalized Hyperplane Tree (GHT*) [5] is the first distributed data structure proposed in the literature based on the metric indexing principles. It is a distributed version of the Generalized Hyperplane Tree (GHT) [44], which is a binary tree built by a recursive selection of two pivots and partitioning of a set of objects by the generalized hyperplane schema (refer to Fig. 12.5a). The process of partitioning starts with the whole dataset and proceeds until the size of the sets gets below a predefined limit. Figure 12.6 depicts an example of a two level GHT built over a set of fourteen objects with the leaf size limit of six objects. As well as the partitioning schema, the tree is not necessarily balanced.

The basic indexing schema of the GHT* is similar to GHT: each peer maintains a replica of the tree structure with internal nodes containing the routing information by means of two pivots. The main difference is that leaf nodes hold a pointer to either a local bucket or to a remote peer storing other buckets (belonging to different leaf nodes of the tree). Buckets represent a set of storage areas of limited capacity labeled uniquely within the peer by BID identifiers. The peers themselves are globally identified by labels denoted as NNID (Network Node ID). The architecture of the system and its navigation schema are determined by a binary Address Search Tree (AST) based on the GHT principles. Figure 12.7 provides an example of the overall GHT* structure.

In order to preserve the requisite of locality of updates, which is essential in a distributed environment such as the one of the GHT*, a certain misalignment of the tree replicas of the peers is tolerated. Therefore, every peer maintains only those root-leaf branches that lead to one of its local buckets and the remaining pointers are substituted by NNIDs of peers responsible for the respective parts of the AST. For this reason, only a limited number of peers are contacted and updated when the system structure changes. However, the GHT* provides a mechanism called *image adjustment* for automatically updating the imprecise parts of the tree structure.

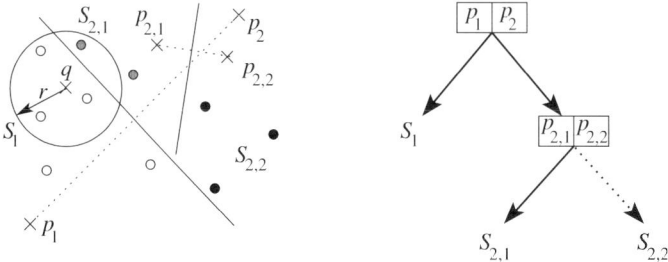

Fig. 12.6. Example of a Generalized Hyperplane Tree, tree branches accessed by the query are emphasized.

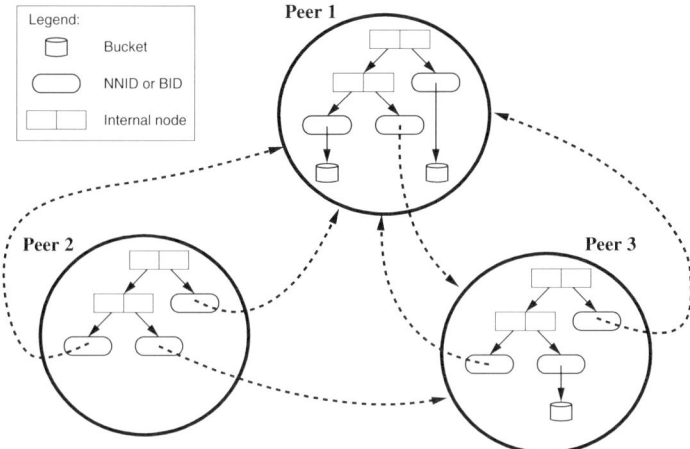

Fig. 12.7. Architecture of the GHT* system – the Address Search Tree.

Any peer of the system may initiate an insert operation. It can also issue similarity range and nearest neighbor queries. All these operations use their local ASTs to navigate within the network. Due to the independence of peers, parallel execution is achieved.

Given a range similarity query $R(q,r)$, the GHT* search algorithm traverses the tree from the root to leaves. In each internal node with pivots p_1, p_2, the distances $d(q, p_1)$ and $d(q, p_2)$ are computed. These values are used in the following step in order to skip accessing the subtree that certainly does not contain any object from the query scope. The distances between object q and any object in the subtree may be estimated by means of the Double-Pivot Distance Constraint [19, 54] based on the triangle inequality property of metric function d.

Lemma 1. *Assume a metric space $\mathcal{M} = (\mathcal{D}, d)$ and objects $o, p_1, p_2 \in \mathcal{D}$ such that $d(p_1, o) \leq d(p_2, o)$. Given a query object $q \in \mathcal{D}$ and the distances $d(p_1, q)$, $d(p_2, q)$, the distance $d(q, o)$ is lower-bounded as follows:*

$$\max\left\{\frac{d(p_1,q)-d(p_2,q)}{2},0\right\} \leq d(q,o).$$

The GHT* search algorithm does not access a subtree if this lower bound is greater than the search radius r. Please, note that both subtrees can be accessed – see an example in Fig. 12.6 in which both branches are followed from the root node and finally the leaves S_1 and $S_{2,1}$ get visited. Reaching a leaf node, the distance $d(q,o)$ is evaluated for every object o stored in this node and the objects that fulfill the query are returned.

The Distributed Vantage Point Tree (VPT*) is a twin structure of the GHT* sharing the same system architecture. The only difference is in the partitioning schema used and respective space pruning principles since the VPT* employs the ball partitioning (refer to Fig. 12.5b) and builds a distributed version of the Vantage Point Tree (VPT) [51].

Figure 12.8 provides an example of a VPT structure which recursively applies the ball partitioning to the indexed set until a predefined storage size limit for leaves is reached. The VPT* search algorithm follows the same general strategy as the GHT* and differs in the tree branches pruning schema. To prune the search space, the following Range-Pivot Distance Constraint [19, 54] is used.

Lemma 2. *Given a metric space* $\mathcal{M} = (\mathcal{D},d)$ *and objects* $o,p \in \mathcal{D}$ *such that* $r_l \leq d(p,o) \leq r_h$, *and given some* $q \in \mathcal{D}$ *and an associated distance* $d(q,p)$, *the distance* $d(q,o)$ *can be restricted by the range:*

$$max\{d(p,q)-r_h, r_l-d(p,q), 0\} \leq d(q,o) \leq d(p,q)+r_h.$$

Having a range query $R(q,r)$, this lemma is employed by evaluating the actual lower bounds on the distances from q to objects in the left and right branches independently. If one of these bounds is greater than r, the respective branch is not accessed.

Metric Content Addressable Network

The Metric CAN (MCAN) [17] defines a mapping from a general metric space into an n-dimensional vector space which is then used for data partitioning and navigation by means of the well-known P2P protocol CAN (Content Addressable Network) [32].

Having a preselected set of n pivots $p_1, p_2, \ldots, p_n$ from a sample dataset, the mapping $\Psi: \mathcal{D} \rightarrow \mathbb{R}^n$ is defined as follows:

$$\Psi(o) = (d(o,p_1), d(o,p_2), \ldots, d(o,p_n)), \forall o \in \mathcal{D}. \qquad (12.1)$$

This transformation is *contractive* and uses the L_∞ distance measure for evaluating the dissimilarity between two objects of the $\mathbb{R}^n$ space, i.e., $L_\infty(\Psi(x), \Psi(y)) \leq d(x,y)$ (see [10] for details).

Every peer takes over responsibility for a *zone* (hypercuboid) of the n-dimensional space and stores data objects having Ψ-values within this zone. An

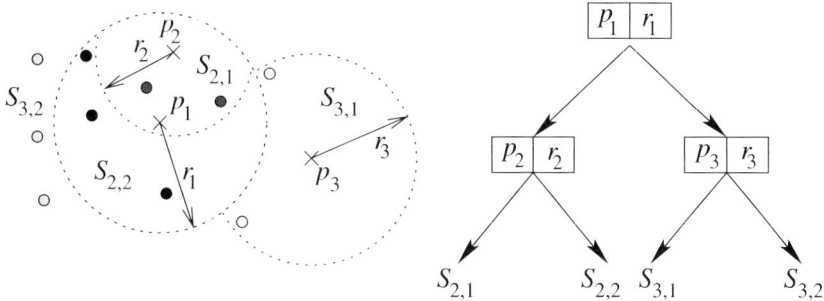

Fig. 12.8. Example of a Vantage Point Tree.

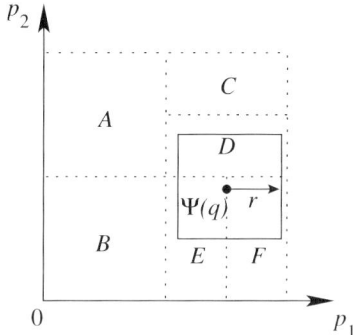

Fig. 12.9. Logical structure of the Metric CAN and the range query $R(q,r)$ transformed by the mapping Ψ.

example of such a zoning of two-dimensional space is depicted in Fig. 12.9. This partitioning as well as the routing algorithm follows a protocol similar to the one of the original CAN. Every peer maintains a routing table that contains the network identifiers and the coordinates of its neighbors' regions in the vector space. In order to locate the peer responsible for a given key $k \in \mathbb{R}^n$, the routing algorithm recursively passes the query to the neighboring peer that is geometrically the closest to the target point k in the space. The average number of neighbors per peer is proportional to the space's dimension n while the average number of hops to reach a peer is inversely proportional to this value.

The insertion algorithm is straightforward. Given a new object o, the peer that initiates the insert operation first computes the $\Psi(o)$ coordinates using Eq. (12.1). The insertion request, along with the object o, is then forwarded to the peer responsible for the n-dimensional $\Psi(o)$ key, by means of the standard CAN navigation schema. Eventually, the target peer stores the object o. When a peer reaches its storage capacity it performs a split operation if there is a free peer available.

A range query $R(q,r)$ at the level of the metric space $\mathcal{D}$ is transformed into a range query at the level of the n-dimensional space. However, since in this latter space the L_∞ distance is used, the query becomes an hypercube with side $2r$ centered in $\Psi(q)$. In Fig. 12.9, a two-dimensional example is presented. All peers intersecting this hypercube have to be visited in order to complete processing of the range query $R(q,r)$ (the peers D, E, and F in the example). These relevant peers are identified by a CAN-based *multicast algorithm* [21, 33]. Finally, the identified peers are examined to retrieve all qualifying objects.

Metric Chord

As mentioned earlier, the Metric Chord (M-Chord) [30] also uses a mapping of the original metric space into a coordinate space. However, in order to make use of the P2P routing protocol Chord [40], the coordinate space must be one-dimensional. This mapping is achieved by using the vector indexing method iDistance [20, 53], generalized to metric spaces. This technique partitions a vector space into n clusters $(C_0, C_1, \ldots, C_{n-1})$, identifies the cluster centers $(p_0, p_1, \ldots, p_{n-1})$, and maps the data objects according to their distances from the nearest center. Having a separation constant c that avoids clusters' overlaps, the iDistance value for an object $o \in C_i$ is

$$idist(o) = d(p_i, o) + i \times c. \tag{12.2}$$

This mapping schema is visualized in Fig. 12.10a.

Since the iDistance space partitioning and selection of pivots are originally designed for vector spaces, we cannot apply them directly to general metric spaces. To overcome this problem, a set of n pivots $p_0, p_1, \ldots, p_{n-1}$ is selected and the space is partitioned according to these pivots. Specifically, the Voronoi-like partitioning is applied, i.e., every object is assigned to its closest pivot. Except for these adaptations the iDistance approach can be fully utilized in the metric space model.

The original Chord protocol requires that its key space, i.e., the iDistance domain, is *normalized* by an order-preserving hash function h into the domain of size 2^m (where m is a positive integer representing the number of bits for the nodes and the keys identifiers). The parameter m should be large enough to make the probability of hash collisions negligible. In the ideal case, the resulting domain would have a uniform distribution in order to fully preserve the routing performance of the Chord. The function h is defined so that it is uniform with respect to the distribution of a given sample dataset. If the distribution of the indexed dataset significantly differs from the sample set, the Chord performance is damaged. Applying the function h, the M-Chord key-assignment formula becomes, for an object $o \in C_i$, $0 \leq i < n$:

$$m\text{-}chord(o) = h(d(p_i, o) + i \times c). \tag{12.3}$$

Once the data space is mapped into the one-dimensional M-Chord domain, the responsibility for intervals of this domain is divided among active peers of the system. The navigation within the system is supplied by the P2P routing protocol Chord. This protocol presumes that each of the participating peers is assigned a key from the indexed domain. The peers are shaped into a virtual circle (modulo the domain size 2^m) and every peer is responsible for the keys between the key of its predecessor on

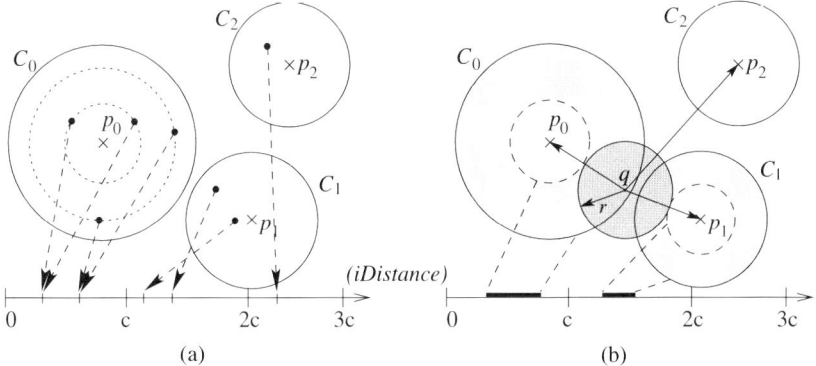

Fig. 12.10. The principles of the iDistance method.

the circle and its own key. The peers maintain information about two neighbors on the circle and about up to m long-distance peers. In this way, we can guarantee (with high probability) that the process of localizing the peer responsible for a given key requires a logarithmic number of forward messages.

Figure 12.11 shows the logical architecture of the system. In (a), a schema of the insert operation of an object $o \in \mathcal{D}$ into the structure is provided. First, the initiating peer N_{ins} computes the m-$chord(o)$ key using Eq. (12.3) and then employs the Chord to forward a store request to the peer N_o responsible for the computed key. Peers store data objects in a B^+-tree according to their M-Chord keys. When a peer reaches its storage size limit it executes a split. A new peer is placed on the M-Chord circle, so that the requester's storage is split evenly.

When a range query $R(q,r)$ is to be processed, several iDistance intervals are specified for the clusters that intersect the query sphere – see an example in Fig. 12.10b. The peer N_q that initiates the query identifies these intervals and the Chord protocol is then employed in order to reach the peers responsible for the midpoints of the intervals. Finally, the request is spread over all peers that cover the whole particular interval (refer to Fig. 12.11b).

12.4 Experience from Performance Trials

The step towards distributed data structures for similarity searching was motivated by insufficient scalability of centralized structures. The inherently heavy computational demands of similarity query processing, as the most critical aspect, are reduced due to parallelism. The number of computations of the distance function is considered as the most important indicator of efficiency of centralized index structures. The equivalent of this quantity in distributed and parallel environments is the *parallel number of distance computations* – the maximum number of distance evaluations performed in a serial manner during query execution.

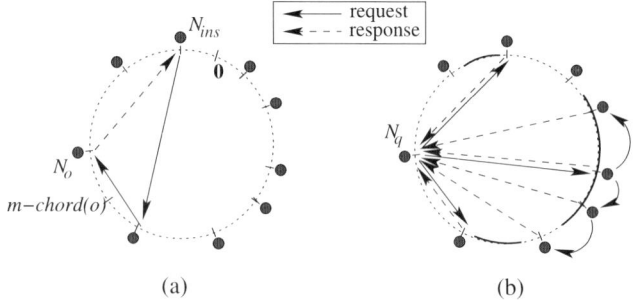

Fig. 12.11. The schema of (a) the insert and (b) range operations in the M-Chord structure.

The price to be paid for the utilization of parallelism is the cost of communication among the nodes of a distributed system. The relative importance of the communication costs depends on the type of underlying infrastructure used. Since all the presented approaches expect the intra-system communication via a message passing paradigm, the following two criteria can be considered in order to measure the communication costs:

- *total number of messages* – the number of all messages (requests and responses) sent during a query execution;
- *maximum hop count* – the maximum number of messages sent in a serial way in order to complete a query.

The results presented in this section have been obtained from performance experiments conducted on prototype implementations of the last four structures described above. A detailed analysis of the experiments is available in [6]. Here, we reduce to the findings related to 45-dimensional vectors representing color image features, compared by a quadratic-form distance function and to protein symbol sequences of length sixteen, compared by a weighted edit distance according to the Needleman-Wunsch algorithm. The datasets are denoted with VEC and DNA, respectively. The structures grow dynamically as the volume of stored data increases – provided sufficient number of network resources is available. In our experiments, the storage capacity of individual peers is 5,000 data objects for all the structures (five buckets with capacity 1,000 in the case of the GHT* and the VPT*). The average storage load ratio was about 66%, which results in approximately 300 active peers for a dataset size of 1,000,000 objects – the maximum file size tested.

Figure 12.12 depicts scalability trends observed while processing similarity range queries $R(q;1,500)$ on VEC and $R(q;15)$ on DNA for the last four structures, increasing the dataset size. The graphs in Fig. 12.12a,d exhibit a quite stable trend of the parallel number of distance computations for all structures but the MCAN() on VEC and M-Chord on DNA. The noticeable fluctuations of the MCAN are caused by cumulations of splits of multiple overloaded peers. On the other hand, the M-Chord's growing behavior can be attributed to the mapping and hashing functions which were struggling to diminish the increasing number of collisions which resulted in over-

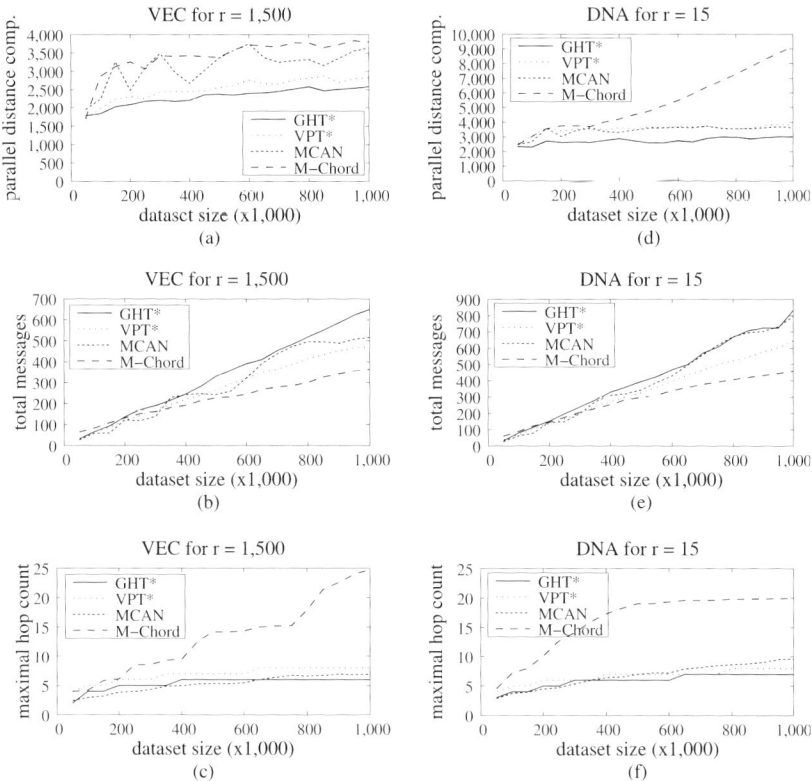

Fig. 12.12. The scalability trends for range queries $R(q, 1,500)$ on VEC (left) and $R(q, 15)$ on DNA (right): (a,d) parallel number of distance computations, (b,e) total number of messages, and (c,f) maximum hop count.

loaded nodes that could not be split. This is caused by the distance function used on the DNA dataset which produced relatively small variety of possible values.

All four algorithms for range queries are designed in such a way that no peer performs significant computations before forwarding requests to other peers. Therefore, the upper limit on the parallel number of distance computations is the maximum number of data objects stored on a single peer, which is 5,000 in our setting. This is not true for M-Chord because of overloaded nodes. The native metric approaches, namely the GHT* and the VPT*, have lower parallel costs than the transformation techniques. The reason is that the usage of buckets spreads the "near" data more widely over peers while the transformation techniques inherently try to preserve the locality of data. The other side of the coin is the number of peers involved in the query processing – the native techniques demonstrate a noticeably higher percentage of visited peers.

Figures 12.12b,e and 12.12c,f show the communication costs in terms of the total number of messages and the maximum hop count, respectively. The total messaging grows with the size of the structure because the space area relevant to the range query is covered by more peers. This indicator grows faster for the GHT* than for the others because it contacts a higher percentage of peers while processing a query. The graphs for M-Chord indicate that the total message costs grow slowly but the major increase is in a serial way of message passing which negatively influences the hop count. This is caused by the currently sequential algorithm for message distribution within M-Chord clusters. The parallel number of distance computations together with the maximum hop count can be considered as the characterization of the actual response time of the query.

Another positive effect brought by the distributive nature of the structures is an ability to simultaneously process multiple queries. Hence, the so-called *interquery parallelism* can be considered as the level of capability of accepting multiple simultaneous queries. In our experiment, groups of 10–100 queries were executed at the same moment – each from a different peer. The *overall parallel costs* of the set of queries were measured as the maximum number of distance computations performed on a single peer of the system. This value can be considered as a characterization of the overall response time of the set of queries. The query objects have been selected at random and the size of the stored data volume has been fixed to 500,000 objects. Figures 12.13a,c show the overall parallel costs, actually quite similar for all the structures.

In order to measure the improvement gained from the simultaneous processing of queries, a baseline for the overall parallel costs has been established as the *sum of the parallel costs* of individual queries. The ratio of this sum to the *overall parallel costs* characterizes the improvement achieved by the interquery parallelism and we refer to this ratio as the *interquery improvement ratio*. This value can also be interpreted as the number of queries that can be handled by a system simultaneously without slowing down the response time of individual queries. The graphs in Fig. 12.13b,d show this ratio and we can see that the improvement is better for the transformation techniques rather than for the native ones – mainly caused by different parallel costs for processing of individual queries.

In summary, the desired scalability of similarity searching has been reached by distribution of query processing over a set of cooperating peers. The native structures spread data and computations more uniformly over the set of peers, thus achieve better response times. On the other hand, the transformation techniques preserve the locality of data and involve fewer peers while answering a query, so they are better for the simultaneous query processing. Depending on the amount of resources available, the behavior of the structures, e.g., the upper bound on the response time, can be tuned by setting the storage capacity of individual peers.

12.4.1 Performance Tuning

Performance tuning of indexing structures is very important because they usually have many parameters that must be properly set in advance, e.g. the bucket capacity, ρ in ρ-split functions in M-Grid, number of pivots in M-Chord or MCAN, etc. The user or administrator of a production system typically has a clear notion about the

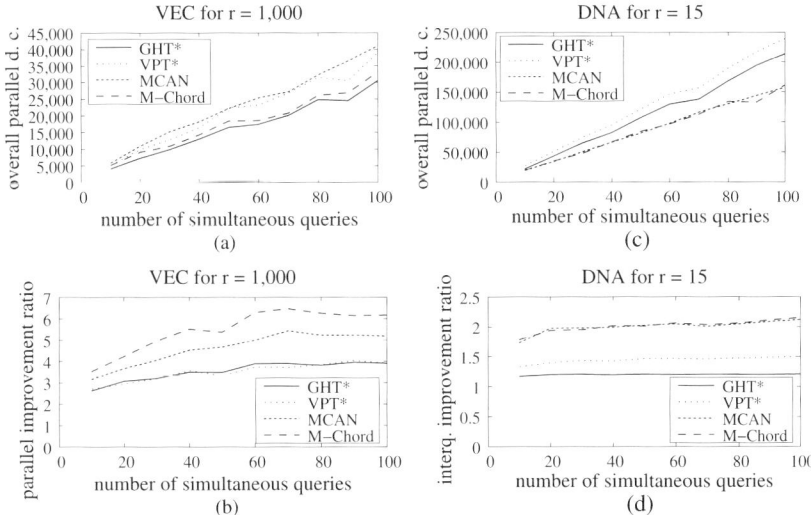

Fig. 12.13. (a,c) The overall parallel costs and (b,d) the interquery improvement ratio for VEC and DNA datasets, respectively.

maximum response time of a query and the total number of queries that will be issued simultaneously. They also suggest maximum memory requirements that are available on individual network nodes and the maximum number of nodes available.

The best setting of individual parameters of indexing structures exploits all available computational resources as efficiently as possible. Nonetheless, finding such a setting is often very exhaustive. Regardless of specifics of an indexing structure, a good utilization of distributed resources can also be reached by replication of heavily loaded nodes and by merging data of under-loaded nodes. In this respect, we introduce *replication* and *grouping* factors. The former denotes how many copies of a single bucket there are in the system, organized on different nodes, of course. The latter represents the number of buckets stored on a single node. In these terms, the maximum parallelization is one bucket per node.

In this section, we study the behavior of the M-Grid structure when the maximum number of simultaneous queries and the maximum response time are given. Our experimental setting was at maximum 64 buckets per node and in total 4,100 Grid nodes available. We used the same dataset containing one million of 45-dimensional vectors and test queries with radius $r=2,000$. Such queries are quite demanding because they return about 20,000 objects. The whole dataset was organized in 1,022 buckets which were afterwards distributed among available Grid nodes.

In order to study the performance of M-Grid, we have temporarily fixed the grouping and replication factors. Figure 12.14 presents costs to answer a batch of 10 or 100 queries for different M-Grid configurations. Different graphics distinguishes individual grouping factors. The horizontal line in each graph constitutes the limit on the query response time. Only the configurations under it satisfy both the user restrictions.

From the figures, we can observe that the most efficient configurations are the ones with the grouping factor of 64. The M-Grid with the grouping factor greater than 64 has the probability of accessing a node equal to 100%. Therefore, all nodes are almost equally loaded and used optimally in this respect. In Fig. 12.14a, the user requires ten simultaneous queries to be completed in 10,000 distance computations. Only configurations running on at least 512 nodes can meet these requirements. The most economical setting uses the grouping factor of 64 and 512 nodes, which leads to 32 replicas[8]. The other configuration almost equivalent in power uses 512 nodes as well, but the grouping factor is eight, which results in four replicas. Nonetheless, such a configuration exceeds the user's requirement by 1,400 distance computations.

Figure 12.14b depicts the same general behavior but the user specified the threshold of 100,000 distance evaluations and 100 simultaneous queries. The results for various configurations are the same but shifted up. The two configurations emphasized above both are the most efficient solutions again. The latter configuration, however, needed 102,123 distance computations.

The trends in all these graphs have also shown that doubling the number of Grid nodes improves the distributed power of the system nearly twice, i.e., a query is answered in the half number of distance computations. From the memory consumption point of view, configurations with smaller grouping factors are preferable if nodes cannot maintain too much data for some reason.

The advantage of M-Grid's addressing schema is that it is based on principles of linear hashing. Hence, new buckets are allocated as the data volume is increasing. By monitoring performance indicators, the M-Grid can increase the grouping factor or the replication factor gracefully to adjust the performance automatically.

Our experiments revealed that the M-Grid can be tuned to meet even very tight performance conditions. We used queries with the radii $r=2,000$ each returning around 20,000 objects. Such a setting is rather high. In practice, smaller queries giving tens of similar objects are more likely. Also the requirement of 100 simultaneously executed queries is immoderate implying a heavy-loaded system. The response time equivalent to 100,000 distance evaluations was about 8s in the worst case, which is reasonable. On the other hand, the experiment with more relaxed requirement of 10 concurrent queries had to be completed in 10,000 distance computations (equals to 0.8s), which is real-time processing. According to the experiments with one million data items, such high expectations can be fulfilled with 512 Grid nodes. Assuming more likely requirements of radii $r=1,000$ and the response time less than 2.5s, the system would require only 30-35 nodes, which is a feasible environment for any institution.

To sum up, by monitoring performance indicators the structures can adapt to changes in load usually caused by updating data or by altering user needs. Future research directions include development of more sophisticated and general load-balancing strategies which would be able to monitor and distribute the load of more

---

[8] $replicas = \frac{nodes \times grouping}{buckets}$, i.e., $\frac{512 \times 64}{1022}$

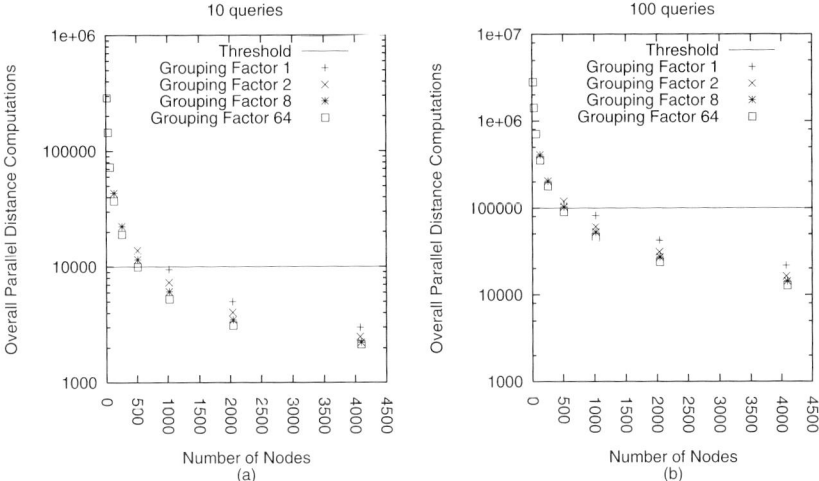

Fig. 12.14. Response times in distance computations for different configurations of M-Grid: (a) 10 simultaneous queries and (b) 100 simultaneous queries.

index structures (overlays) running on the same hardware. Such a direction is also supported by further development of indexing methods able to answer complex similarity queries combining more predicates.

12.5 Conclusions

Metric spaces have become an important paradigm for similarity search in several application domains. In this chapter, we have shown that the principles of metric space paradigm have been used to solve also problems in Bioinformatics, especially in the fields of comparative genomics and proteomics. The advantage of expressing the similarity in terms of metric distances becomes appealing also for Bioinformatics application. For example, in the sequence alignment problem, the distance is the number of changes that must be made to convert one sequence into the other and represents the number of mutations that will have occurred following separation of the genes during evolution; the greater the distance, the more distantly related are the sequences in evolution [27].

One of the major obstacles in applying metric distances to Bioinformatics is due to the violation of the triangle inequality. For this reason, popular exhaustive sequence searching tools, such as FASTA and BLAST require a linear scan of the entire database for each search [50]. On the other hand, users searching in large datasets require construction of efficient access methods to speedup retrieval due to poor performance of the linear scan. Most of the existing index structures are limited to operate in main memory only, so they do not scale up to high volumes of data. Therefore, we first concentrated our attention on centralized accessed methods where indexed data are stored in secondary memory (disks). We provided an introduction to metric structures to allow an understanding of their functionalities. We also reported results from practical experiments which illustrate the limited capabilities of single-computer implementations.

However, the concept of large data is relative: the growth of computational and storage resources of computers is so impressive that even a laptop can nowadays store and process amounts of data that only a mainframe computer would have been able to organize in the past. Nevertheless, the key issue is not the dataset size itself but its growth rate, which implies that also processing time has to scale accordingly. The consequent degradation in performance of centralized access methods requires investigation of new search methods that organize the database in parallel in order to speed up on-line searching. With such an infrastructure, parallel distance computations would enhance the search response time significantly.

In this chapter, we have presented the latest efforts in developing distributed approaches to similarity searching in metric spaces. We have described several distributed index structures, namely the M-Grid exploiting a centralized directory and the GHT*, the VPT*, the MCAN and the M-Chord representing pure peer-to-peer based approaches without any central control. We have also focused on their scalability by studying their performance on executing similarity queries from two different points of view: growing data volume, and accumulating queries evaluated concurrently.

Though all of the considered approaches have demonstrated a strictly sub-linear scalability in all important aspects of similarity searching for complex metric functions, the most essential lessons we have learned from the experiments can be summarized in the following table.

	single query	multiple queries
M-Grid	excellent	poor
GHT*	excellent	poor
VPT*	good	satisfactory
MCAN	satisfactory	good
M-Chord	satisfactory	very good

In the table, the *single query* column expresses the power of a corresponding structure to speed up the execution of one query. This is especially useful when the probability of concurrent query requests is very low (preferably zero), so only one query is executed at a time and the maximum number of computational resources can be exploited. On the other hand, the *multiple queries* column expresses the ability of structures to serve several queries simultaneously without degrading their performance by waiting.

We can see that there is no clear winner considering both the single and the multiple query performance evaluation. In general, none of the considered structures has a poor performance of single query execution, but the GHT* and the M-Grid are certainly the most suitable for this purpose. However, they are the least suitable structures for concurrent query execution – queries solved by the GHT* are practically executed one after the other. The M-Grid is slightly better in this respect. Such a behavior is caused by tuning the M-Grid to exploit available resource equally. However, the M-Chord structure exhibits the opposite behavior. It can serve several queries of different users in parallel with the least performance degradation, but it takes more time to evaluate a single query.

Within the chapter, we have presented a suitable solution for indexing data produced in Bioinformatics area. The advantage of metric access structures is their universality in applying to various data. We have also explained the issue of data scalability and pointed out weaknesses of centralized solutions. We have mainly focused on distributed structures which are capable of providing good enough querying performance.

References

[1] A. Alpkocak, T. Danisman, and T. Ulker. A parallel similarity search in high dimensional metric space using M-Tree. In D. Grigoras, A. Nicolau, B. Toursel, and B. Folliot, editors, *Proceedings of the NATO Advanced Research Workshop on Advanced Environments, Tools, and Applications for Cluster Computing-Revised Papers (IWCC 2001), Mangalia, Romania, September 1-6, 2001*, volume 2326 of *Lecture Notes in Computer Science*, pages 166–171. Springer, 2002.

[2] S. F. Altschul and B. W. Erickson. Locally optimal subalignments using nonlinear similarity functions. *Bulletin of Mathematical Biology*, 48:633–660, 1986.

[3] G. Amato, F. Rabitti, P. Savino, and P. Zezula. Region proximity in metric spaces and its use for approximate similarity search. *ACM Transactions on Information Systems (TOIS 2003)*, 21(2):192–227, April 2003.

[4] M. Batko, V. Dohnal, and P. Zezula. M-Grid: Similarity searching in Grids. In *Proceedings of ACM International Workshop on Information Retrieval in Peer-to-Peer Networks (P2PIR 2006), Arlington, VA, USA, November 11, 2006*, page 8. ACM, 2006.

[5] M. Batko, C. Gennaro, and P. Zezula. A scalable nearest neighbor search in P2P systems. In *Proceedings of the 2nd International Workshop on Databases, Information Systems and Peer-to-Peer Computing (DBISP2P 2004), Toronto, Canada*, volume 3367 of *Lecture Notes in Computer Science*, pages 79–92. Springer, February 2005.

[6] M. Batko, D. Novak, F. Falchi, and P. Zezula. On scalability of the similarity search in the world of peers. In *Proceedings of First International Conference on Scalable Information Systems (INFOSCALE 2006), Hong Kong, May 30 - June 1*, pages 1–12. ACM Press, 2006.

[7] A. Baxevanis and B. Ouellette. *Bioinformatics. A Practical Guide to the Analysis of Genes and Proteins (Second Edition)*. Wiley-Interscience, 2001.

[8] D. A. Benson, I. Karsch-Mizrachi, D. J. Lipman, J. Ostell, and D. L. Wheeler. Genbank: update. *Nucleic Acids Research*, 32:Database Issue D23–D26, 2004.

[9] S. Brin. Near neighbor search in large metric spaces. In U. Dayal, P. M. D. Gray, and S. Nishio, editors, *Proceedings of the 21th International Conference*

on *Very Large Data Bases (VLDB 1995), Zurich, Switzerland, September 11-15, 1995*, pages 574–584. Morgan Kaufmann, 1995.
[10] E. Chávez, G. Navarro, R. A. Baeza-Yates, and J. L. Marroquín. Searching in metric spaces. *ACM Computing Surveys (CSUR 2001)*, 33(3):273–321, September 2001.
[11] P.-H. Chi, C.-R. Shyu, and D. Xu. A fast scop fold classification system using content-based e-predict algorithm. *BMC Bioinformatics*, 7:362+, July 2006.
[12] P. Ciaccia and M. Patella. Bulk loading the M-tree. In *Proceedings of the 9th Australasian Database Conference (ADC 1998), Perth, Australia, February 2-3, 1998*, volume 20(2) of *Australian Computer Science Communications*, pages 15–26. Springer, 1998.
[13] P. Ciaccia, M. Patella, and P. Zezula. M-tree: An efficient access method for similarity search in metric spaces. In M. Jarke, M. J. Carey, K. R. Dittrich, F. H. Lochovsky, P. Loucopoulos, and M. A. Jeusfeld, editors, *Proceedings of the 23rd International Conference on Very Large Data Bases (VLDB 1997), Athens, Greece, August 25-29, 1997*, pages 426–435. Morgan Kaufmann, 1997.
[14] V. Dohnal. *Indexing Structures for Searching in Metric Spaces*. PhD thesis, Faculty of Informatics, Masaryk University in Brno, Czech Republic, May 2004. http://www.fi.muni.cz/~xdohnal/phd-thesis.pdf.
[15] V. Dohnal, C. Gennaro, P. Savino, and P. Zezula. Separable splits in metric data sets. In A. Celentano, L. Tanca, and P. Tiberio, editors, *Proceedings of the 9th Italian Symposium on Advanced Database Systems (SEBD 2001), Venezia, Italy, June 27-29, 2001*, pages 45–62. LCM Selecta Group - Milano, 2001.
[16] V. Dohnal, C. Gennaro, P. Savino, and P. Zezula. D-Index: Distance searching index for metric data sets. *Multimedia Tools and Applications*, 21(1):9–33, 2003.
[17] F. Falchi, C. Gennaro, and P. Zezula. A content-addressable network for similarity search in metric spaces. In *Proceedings of the the 2nd International Workshop on Databases, Information Systems and Peer-to-Peer Computing (DBISP2P 2005), Trondheim, Norway, August 28-29, 2005*, pages 126–137, 2005.
[18] C. Gennaro, P. Savino, and P. Zezula. Similarity search in metric databases through hashing. In *Proceedings of the 3rd ACM Multimedia 2001 Workshop on Multimedia Information Retrieval (MIR 2001), Ottawa, Ontario, Canada, October 5, 2001*, pages 1–5. ACM Press, 2001.
[19] G. R. Hjaltason and H. Samet. Index-driven similarity search in metric spaces. *ACM Transactions on Database Systems (TODS 2003)*, 28(4):517–580, 2003.
[20] H. V. Jagadish, B. C. Ooi, K.-L. Tan, C. Yu, and R. Zhang. iDistance: An adaptive B^+-tree based indexing method for nearest neighbor search. *ACM Transactions on Database Systems (TODS 2005)*, 30(2):364–397, 2005.
[21] M. B. Jones, M. Theimer, H. Wang, and A. Wolman. Unexpected complexity: Experiences tuning and extending can. Technical Report MSR-TR-2002-118, Microsoft Research, December 2002.
[22] R. Mao, W. Xu, S. Ramakrishnan, G. Nuckolls, and D. P. Miranker. On optimizing distance-based similarity search for biological databases. In *Proceed-*

ings of the 4th International IEEE Computer Society Computational Systems Bioinformatics Conference (CSB 2005), Stanford, USA, pages 351–361, 2005.

[23] R. Mao, W. Xu, N. Singh, and D. P. Miranker. An assessment of a metric space database index to support sequence homology. *International Journal on Artificial Intelligence Tools*, 14(5):867–885, 2005.

[24] R. Mao, W. Xu, W. S. Willard, S. R. Ramakrishnan, and D. P. Miranker. MoBIoS index: Support distance-based queries in bioinformatics. In *Proceedings of the 2006 Workshop on Intelligent Computing & Bioinformatics of the Chinese Academy of Sciences (WICB 2006), Hefei, Anhui, China, November 12-14, 2006*, 2006.

[25] D. P. Miranker, W. J. Briggs, R. Mao, S. Ni, and W. Xu. Biosequence use cases in MoBIoS SQL. *IEEE Data Engineering Bulletin*, 27(3):3–11, 2004.

[26] D. P. Miranker, W. Xu, and R. Mao. Mobios: A metric-space dbms to support biological discovery. In *Proceedings of the 15th International Conference on Scientific and Statistical Database Management (SSDBM 2003), Cambridge, MA, USA, July 9-11, 2003*, pages 241–244. IEEE Computer Society, 2003.

[27] D. W. Mount. *Bioinformatics – Sequence and Genome Analysis, Second Edition*. Cold Spring Harbor Laboratory Press, 2004.

[28] E. Myers. A sublinear algorithm for approximate keyword searching. *Algorithmica*, 12(4/5):345–374, 1994.

[29] S. B. Needleman and C. D. Wunsch. A general method applicable to the search for similarities in the amino acid sequence of two proteins. *Journal of Molecular Biology*, 48:443–453, 1970.

[30] D. Novak and P. Zezula. M-Chord: A scalable distributed similarity search structure. In *Proceedings of First International Conference on Scalable Information Systems (INFOSCALE 2006), Hong Kong, May 30 - June 1*, pages 1–10. IEEE Computer Society, 2006.

[31] V. Pestov and A. Stojmirovic. Indexing schemes for similarity search: an illustrated paradigm. *Fundamenta Informaticae*, 70(4):367–385, 2006.

[32] S. Ratnasamy, P. Francis, M. Handley, R. Karp, and S. Schenker. A scalable content-addressable network. In *Proceedings of the 2001 ACM Conference on Applications, Technologies, Architectures, and Protocols for Computer Communications (SIGCOMM 2001)*, pages 161–172. ACM Press, 2001.

[33] S. Ratnasamy, M. Handley, R. Karp, and S. Shenker. Application-level multicast using content-addressable networks. In *Proceedings of the 3rd International COST264 Workshop on Networked Group Communication, London, UK, November 7-9, 2001*, volume 2233 of *Lecture Notes in Computer Science*. Springer, 2001.

[34] P. H. Sellers. On the theory and computation of evolutionary distances. *SIAM Journal on Applied Mathematics*, 26(4):787–793, 1974.

[35] P. H. Sellers. The theory and computation of evolutionary distances: Pattern recognition. *Journal of Algorithms*, 1(4):359–373, 1980.

[36] P. H. Sellers. Pattern recognition in genetic sequences by mismatch density. *Bulletin of Mathematical Biology*, 46:501–514, 1984.

[37] T. Skopal. Pivoting M-tree: A metric access method for efficient similarity search. In V. Snášel, J. Pokorný, and K. Richta, editors, *Proceedings of the Annual International Workshop on DAtabases, TExts, Specifications and Objects (DATESO 2004), Desna, Czech Republic, April 14-16, 2004*, volume 98 of *CEUR Workshop Proceedings*. Technical University of Aachen (RWTH), 2004.

[38] T. Skopal, J. Pokorný, M. Krátký, and V. Snášel. Revisiting M-Tree building principles. In L. A. Kalinichenko, R. Manthey, B. Thalheim, and U. Wloka, editors, *Proceedings of the 7th East European Conference on Advances in Databases and Information Systems (ADBIS 2003), Dresden, Germany, September 3-6, 2003*, volume 2798 of *Lecture Notes in Computer Science*. Springer, 2003.

[39] T. F. Smith, M. S. Waterman, and W. M. Fitch. Comparative biosequence metrics. *Journal of Molecular Evolution*, 18:38–46, 1981.

[40] I. Stoica, R. Morris, D. Karger, F. Kaashoek, and H. Balakrishnan. Chord: A scalable Peer-To-Peer lookup service for internet applications. In *Proceedings of ACM Special Interest Group on Data Communications (SIGCOMM 2001), San Diego, USA*, pages 149–160. ACM Press, 2001.

[41] A. Stojmirovic and V. Pestov. Indexing schemes for similarity search in datasets of short protein fragments. *ArXiv Computer Science e-prints*, September 2003.

[42] C. Traina, Jr., A. J. M. Traina, R. F. S. Filho, and C. Faloutsos. How to improve the pruning ability of dynamic metric access methods. In *Proceedings of the 2002 ACM CIKM International Conference on Information and Knowledge Management (CIKM 2002), McLean, VA, USA, November 4-9, 2002*, pages 219–226. ACM, 2002.

[43] C. Traina, Jr., A. J. M. Traina, B. Seeger, and C. Faloutsos. Slim-Trees: High performance metric trees minimizing overlap between nodes. In C. Zaniolo, P. C. Lockemann, M. H. Scholl, and T. Grust, editors, *Proceedings of the 7th International Conference on Extending Database Technology (EDBT 2000), Konstanz, Germany, March 27-31, 2000*, volume 1777 of *Lecture Notes in Computer Science*, pages 51–65. Springer, 2000.

[44] J. K. Uhlmann. Satisfying general proximity/similarity queries with metric trees. *Information Processing Letters*, 40(4):175–179, 1991.

[45] M. R. Vieira, C. Traina, Jr., F. J. T. Chino, and A. J. M. Traina. DBM-Tree: a dynamic metric access method sensitive to local density data. In *Proceedings of the 19th Brazilian Symposium on Databases (SBBD 2004), Brasília, Distrito Federal, Brasil, October 18-20, 2004*, pages 163–177. University of Brasília, 2004.

[46] J. T.-L. Wang, X. Wang, D. Shasha, and K. Zhang. MetricMap: an embedding technique for processing distance-based queries in metric spaces. *IEEE Transactions on Systems, Man, and Cybernetics, Part B: Cybernetics*, 35(5):973–987, 2005.

[47] M. S. Waterman and M. Eggert. A new algorithm for best subsequence alignments with application to tRNA - rRNA comparisons. *Journal of Molecular Biology*, 197:723–728, 1987.

[48] M. S. Waterman, T. F. Smith, and W. A. Beyer. Some biological sequence metrics. *Advances in Mathematics*, 20:367–387, 1976.
[49] W. Xu, W. J. Briggs, J. Padolina, R. E. Timme, W. Liu, C. R. Linder, and D. P. Miranker. Using MoBIoS' scalable genome join to find conserved primer pair candidates between two genomes. In *Proceedings of the 12th International Conference on Intelligent Systems for Molecular Biology/Third European Conference on Computational Biology (ISMB/ECCB 2004), Glasgow, UK*, pages 355–362, 2004.
[50] W. Xu, D. P. Miranker, R. Mao, and S. Wang. Metric-space search of protein sequence databases. Technical Report TR-04-06, The University of Texas at Austin, Department of Computer Sciences, October 2003.
[51] P. N. Yianilos. Data structures and algorithms for nearest neighbor search in general metric spaces. In *Proceedings of the 4th Annual ACM Symposium on Discrete Algorithms (SODA 1993), Austin, Texas, USA, January 25-27, 1993*, pages 311–321. ACM Press, 1993.
[52] P. N. Yianilos. Excluded middle vantage point forests for nearest neighbor search. Technical report, NEC Research Institute, Princeton, NJ, July 1998.
[53] C. Yu, B. C. Ooi, K.-L. Tan, and H. V. Jagadish. Indexing the distance: An efficient method to knn processing. In P. M. G. Apers, P. Atzeni, S. Ceri, S. Paraboschi, K. Ramamohanarao, and R. T. Snodgrass, editors, *Proceedings of 27th International Conference on Very Large Data Bases (VLDB 2001), Roma, Italy, September 11-14, 2001*, pages 421–430. Morgan Kaufmann, 2001.
[54] P. Zezula, G. Amato, V. Dohnal, and M. Batko. *Similarity Search: The Metric Space Approach*, volume 32 of *Advances in Database Systems*. Springer, 2005.
[55] P. Zezula, P. Savino, G. Amato, and F. Rabitti. Approximate similarity retrieval with M-Trees. *The VLDB Journal*, 7(4):275–293, 1998.
[56] P. Zezula, P. Savino, F. Rabitti, G. Amato, and P. Ciaccia. Processing M-trees with parallel resources. In *Proceedings of Eight International Workshop on Research Issues in Data Engineering: Continuous-Media Databases and Applications (RIDE 1998), Orlando, Florida, USA, February 23-24, 1998*, pages 147–154. IEEE Computer Society, 1998.

13

Computational Modelling of the Biomechanics of Epithelial and Mesenchymal Cell Interactions During Morphological Development

Jiří Kroc[1,2]

[1] Department of Mechanics, University of West Bohemia, Univerzitni 22
  306 14 Pilsen, Czech Republic
  E-mail address: kroc@c-mail.cz, URL: http://www.c-mail.cz/kroc
[2] Corresponding address: J. Kroc Ph.D., Havlíčkova 482, 332 03 Šťáhlavy, Czech Republic

Summary: Computational modelling of morphological development of tissues based on complex systems and cellular automata can be decomposed into three interdependenent processes. Those three crucial parts are mechanical response of tissues, diffusion of signalling molecules, and gene regulatory network. It is shown that development of an adequate mechanical model of living tissues provides the morphological model with sufficient flexibility necessary to achieve expected morphological development scenarios. In this contribution, the attention is focussed to development of mesenchymal and epithelial tissues which, e.g., creates the basic mechanism of tooth development. The future development of the model is discussed with emphasis on open questions.

13.1 Introduction

Morphological development and growth of living tissues is realized by fundamental biological processes occurring in multicellular tissues, organs, and organisms [1]. They typically operate during growth of tissues, but they also occur during healing processes, re-modelling issues, etc. Therefore, a better understanding of morphological development of living tissues and related processes is required by developmental biology, morphology, genetics, human medicine, and other scientific disciplines.

When dealing with the growth of living tissues, it is not a good idea to omit the single-cell-level which creates tissues. To be more precise the greatest difficulties in tissue modelling are caused by the well known fact that tissues are processing information and maintain themselves in many physical and biological levels simultaneously—starting from the level of chemicals and DNA, going through polypeptides, proteins, cellular infrastructures and cycles, further going through cells, and finishing at the level of tissues, organs, and bodies. There are difficulties with building of single scale models without including fundamental properties of living tissues at other scales. It is very different from the situation occurring in modelling of non-living matter, e.g., mechanical properties of metallic materials where the overall mechanical response directly results from properties of atoms of given metal [2].

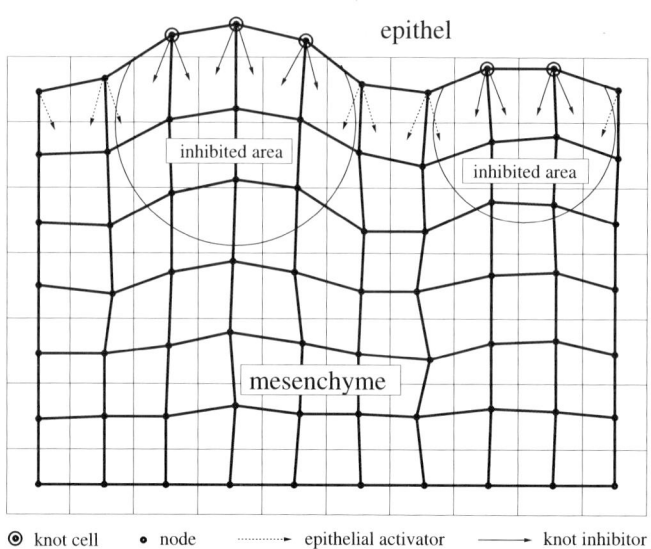

Fig. 13.1. An example network made of nodes interconnected by fibers where epithelial nodes are—located at the upper surface layer—producing activator (doted arrows), knot cells producing inhibitor (solid arrows), and mesenchymal cells are represented by the rest of nodes.

It is not difficult to imagine that a mathematical and computational description of all processes involved within a single living cell is far beyond the scope of any man-made computational device so far developed. We know that in one cubic centimeter of tissue there are $10^5 - 10^6$ cells if we expect that one cell has the diameter of $100 \mu m$. The number of cell parts such as proteins and organelles, etc. which creates one cell is about the order of 10^9. Hence, there is an evident need of simplifications in models of living tissues—which are composed of an enormous number of living cells. It is not a straightforward process to find such simplifications describing behaviour of real tissues, which are fundamental and have to be incorporated in a model.

A mathematical model of morphological development realized by epithelial and mesenchymal interaction is built using theories of complex systems. Cellular automata (CAs) method [3–8] is used as the computational tool to solve a model of mesenchymal and epithelial interaction which is decomposed into three distinct but inter-dependent parts, i.e. growth by cell division, signalling to neighbouring cells by chemicals and transformation of cells into different cell types due to gene regulatory network. The cellular automata method enables a detailed—spatial and temporal—

definition of behaviour of every part of the simulated topology. Some models of morphological development are already known but the problem is that they do not fully reflect biologically observed behaviour, e.g. some non-local computations of mechanical interactions are used what is not coherent with biological observations. Those models typically use simplified gene regulatory networks, but they do not work with relevant mechanical interactions of cells, and use some other simplifications which might lead to erroneous biological results.

The motivation of the CA-model of mechanical behaviour of mesenchyme and epithelium presented here comes from the tensegrity models [9–13] where—generally—the structure is composed from a set of two generic types of elements, one is under compression load (bars) and the other one under tensile load (strings). Spatial combination of those two types of elements leads to light and stable structures which are able to sustain large loads compared to classical structures. In the model, we work only with bars, named as fibres, interconnecting nodes—originally located in the center of each cell—where one node belongs exactly to one cell as shown in Figure 13.1.

Structural design based on CAs proved that it is easy to define a computational approach, which is capable to optimize shapes and weights of structurally fairly complicated components. It is proven [14, 15] that this new approach leads to better solutions compared to other methods such as are generated by combination of partial differential equations (PDE) and genetic programming. The main advantage of such CA-approach is the local definition of the optimization conditions which are incorporated in the local function driving CA evolution. Use of CAs saves a lot of computational time compared to genetic programming techniques where many instances of the optimized structures have to be evaluated in parallel. In such CA approach the only one instance of the optimized structure is evaluated.

We employ knowledge achieved in structural design [14–16] to model mechanical properties of mesenchyme and epithelium in this contribution. Involvement of gene regulatory network and diffusion of chemicals is widely discussed. It should be emphasized that there exists a strong distinction between living cell and a part of a cellular automaton called CA-cell within the whole text. Either of them is typically called cell.

This book chapter is structured as follows. Initially, important biological properties of living cells and tissues are briefly reviewed with special attention to one type of morphological development of tissues realized epithelial–mesenchymal interaction. This part is fundamental for understanding of the whole problem presented in this chapter. Then simplifications applied in the proposed model are discussed, followed by information about the general structure of models of mesenchymal and epithelial interaction. In the section dealing with the model, three different model components are defined. Namely, mechanical interactions of mesenchyme and epithelium, tissue growth, signalling based on diffusion, and cell differentiation based on gene regulatory network are shown. Then results are presented and thoroughly discussed with their relation to experimental observations. Finally, the future development of this type of models is discussed followed by the conclusions.

13.2 Introduction to Cell and Tissue Biology

First, it is necessary to start with a description of single cell functioning [1]. Morphological development realized by interaction of epithelium and mesenchyme is described in the next subsection. Simply said, a cell is a fairly complicated complex structure maintaining itself and influencing its surrounding using DNA, proteins, and chemicals. Those cellular components are mutually interconnected using a complicated network of chemical, signalling, and metabolic paths. DNA is stored in cellular nucleus. RNA is a copy of a DNA sequence defining a single gene (this process is called transcription). RNA goes out from the cellular nucleus. A protein is produced by translation of RNA in ribosomes ('factories' that make proteins according to the plan provided by RNAs; this process is called translation) which are located around cell nucleus. Proteins serve as building blocks of every cell, and as signalling media. Higher level building blocks of each cell are made from proteins, e.g., cellular organella, mitochondria, cellular membrane, intermediate filaments (defined later), tubulin and actin fibres, extracellular matrix, etc.

Each cell state is resulting from mutual interactions of all its parts, at the same time the cell state decides which operations—inner processes—are going to be activated and/or deactivated. It is done by switching on or off genes relevant to a current cell state; this process is called gene expression. Detailed description of behaviour of cells and tissues goes beyond the scope of this chapter, see for details [1]. Hence, we focus our attention to important processes which are used—in their simplified forms—to describe a computational model of morphological growth. Let us start with mechanical properties of cells.

We focus our attention only to vertebrate cells—which belong to Eukaryotic cell type—in this text. It is worth to point out at this moment that different species could have more or less different cell functioning, and hence, different mechanical, signalling, and maintaining parts!

As mentioned above, the essential part of cellular machinery is expression of genes maintained by RNA and production of proteins in ribosomes. Produced proteins are used for several different purposes which might operate simultaneously, e.g. they might built a cell infrastructure and serve as a part of cellular regulatory path. They could mechanically construct cell, they could become a part of a regulatory path, they could be involved in the cellular metabolism, and finally they could serve as a signalling medium which influences cellular regulatory cascades. It is quite often that one particular protein falls in more than one category.

As a first approximation, vertebrate cells are from the mechanical point of view composed from a membrane—which is mechanically unstable—, from intermediate filaments, actin fibers, and from tubulin fibers. Intermediate filaments themselves could sustain great loads. They create building parts of the intracellular structure called cytoskeleton which enables cells to sustain a large mechanical load without its mechanical failure. Intermediate filaments are passing through cellular membranes by desmosomes where those filaments are anchored. Collagen as a part of extracellular matrix bear extracellular mechanical loads, and is anchored in desmosomes in cell membranes from outside, and desmosomes are—as we know—anchored to intermediate filaments contained inside cells.

Intermediate filaments cross intracellular volume contrary to actin fibers which are located inside cells but in the close vicinity of cell membranes. Actin fibers enables cells to actively change their shapes, their locomotion, and to mechanically interact with intracellular organelles and surrounding of cells. Tubulin fibers create intra-cellular structure inside a cell which serves to deliver proteins and other building blocks to its destination within cell interior. Tubulin fibres do not influence mechanical properties of cells.

Chemicals and signalling proteins operating within and outside cells are serving as messengers bringing information from one site to another one. Those messengers are fundamental for maintaining cellular and tissue machinery. The whole cell is informed what it has to do due to information mediated by chemicals and signalling proteins which is propagated inside the cell (intracellular) and among surrounding cells *via* extracellular liquid. Signalling/regulatory paths are mediated by chemicals and signalling proteins which are switching on and off different cellular processes. Typically, different signalling paths are operating in different cellular types (see mesenchymal and epithelial cell types defined later).

A cell could be switched from one cell type to another by activation of different signalling and regulatory paths which in turn affects gene expression—, i.e., different sets of proteins are created. Switching of the cell could be triggered internally or externally. For simplicity, we mention only external switching here which could be realized by chemicals and/or proteins diffusing through extracellular matrix to given cell or by mutual contact of specialized parts of cell membranes. In the following we expect only switching of cell type by diffusing chemicals or proteins (see creation of enamel knots and proliferation of epithelial and mesenchymal cells in the next section).

13.3 Overview of Morphological Development of Tooth Resulting from Interaction of Epithelium and Mesenchyme

The morphological development of vertebrate organisms is composed from many developmental mechanism, see [17]. The knowledge is still incomplete but basic understanding is achieved. It is reported that there are three basic groups mechanisms acting during morphological development: autonomous, inductive and morphogenetic. In the autonomous mechanisms cells enter a specific state arrangement without interaction. Inductive mechanisms of cellular development results from mutual inter-cellular communication, which leads to change of cellular state. Finally, morphogenetic mechanisms are resulting from cellular interactions without any change of states of involved cell.

Autonomous developmental mechanisms involve division of heterogeneous egg, asymmetric (cell division) mitosis, and temporal dynamics with mitosis. Inductive developmental mechanisms are hierarchic and emergent. The largest group of developmental mechanisms is the morphogenetic one. It involves directed mitosis, differential growth, apoptosis, migration, differential adhesion, contraction, and matrix modification, see [17] for details.

There exists different types of biological models focussing their attention to different scales of biological tissues. Macroscopic models such as Physiome[3] treating tissues as continuum quantities have the capability to describe many biological phenomena but fail when describing cell behaviour and morphological development. There are molecular and subcellular models such as V-cell[4] or BioSym[5] that work well for description of processes operating within a single cell. It is worth to mention the multiscale model of morphogenesis [18], which is based on the Metropolis algorithm for Monte-Carlo Boltzmann dynamics describing cell membrane movement as thermal fluctuations of surfaces, which minimize surface energy [19, 20]. Signalling is modelled by partial differential equations of diffusion in three-dimensions and signalling by a simple automaton.

Modelling of morphological development of the whole organism is a quite complex process that is far beyond our knowledge and simultaneously beyond capacity of any computer. Therefore, we focus our attention to one special case, i.e. to tooth development [17, 18, 21–24]. It is well known fact that in tooth development, the key process is mechanical and chemical interaction of mesenchyme and epithelium, which is accompanied by creation and influence of enamel knots.

The most important tooth developmental stages of mammalian cheek tooth is having crown (often called molar tooth), which is composed from various combination of shapes and cusps as depicted in Fig. 13.2. Tooth shapes are created by combination of localized growth and invagination of epithelium into mesenchyme during development [22, 25]. Cusps start to be formed at their tips; all is mediated by creation of epithelial signalling centers called enamel knots. The first and second order knots are created from non-proliferative cells but they stimulate proliferation of the surrounding areas of them [22, 26–28] *via* expression of signalling molecules, see Figs. 13.1 and 13.2. It is believed that tooth development is done by induction and morphogenesis inter-dependently, see [17] for details.

The tooth development is initiated from layers of epithelium and mesenchyme. Then growth of epithelium creates a tooth bud, which grows. At a certain moment—determined by the amount of given growth factor—a primary enamel knot is created. This knot stimulates growth of mesenchymal cells in its vicinity and suppress growth of mesenchyme what leads to creation of cup stage. Further growth activates occurrence of the second order knots, again activated by exceeding of a threshold concentration of the growth factor. Secondary knots leads to further modulation of tooth invagination and creates bell tooth developmental stage. In the late bell stage, enamel is created at the epithelial layer, which is touching mesenchyme. At this stage, the original epithelial layer is disconnected from tooth. The development of tooth is finished by creation of tooth roots and by its eruption.

---

[3] http://www.physiome.org
[4] http://www.ibiblio.org/virtualcell/index.htm
[5] http://www.accelrys.com/about/msi.html

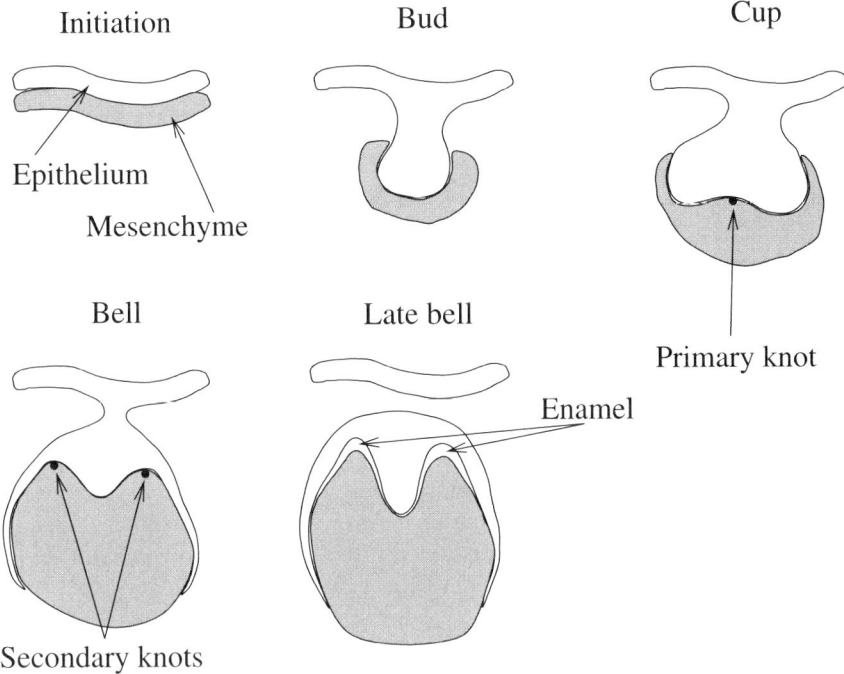

Fig. 13.2. Tooth development resulting from mesenchyme and epithelium interaction moderated by occurrence of enamel knots depicted in a series of developmental stages: initiation, bud, cup, bell, and late bell. In this chapter, the attention is focussed to description of tooth development going from bud, through cup, to bell stage, for details see [21].

From the mathematical and computational point of view, mechanical, signalling, and gene regulatory components of living cells and tissues are closely linked to each other. All are from one perspective independent—and hence, could be defined separately in a model—but at the same time they are interdependent. Therefore, it is impossible to describe the overall tissue behaviour during morphological development without detailed knowledge of each component and its dependence on other components.

All information provided here—see for details [1, 17, 21]—enables us to propose an abstract computational model of living tissues described step-by-step in the following sections.

13.4 Simplifications used in model of morphological growth

Biological processes within cells and tissues could be—from biological and consequently from the computational point of view—decomposed into two distinct groups without a clearly defined border. The first and much greater group of processes deals with common functioning of cells and tissues, i.e. all processes taking place within cells which serve to its reproduction and survival. The second and for us more important group deals with processes which are directly involved in morphological development of cells and tissues. Morphological development of simple tissues could be at the first approximation described by a relatively small set of genes creating a gene regulatory network. The size of such gene regulatory network could substantially increase within more complicated tissues or organs.

The main reason why all processes operating within cells are decomposed into those two groups is forced by the computational load which is required to simulate all biological processes within cells and tissues as discussed above. The border between those two distinct groups of processes could be—and in the near future will be for sure—moved towards involvement of not only morphologically critical processes, as is done in the work presented here, i.e. it means that less morphologically important processes become part of developmental models as well.

The key idea of modelling based on the above mentioned decomposition of cell functioning is to neglect all processes from the group maintaining common functioning of cells and to model only processes from the group describing morphological growth. Such neglecting of computationally 'unnecessary' processes dramatically decrease the computational load required for simulation of morphological growth what in turn leads to computationally tractable models. 'Unnecessary' processes—maintaining ones—are going on in all cells automatically at any moment. It is expected that they do not interfere with processes involved in morphological growth. If some interaction of a process belonging to the group of maintaining processes—and not yet involved within group of morphological ones—is detected to interact with morphological growth then such process could be easily involved in the model by mere shifting it from the group of maintaining processes to the group of morphological processes.

Therefore, this strategy of model design is open for future development and enables us to capture the essential processes occurring during morphological development without necessity to use extreme or unavailable computational power. We could from a certain point of view say that the overall functioning of cells is projected into a small subspace where only morphologically important processes are projected.

As discussed in the previous text, a precise and detailed computational model of living tissues—even a model of one living cell—is far beyond the computational capacity of the best available computers. There is a way how to overcome such deficiency. In modelling of morphological growth, we could employ substantially simplified models—which involve only those morphologically fundamental and generic processes operating in living cells and tissues. If we are able to localize such essential processes playing the key role during morphological development of tissues then we could succeed in building simple models of morphological growth. However, this is not an easy task because the knowledge of living matter is still not covering the whole field and there is much hidden information

In the remainder of this section, simplifications used in the design of the proposed model are briefly reviewed. There are three fundamental groups of processes observed within morphologically developing tooth tissues–made by interaction of mesenchyme and epithelium–which are creating cornerstones of the proposed model. They are, namely, mechanical interaction, signalling, and cell type switching. By mechanics we mean a mechanical model of living tissue working fairly above the level of single cells. Signalling is represented by diffusion of chemicals and signalling proteins through the tissue—here we employ only diffusion but proteins within living cells could be actively 'delivered' attached to myosin walking on tubulin fibers, or by proteins incorporated in the cell membranes could serve as signalling ones as well. Finally, cell type switching is handled by a gene regulatory network—which is represented by a tiny part from the set of all genes—where this network includes only morphogenetically necessary genes, and therefore, its size is easy to handle.

Only those chemicals and signalling proteins which are fundamental for maintaining all actions of used gene regulatory network are involved in the model. It is worth to stress out that within cells and tissues could be operating an enormous number of signalling chemicals and signalling proteins. A vast number of them is switched off during the greater part of cellular life and most of those genes in operation are maintaining survival and mitosis of the cell. Therefore, only a small fraction of genes is employed during morphological development.

The mechanical model of tissues is built from nodes interconnected by deformable fibers at a mesoscopic level, i.e. far above the size of single cell and below the size of tissue. Hence, the model is substantially simplifying mechanical structure of cytoskeleton and extracellular matrix—made of intermediate filaments, actin fibres, collagen, etc.—as previously discussed. The model enables to capture the following features: localization of mechanical strains and stresses caused by deformation, local tissue and cell remodellation, local tissue growth, creation of epithelial forces deforming mesenchyme, and changes of cell/tissue type due to signalling. In the following section, all three model parts are defined and explained in detail along with results.

13.5 Model

The model of the mesenchymal and pseudo-epithelial interaction is built step by step. Firstly, a one-dimensional model of mesenchyme and pseudo-epithelium is defined, studied, and carefully tested on tensile and compressible deformation. Then a two-dimensional model is proposed with special attention to mechanical properties of mesenchyme where mechanical properties of epithelium are simplified. Details—where and how mechanical forces could be created within living cells and tissues—are discussed in [1, 29–32]. It is a quite well known fact that cells are operating with small local actions, generated by actin fibres, which is leading to large global shape changes of tissue.

13.5.1 Three inter-dependent parts of the model

The model itself is divided into three distinct biological and computational parts—explained in the previous text—which are handling mechanical, signalling, and switching processes within evolving tissues. The first version of the mechanical model is published in [33] extended in [34] where mechanical interaction of mesenchyme and epithelium is described using a model of network made from a set of nodes interconnected by deformable fibers. Signalling is described by diffusion of signalling proteins/chemicals. Diffusion is implemented by distribution of amount of signalling protein among neighbouring nodes. It is a CA-analog of discretization scheme solving partial differential equation of diffusion working with the Laplace operator, see the definition of diffusion controlled cellular automaton [35] for details. Distribution of chemical content among neighbouring nodes leads to the same result as the finite difference scheme does. Switching of cell types is done using a simple Boolean network which handles change of one cell type into another one.

13.5.2 Mechanical interaction of epithelium and mesenchyme

The model works with a network of nodes interconnected by deformable fibers. Each cell from a rectangular domain—made of square cells—manages one node, see Figure 13.1. It is assumed that fibers are deformable by tension and compression. Strain is defined as

$$\varepsilon(t) = \frac{L(t) - L_0}{L_0}, \qquad (13.1)$$

where L_0 is the initial length and $L(t)$ [m] is its actual value at given time t, see Figure 13.3. Please, be aware that the initial length L_0 could evolve during growth of tissue as well as in explained in the following subsection. Use of Equation 13.1 allows to work with relative values used in Hook's law.

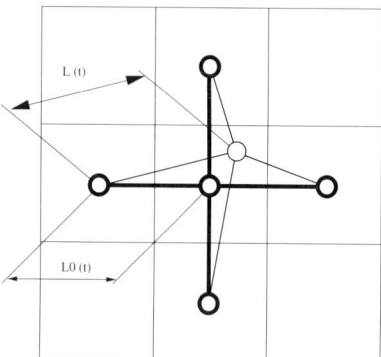

Fig. 13.3. An idealized figure depicting the way how strain $\varepsilon(t)$ is computed using the initial undeformed fiber length L_0 and the actual deformed value $L(t)$ of it. Deformation is computed for each fiber independently.

Hook's law representing the linear dependence of force or stress on strain is defined as

$$\sigma(t) = \frac{F(t)}{A} = E \cdot \varepsilon, \tag{13.2}$$

where $\sigma(t)$ is stress [N/m^2], $F(t)$ is force [N], and A is the cross-section of fibers [m^2]. This equation is ideally elastic—i.e., linear—for the whole range of strain ε what is rather physically unrealistic because it allows to compress material to physically impossible strains.

Therefore, the incompressibility of tissue deformation is incorporated in the model by the use of a modified Hook's law where the dependence of force F on deformation ε is composed from two distinct parts. One is defined by the Hooks law for tensile and compressible deformation which has the form of Equation 13.2, and the other one represents incompressibility of material. In our case, we expect that material could not be compressed below $\varepsilon = -0.8$ of its original length (see Figure 13.4 for details)

$$\begin{aligned} F &= E \cdot A \cdot \varepsilon, & \varepsilon &\in (-0.8, +\infty), \\ \varepsilon &= -0.8, & F &\in (-\infty, E \cdot A \cdot (-0.8)), \end{aligned} \tag{13.3}$$

There is linear dependence of force F on strain ε above $\varepsilon = -0.8$, and the only value of $\varepsilon = -0.8$ is taken for force below the value of $E \cdot A \cdot (-0.8)$ due to incompressibility. Dependence of the force F on deformation ε is depicted in Figure 13.4 with the incompressibility threshold at $\varepsilon = -0.8$.

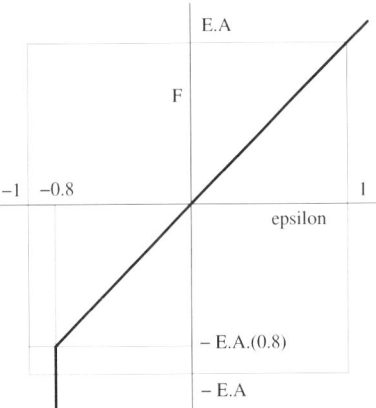

Fig. 13.4. Plot of the non-linear dependence of the force F on deformation ε with the incompressibility threshold at $\varepsilon = -0.8$ is depicted here. Force F below $-E \cdot A \cdot 0.8$ does not cause any further compression of deformed fibers.

The main reason why—as a first approximation—such dependence of force F on strain ε is used is strictly defined by one well known physical constrain. Compressibility of solids and liquids has a limit which states that they could not be compressed below $\varepsilon = -1$. It stems from the mass conservation law because mass could not be compressed to negative volumes. Hence, there is a good reason to use some kind of nonlinear law describing dependence of stress on strain for compression as in our case.

If one uses the linear dependence of stress on deformation then the following sequence of values of L which is derived from L_0 by multiplying it by a factor of $2, 1.1, 0.9, 0.5,$ and 0.01 and by inserting into the Equation 13.1 gives ε equal to $1, 0.1, -0.1, -0.5,$ and -0.99, respectively. There is an obvious limit in compression equal to $\varepsilon = -1$.

The following set of three Equations 13.4, 13.5, and 13.6 represents local equilibria for three types of cells used in the two-dimensional model, i.e. for the top nodes or surface ones (Equation 13.4), bulk nodes (Equation 13.5), and bottom fixed nodes (Equation 13.6)—where similar equations to Equation 13.6 are valid for the left and right nodes

$$\sum_{(k,l)\in\{(-1,0),(0,-1),(1,0)\}} F^{(k,l)} + {}^{ext}F_{surf}^{(k,l)} = 0, \qquad (13.4)$$

$$\sum_{(k,l)\in\{(-1,0),(0,-1),(1,0),(0,1)\}} F^{(k,l)} + {}^{ext}F_{bulk}^{(k,l)} = 0, \qquad (13.5)$$

$$\sum_{(k,l)\in\{(1,0),(0,1),(-1,0)\}} F^{(k,l)} + {}^{fix}F^{(k,l)} = 0, \qquad (13.6)$$

where F^{ext} represents an externally applied force to the cell in our case (see the principle in Figure 13.5), F^{fix} represents fixing force applied at the bottom, left, and right border cells, and indexes k,l represents the relative x,y coordinates of neighbouring cells of the cell under consideration. The last Equation 13.6 represents the situation where cells are fixed for the whole time to initially defined locations. Force F^{fix} balance the other forces, and therefore, no movement of those cells occurs. It could be simply done by keeping all those border cell coordinates fixed through the whole simulation. In the one-dimensional case—where a column of cells/bars is taken and the only allowed deformation works vertically—, no equilibrium is computed at the bottom cell. The position is simply kept constant with the coordinate y fixed.

The vertical displacement of the top node y_N in the one-dimensional case computed according to Equations 13.1, 13.2 and the simplified version of Equation 13.4 in the form $\sum_{(k,l)\in\{(0,-1)\}} F^{(k,l)} + F_{surf}^{ext} = 0$. After some rearrangement, it yields the following formula for tensile deformation

$$y_N(t+1) = F^{ext} \cdot L_0/(E \cdot A) + y_N(t) + L_0. \qquad (13.7)$$

Whereas the vertical displacement of i-th bulk node in the one-dimensional case computed from Equations 13.1, 13.2, and the simplified version of Equation 13.5 in the form $\sum_{(k,l)\in\{(0,1),(0,-1)\}} F^{(k,l)} + F_{bulk}^{ext} = 0$, after some rearrangement, leads to simple averaging of positions

$$y_i(t+1) = \frac{1}{2}(y_{i+1}(t) + y_{i-1}(t)). \qquad (13.8)$$

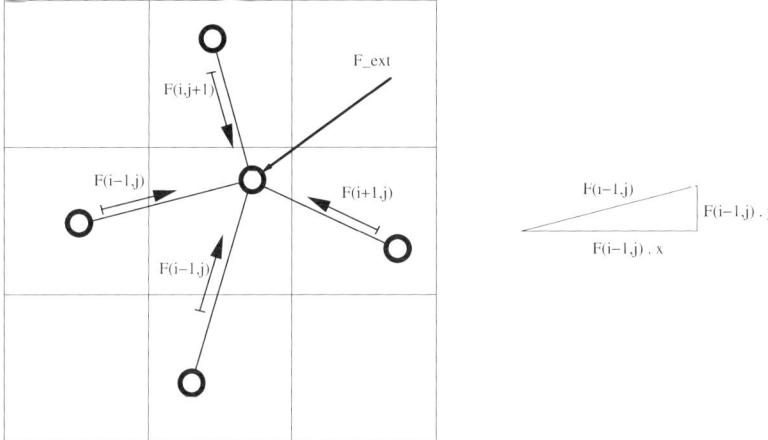

Fig. 13.5. The principle of how forces—in two dimensions—defining the equilibrium are computed for each node is depicted here. All acting forces are split into vertical and horizontal directions and equilibria in both directions are computed independently.

where such simple averaging procedure is possible only in the one-dimensional case contrary to higher dimensional cases. It could be done due to use of the linear Hook's law in compression and it is valid for small deformations. Please, note which simulation steps are taken on the left and right sides of the equation. Vertical displacement of all nodes in the case of compression works with the same equation as in the case of tensile deformation.

Computations of node displacements in the two-dimensional case are definitely more complicated than in the one-dimensional case. The main idea of the algorithm is explained in Figure 13.6. Whereas in the one-dimensional case a new position of the central node could be simply computed by mere averaging of positions of upper and lower nodes, in the two-dimensional case we have to use an iteration method to find an estimated position.

In Figure 13.6, the original position of the bulk node at time t managed by the updated cell (i, j) is expected to be moved to the estimated position—given by the solution of the equilibrium equations—which is the optimal solution of the problem with respect to forces applied by the neighbouring nodes $(i-1, j),(i, j-1),(i+1, j)$, and $(i, j+1)$ and—if they exists—to external forces. If the node is moved to this estimated position then a local change of position could be too fast and the updating algorithm looses its stability. Such instability could be removed by taking some value laying on the line interconnecting the original and estimated positions. This value is called the final position at time $t+1$. The distance from original point to the final one is a predefined fraction p of the distance of original and estimated points. The situation at the top cells is similar to the situation explained for the bulk cells except for the fact that only three neighbouring cells are presented there, i.e. $(i-1, j),(i, j-1)$, and $(i+1, j)$.

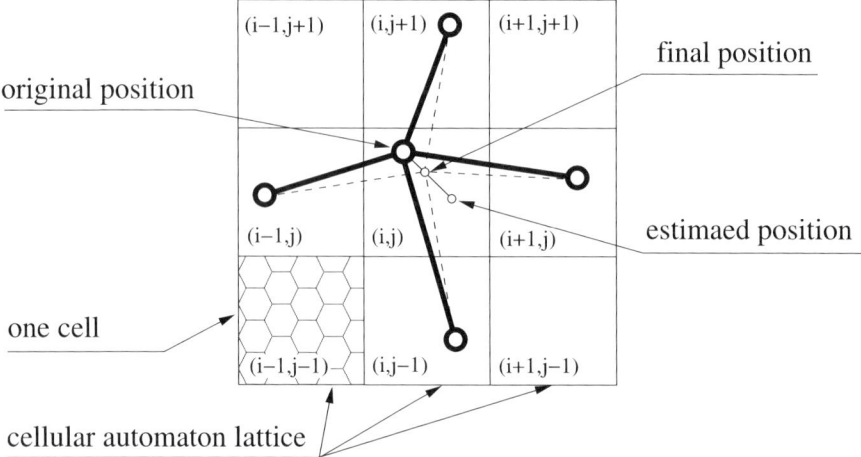

Fig. 13.6. Figure depicting the principle of the used algorithm. The original position of the node managed by the updated cell (i, j) is moved to the final position—computed by the algorithm—according to values provided by four neighbouring cells which lays on the line connecting the original position with the estimated one.

Initially, the position of the node under consideration is estimated using Equations 13.4, 13.5 or 13.6 representing the local equilibrium of given node. The algorithm used to find new position of nodes works by halving of intervals in two dimensions. Then deformation limits are tested and the value called estimate obtained, i.e. compression could not go below $\varepsilon = -0.8$. Finally, $p\%$ shift of the old position towards the estimated position of the cell under consideration is taken where $p = 0.1$. One of the reasons to take a part of the shift towards the estimated value from the initial node (i,j) position is coming from the fact that the model is not dynamical one but only a quasi-statical one. Hence, damping of oscillations of nodes which is present in the model could not be eliminated. Therefore, only a fraction from the possible node shift have to be taken into account. Otherwise, the oscillatory behaviour of the simulated structure might become dominant, could cause node mixing, and hence leading to computational failure.

13.5.3 Tissue growth

Tissue growth is implemented by growth of fibers—which are interconnecting nodes—i.e. by a change of their initial length L_0. It is expected that length L_0 depends on time t and on the growth pre-factor g as follows

$$L_0(t) = g \cdot t \cdot L_0(0) + L_0(0) = L_0(0) \cdot [g \cdot t + 1] \tag{13.9}$$

where $L_0(0) = const$ and $g \geq 0$. Evolution of $L_0(t)$ represents local tissue growth. We have to keep in mind that tissue growth is realized by proliferation of tissue cells.

It means that the number of cells is locally doubled, and hence, the local volume occupied by those cells increases.

The model is mesoscopic and operates at a level which is above the level of single living cells (do not exchange terms 'living cell' with 'cell' where 'cell' means computational unit of the CA model). Therefore, nodes and fibers are representing properties of a certain portion of the tissue. Hence, proliferation of cells within the tissue could be implemented by increase of the length of fibers L_0. As we know, the initial undeformed fiber length L_0 is increased due to local increase of the number of cells due to their proliferation. Some parts of the tissue are imposed to higher strains as L_0 increase there. It naturally causes relaxation of those highly strained tissue parts, and hence, the surface located above it could be shifted upwards. We could say that some kind of 'hills' appear above those proliferating locations. It is a well known fact that a place where a faster proliferation of mesenchyme occurs is determined by competition of signalling proteins. Only the homogeneous tissue growth is applied in this study.

13.5.4 Implementation of diffusion by two computational sub-steps

Diffusion is implemented using two computational sub-steps where completion of both of them is equivalent to one physical diffusion step. In the first diffusion sub-step, signalling molecules located at the updated node are divided into all neighbouring nodes including the one under consideration:

a) The number of neighbouring nodes N_n interconnected with the node under consideration—and where signalling molecules have to be migrated—is counted.
b) The total amount of signalling molecules belonging to the node under consideration is divided into parts having the same size where the number of parts is equal to the number of neighbouring nodes N_n counted at the point a) plus the node under consideration, i.e. the divisor is equal to $N_n + 1$.
c) Signalling chemicals are dispersed into the variable disp[i], where i = 0, 1, ..., N_n. Each variable disp[i] is linked with one neighbouring node among all neighbours N_n under consideration.

Please, note that the rest of the division is not necessary equal to zero. The rest of the division stays whole in the node under consideration, i.e. at the cell from which signalling molecules are migrated to neighbouring cells/nodes. This ensures conservation of the total amount of diffusive agent.

In the second diffusion sub-step, all signalling molecules—located in the variables disp[i] of nodes from the list on neighbouring nodes N_n and pointing to the node under consideration—are migrated towards the node under consideration. Sum of those signalling chemical migrated to the node under consideration plus the amount located within it is taken as the new value of signalling chemical in the next evolution step. Details and implementation of the two-step diffusion algorithm for the square lattice can be found in [35].

13.5.5 Signalling, switching and cell differentiation

Initially the model contains layer of epithelial cells located above the volume of mesenchymal cells. All cells are susceptible to two signalling molecules called activator and inhibitor. The activator leads after exceeding a threshold to non-proliferative change of epithelium cells to knot cells, i.e. a cell type differentiation is activated in this way. On the other hand, the inhibitor produced by knot cells suppress differentiation of epithelial cells and stimulates mesenchymal growth. This model structure is proposed according to experimental observations made on developing teeth.

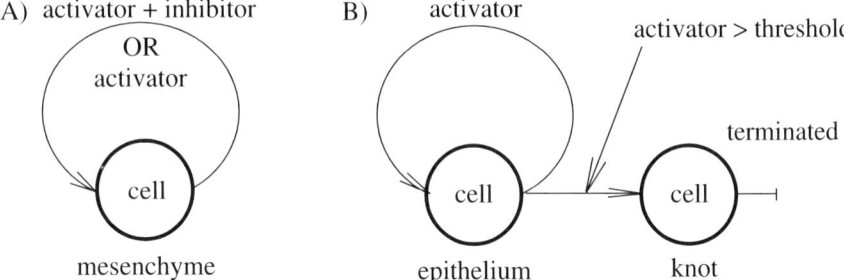

Fig. 13.7. Proliferation—and its link to signalling molecules—of mesenchymal and epithelial cells is depicted here. Epithelial cells has two possible evolutionary scenarios: a) proliferation to an epithelial cell, or b) change to a terminal non-proliferative knot cell.

Morphological change of one cell type into another is handled by a simple gene regulatory network, see Figure 13.7. It is expected that mesenchymal cells could proliferate only into mesenchymal cells. On the other hand, epithelial cells have two possible ways of evolution. The first one is simple, an epithelial cell proliferate into epithelial cells. Nevertheless, the other possible scenario is critical for the molar tooth evolution. If activator produced by epithelial cells exceeds some threshold then a single epithelial cell transforms itself into a knot cell which starts to produce an inhibiting signalling molecule. Production of inhibitor in knot cells locally suppress surrounding epithelial growth and enhance mesenchymal growth. Additionally, activator produced by epithelial cells cause mechanical response of neighbouring epithelial cells. This response—resulting from action of actin fibers—leads to invagination of epithelium into mesenchyme what in combination with mesenchymal growth creates typical molar shape of a mammal tooth.

We could say that involvement of the growth into the tissue model—which is locally influenced by production of activator and/or inhibitor—substantially changes the overall mechanical response of the tissue. In another words, we could conclude that production of activator by epithelium generates epithelial forces, which are in turn applied to the underlaying mesenchyme, and finally enhances invagination of epithelium into mesenchyme. On the other hand, knots producing inhibitor suppresses invagination of surrounding epithelium and stimulates mesenchymal growth, see Figure 13.1.

13.6 Results and Discussions

To ensure that the model is designed and programmed correctly, the analytical solution of the vertical displacement of the top cell y_N was compared—for several different external forces F^{ext}—to values which were computed according to Equation 13.7 for tensile deformation and for compression in the one-dimensional case. Simulations give the theoretically expected values. Testing of the two-dimensional case was done for unloaded and loaded cases. We have to stress that analysis of results in the two-dimensional case is not as simple and straightforward as in the one-dimensional case due to the simple fact that an iterative method finding a solution of the local equilibria has to be used. It is caused by the well known fact that an analytic solution of equilibria equations 13.5, 13.8, and 13.6 does not exist in general.

The topology used in the two-dimensional case is created by a block of 15×10 nodes in x, y directions. The block of those nodes is anchored by cells laying at the left, bottom, and right sides of this block. Anchoring of nodes is fundamental because we do not use epithelium around the whole bulk of mesenchymal nodes. In such case where the epithelium surrounds mesenchyme, the structure made of all interconnected nodes could not collapse as in the case where such surrounding epithelium is not used. The epithelium has fixing properties—caused by actin fibres operating within it—which do not allow the whole structure to collapse. Hence, in our case, we allow only top nodes to move in the topology used in this contribution. The only border cells allowed to move are those laying at the top edge of the block including all bulk cells. Cells number 7, 8, and 9 located at the top edge of the block of cells—counted from the left to the right—are subjected to the external forces $F = -2.5, -5, -10,$ and -20 acting downwards, see Figures 13.8 – 13.14. Fibers have the Young modulus $E = 10^5$; the cross-section of them is $A = 0.01 \cdot 0.01 = 10^{-4}$, the incompressibility threshold is set to $\varepsilon = -0.8$, and the initial distance of nodes $L_0 = 0.1$. Results of simulations dealing with non-growing tissues are published elsewhere [33].

The overall mechanical response of the tissue model—resulting from a combination of epithelial forces and/or growth of tissue due to cell proliferation—is tested for several different deformation conditions, where those combinations are given by the applied mesenchymal force F—where F could be equal to $-2.5, -5, -10, -20$—and by the growth pre-factor g with two options equal to 0 and 0.0002. All combinations of applied forces F and the growth pre-factor g are discussed thoroughly with special attention to the influence of tissue growth on tissue mechanical response. To enable a simple orientation, there are always figures—displaying snapshots of evolving tissues taken in different simulation steps for given force F—presented in two columns. The left one represents the situation where the growth pre-factor $g = 0$ whereas the right column represents snapshots where $g = 0.0002$. The influence of

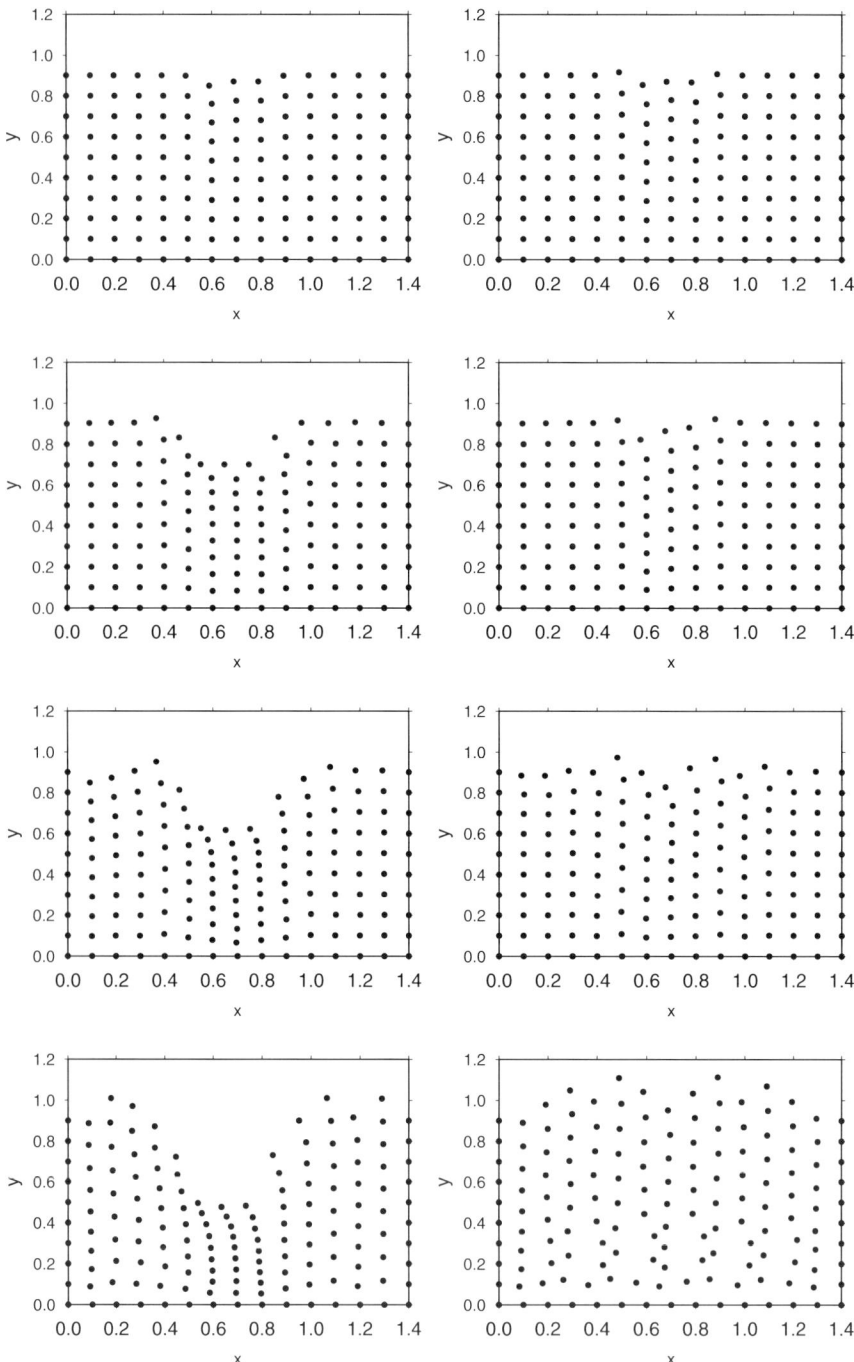

Fig. 13.8. Snapshots of tissue topologies stressed by force $F = -2.5$ and growing with the growth pre-factor $g = 0$ (left column) and $g = 0.0002$ (right column) which are taken at simulation steps 50, 100, 150, and 250 (from the top to bottom).

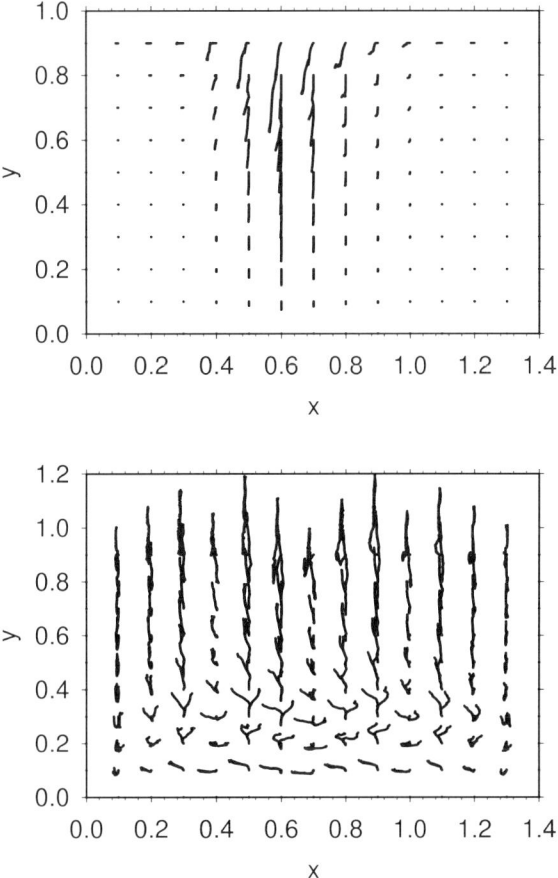

Fig. 13.9. Cumulative plots of node positions for deformation force $F = -2.5$ (steps from 0 to 300) for $g = 0$ (top) and $g = 0.0002$ (bottom) where selected snapshots are shown in Figure 13.8.

growth of tissue on the overall tissue behaviour becomes apparent in such presentation.

Deformation conditions are selected to be close to deformation conditions which are present during morphological growth of tissues of molar teeth, i.e. to the situation where growth of mesenchyme—in the bulk—is accompanied by production of epithelial forces compressing underlaying mesenchyme. It should be stressed out that—despite the fact that no signalling is involved in those simulations which is created by signalling chemicals in epithelium and epithelial knots—evolution of the used model structure resembles deformation response observed in teeth tissues.

Involvement of localized tissue growth would serve as a fine tuning of the already observed tissue overall response.

In the first case, deformation of the 7th, 8th, and 9th upper nodes (computed from the left-side) by force of $F = -2.5$ is applied along with the growth pre-factors $g = 0$ and $g = 0.0002$—numbers of those externally deformed nodes are kept equal through all simulations presented here—, see Figs. 13.8 and 13.9. In all figures taken from the simulations, nodes are depicted without fibers which are interconnecting nearest neighbours. In the case where the growth pre-factor is equal to zero, an invagination in the center of deformed tissue occurs. A more interesting observation is the situation where the growth pre-factor is equal to 0.0002 and where all nodes are going more or less upwards—tissue starts to behave as a swelling one. Additionally, what is even more interesting for us, it behaves as tissue around knot cells where lower forces coming from epithelial cells acts in combination with mesenchymal growth—all is stimulated by higher content of inhibitor produced by knot cells. Such tissue response substantially differs from the situation where a greater epithelial force is applied. A small invagination is still present in the center of epithelium which is less pronounced than in the cases of higher applied forces as shown later. The epithelium forms two hills located at both of its sides of that small invagination at its center. The vertical position of the node in the center of the invagination is still located above its initial value.

In the second case, force $F = -5$ is applied along with the growth pre-factors $g = 0$ and $g = 0.0002$, see Figs. 13.10 and 13.11. The combination of deformation and growth of $g = 0.0002$ represents the case where both invagination of some tissue part and growth of another one are observed simultaneously. There is pronounced invagination of the central part of deformed tissue accompanied by pronounced elevation of tissue nodes at both sides of deformed tissue. Applied force squeezes the central part of tissue where tissue deformation created by it is transmitted by fibres to surrounding externally undeformed tissue. That leads to an elevation of nodes located on the left and right sides from the central area of deformed nodes—what perfectly fits expectations about behaviour in such deformation and growth context. This case with its deformation and growth conditions is very close to observations made upon evolving mesenchymal and epithelial tissue within molar teeth. In other words, growth of 'hills' located around knots and invagination between them, see the Sub-chapter 13.4 for details.

In the third case, force $F = -10$ is applied along with the growth pre-factors $g = 0$ and $g = 0.0002$, see Figs. 13.12 and 13.13. The simulation results in a deep invagination ('valley') in the center of deformed epithelium. The depth of this invagination depends on the applied force F as could be compared with invaginations produced by lower applied forces. As F increase, the depth of the invagination increases but only up to some threshold where no further increase of its depth occurs for the applied force due to incompressibility of fibers what is demonstrated by comparison of mechanical responses of tissue deformed by force $F = -10$ and -20 where no difference in the resulting mechanical response of the deformed tissue is observed.

Note that if we add tissue growth having the growth pre-factor of $g = 0.0002$ to applied force $F = -10$ then we get a different tissue response, see Figs. 13.12

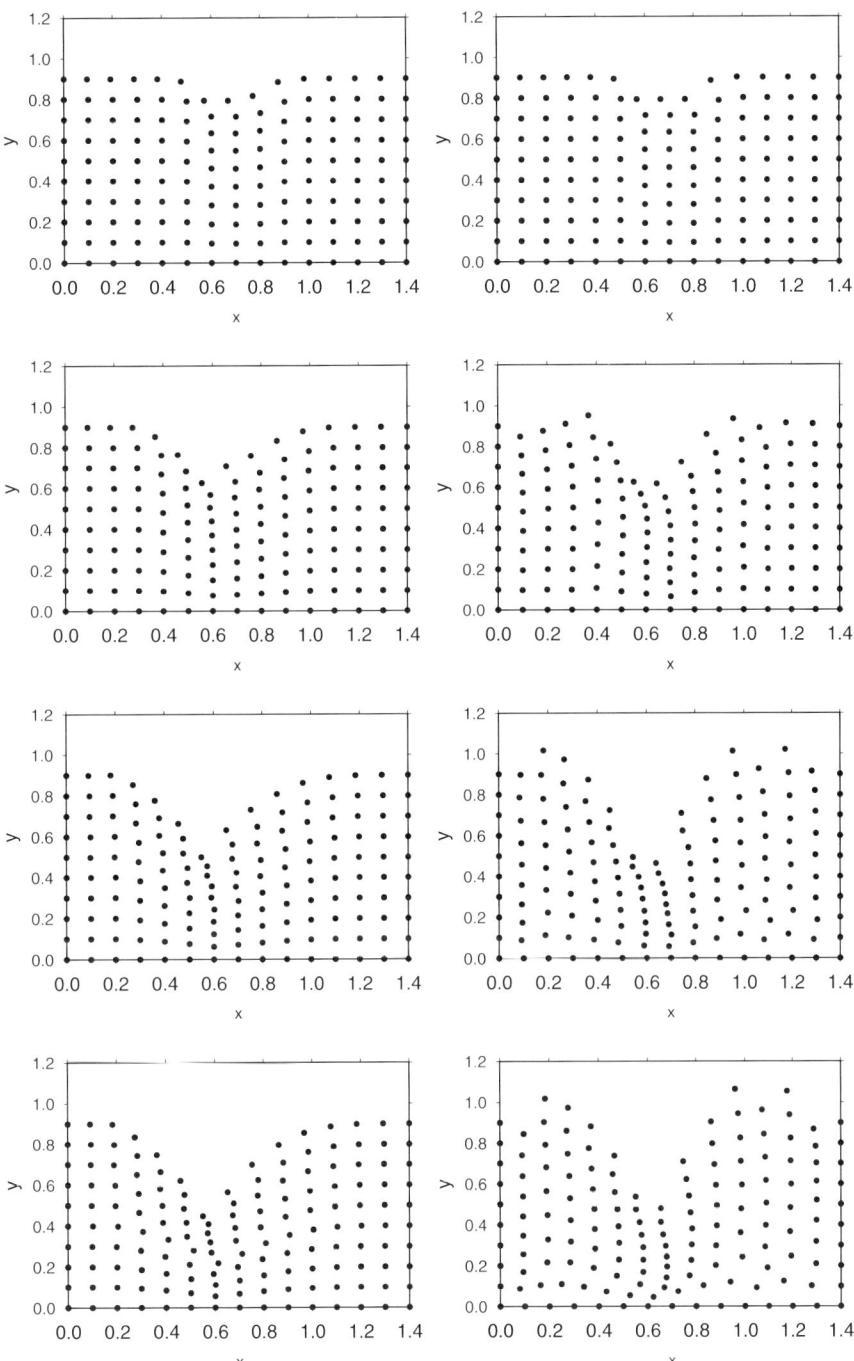

Fig. 13.10. Snapshots of tissue topologies stressed by force $F = -5$ and growing with the growth pre-factor $g = 0$ (left column) and $g = 0.0002$ (right column) which are taken at simulation steps 50, 150, 250, and 300 (from the top to bottom).

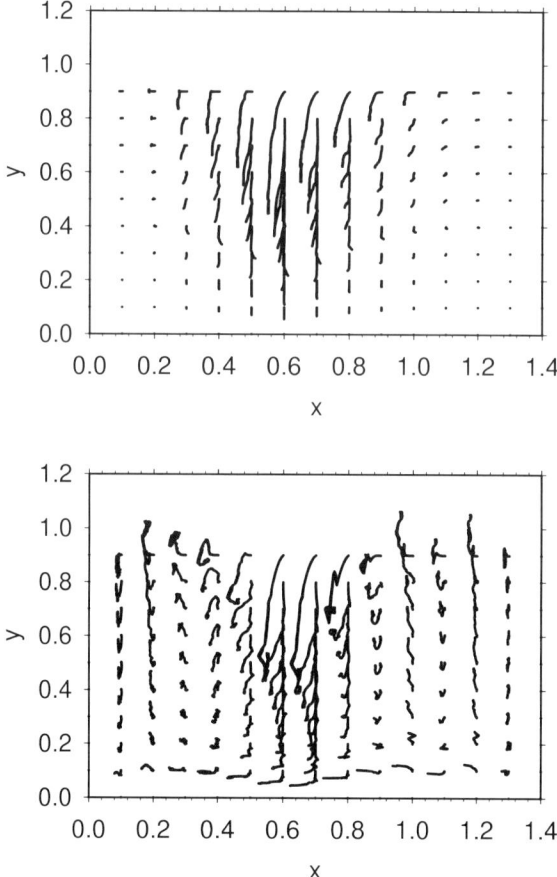

Fig. 13.11. Cumulative plots of node positions for deformation force $F = -5$ (steps from 0 to 300) for $g = 0$ (top) and $g = 0.0002$ (bottom) where selected snapshots are shown in Figure 13.10.

and 13.13. The original downward deformation in the case where the growth prefactor $g = 0$ is removed by a combination of downward and upward deformations. Upward deformation is localized to the left and right sides of epithelium which leads to creation of 'hills' there. Hence, an insertion of the homogeneous growth in the tissue causes quite complex change of the overall tissue behaviour. It is expected that once inhomogeneous growth—handled by gene regulatory network with diffusion of chemicals—will be included in the model then an even more complex response of the deformed and growing tissue will appear. It has to be stressed out that homogeneous mesenchymal growth do not allow so deep invagination of tissues in the center of it as in the previous case where $g = 0$.

13 Biomechanics of Epithelial and Mesenchymal Cell Interactions 287

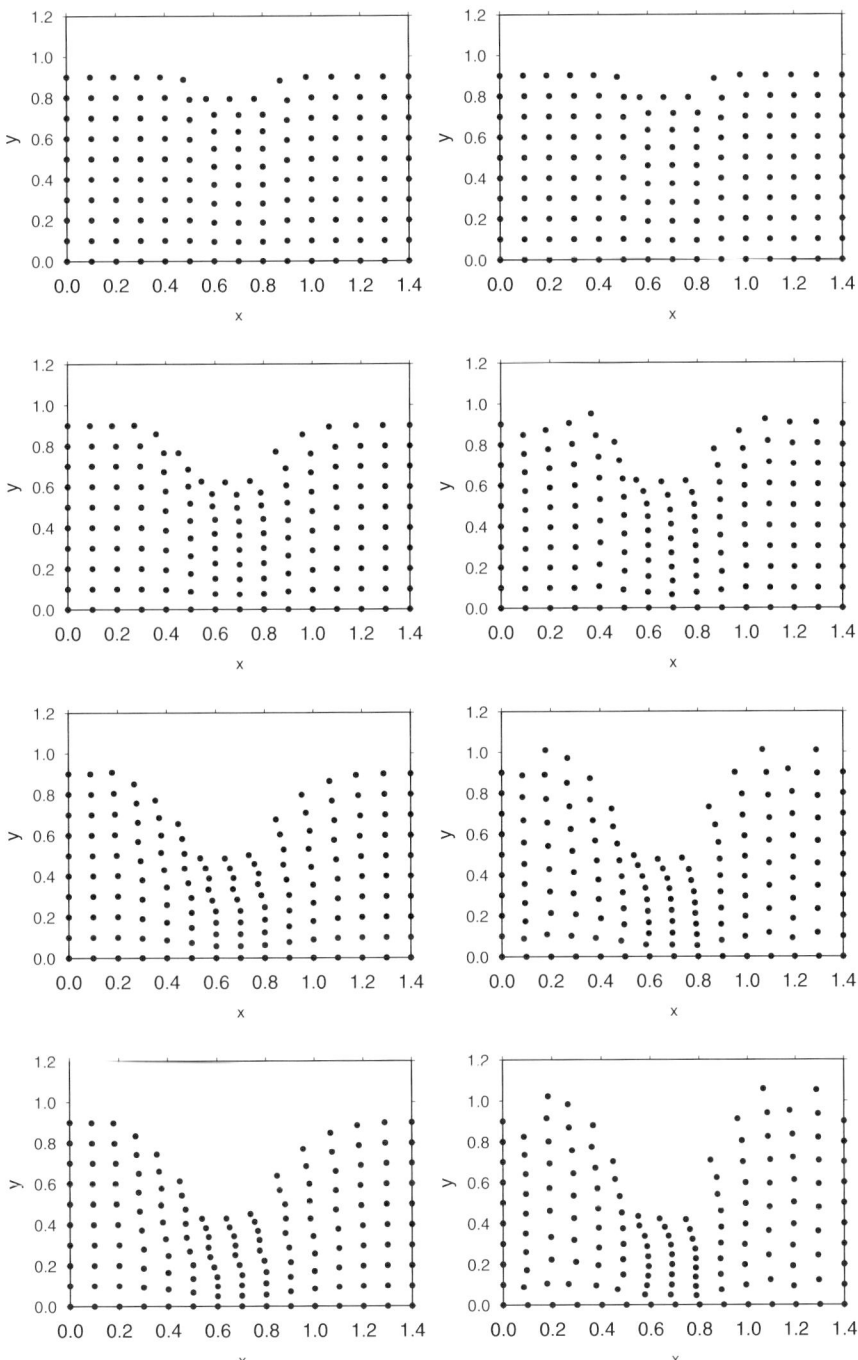

Fig. 13.12. Snapshots of tissue topologies stressed by force $F = -10$ and growing with the growth pre-factor $g = 0$ (left column) and $g = 0.0002$ (right column) which are taken at simulation steps 50, 150, 250, and 300 (from the top to bottom).

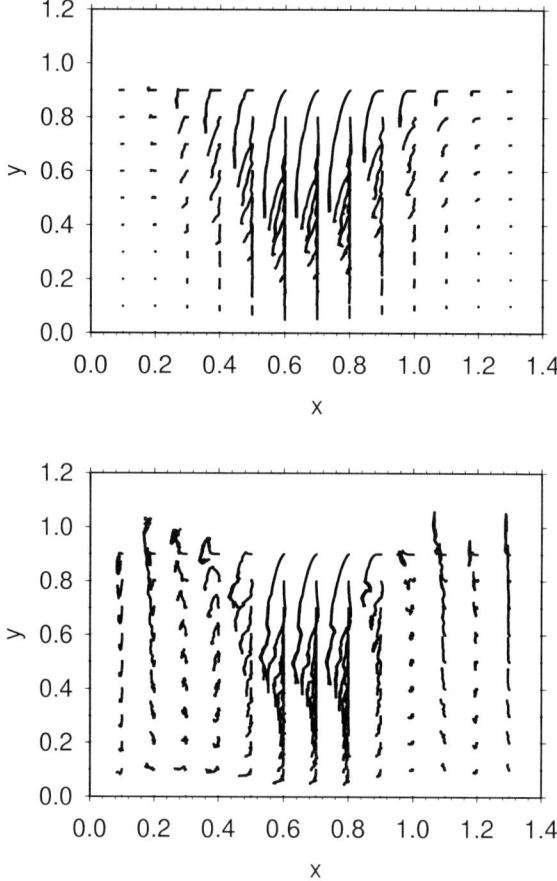

Fig. 13.13. Cumulative plots of node positions for deformation force $F = -10$ (steps from 0 to 300) for $g = 0$ (top) and $g = 0.0002$ (bottom) where selected snapshots are shown in Figure 13.12.

In the last case, deformation by the highest used force $F = -20$ N is applied along with the growth pre-factors $g = 0$ and $g = 0.0002$, see Figs. 13.14 and 13.15. This deformation force produce no difference compared to the case of applied force $F = -20$. The explanation that was given in the case of $F = -10$ is valid for this case as well. This deformation case is presented here to explicitly point out the existence of a deformation limit above which no change in deformation response is observed. It is a direct result of the existence of the incompressibility threshold. Increase of deformation force do not produce any deformation effect above the incompressibility threshold.

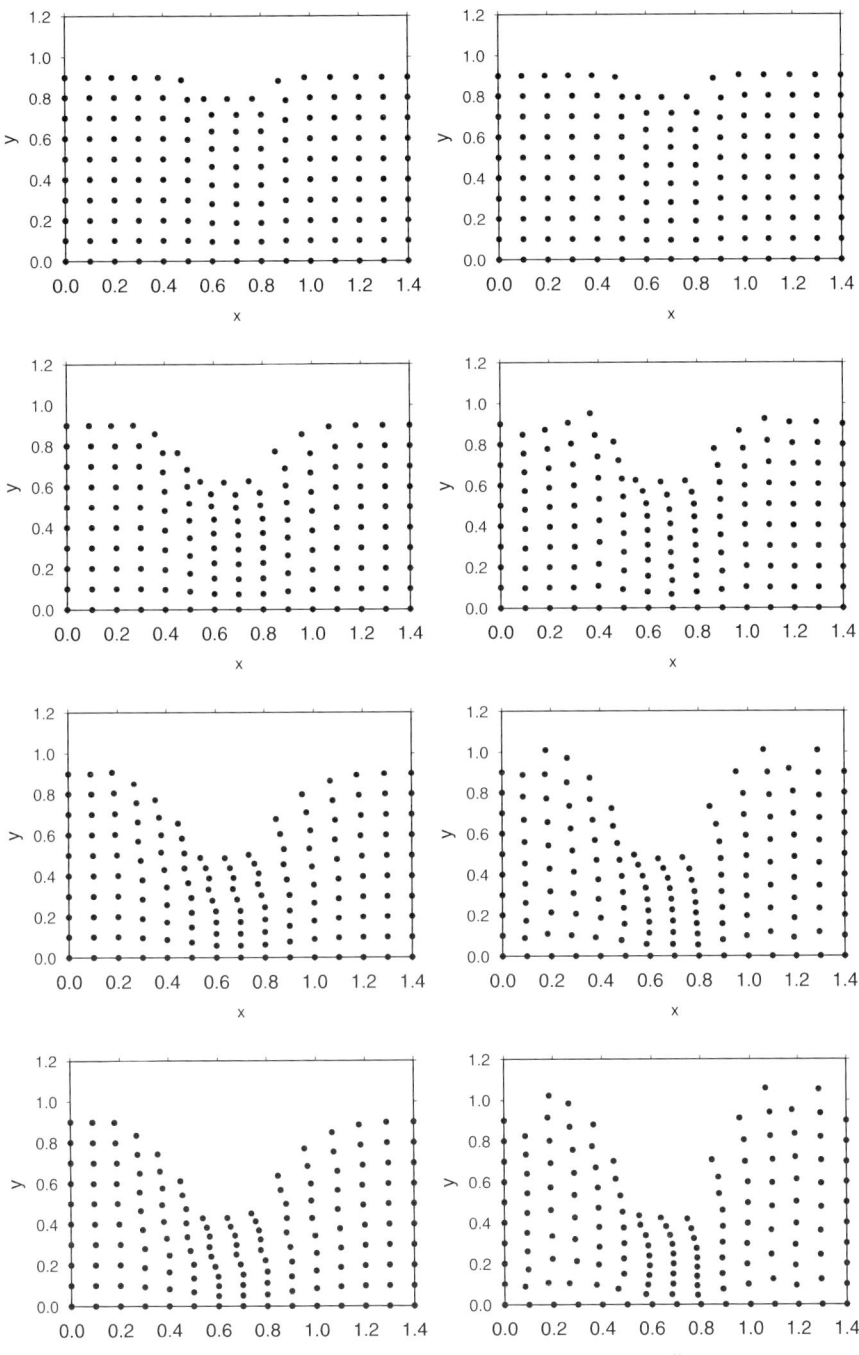

Fig. 13.14. Snapshots of tissue topologies stressed by force $F = -20$ and growing with the growth pre-factor $g = 0$ (left column) and $g = 0.0002$ (right column) which are taken at simulation steps 50, 150, 250, and 300 (from the top to bottom).

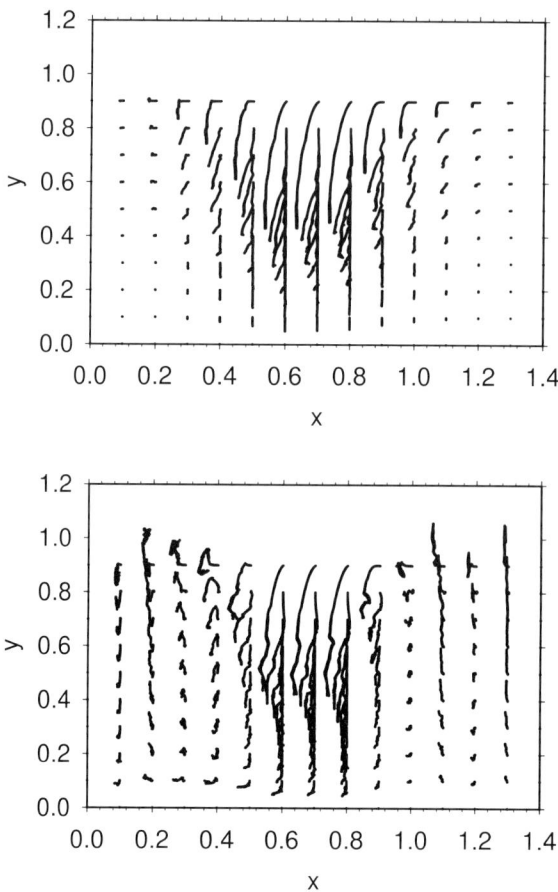

Fig. 13.15. Cumulative plots of node positions for deformation force $F = -20$ (steps from 0 to 300) for $g = 0$ (top) and $g = 0.0002$ (bottom) where selected snapshots are shown in Figure 13.14.

Symmetry breaking observed in simulations is caused by the used algorithm. New position of a node is found by a method that works by halving of intervals in two dimensions. There could be two, three, or at most four equal solution but the algorithm systematically prefer one of them, i.e. in other words, it prefers one direction given by the used algorithm. Hence, in the algorithm used in this model, a small initial systematic deviation could be amplified during the course of deformation. Such preferential choosing of the solution could be simply removed by random choice among equal solutions.

Solution of the local equilibria Equations 13.4, 13.5, and 13.6 is found by an iterative formula because it is a well known fact that there does not exist, in general, an analytical solution of a set of two or more nonlinear equations. It is found that the presented algorithm fails when large simulation steps are used, i.e. when the value of p is approaching or equal to one. The reason of this failure is simple. The algorithm could—when large simulation steps are used—exchange positions of neighbouring nodes, which is not physically acceptable. It automatically leads to mixing of nodes and consequently to loose of stability of simulation. Other possible reasons are discussed earlier.

The advantage of the proposed CA-model is due to the fact that it works with physically relevant dependencies and values. From the designing point of view, it is not much similar to models working with partial differential equations solved by the finite element method (FEM). PDE models are often based on homogenization of intrinsically inhomogeneous properties of living tissues. This might be in some situations misleading and yields artifacts which do not reflect biologically observed properties of living tissues. On the other hand, such discrete modelling as the one presented here might be able to capture special material properties which are 'erased' during homogenization of mechanical properties of tissues used in PDE.

It is necessary to stress that all CA-models are in principle easy to parallelize—and consequently to compute—because they work from the definition with a limited number of local interactions. All computations are simply realized locally using data from the neighbourhood of an updated node. That is a big advantage compared to solution of partial or ordinary differential equations where we do have to typically work with sparse matrices, e.g. there is no necessity to invert matrices in CA-based models contrary to FEM and so on.

13.7 Future development

This contribution provides the necessary biological and conceptual background for the development of a computational model of morphological growth of tissues based on interdependent development of epithelium and mesenchyme. The model operates at the level of tissues rather than at the level of single cells. Such information enables us to formulate a CA-model where influence of pseudo-epithelial force and tissue growth on a deformed tissue—having the form of a structure made from nodes and fibres—is studied. The model responses resulting from the internal mechanical loading—produced by actin fibres operating within epithelial cells and tissue growth—gives background information of what one might expect in the case of use of advanced models.

As is demonstrated, insertion of tissue growth substantially changes the overall tissue response. It does not matter that only the uniform tissue growth is used in the simulations. In future models, localized tissue growth would have even more pronounced impact on tissue development. This localized growth of epithelium, mesenchyme, and creation of knot nodes substantially rely on insertion of diffusion of two signalling proteins which are produced according to a gene regulatory network.

A three-dimensional version of the model has to be developed after inserting diffusion of signalling proteins and gene regulatory network into the model. Along with increase of the number of modelled dimensions, a change of topology to a more realistic one should be done as well. The pseudo-epithelium should be replaced by relevant model of epithelium with a special attention to topology of the growing structure.

The crucial part of the model, not solved in this contribution, is related to the extra large growth of tissues. It seems to be that when tissue growth is simulated from its very beginning to the terminal stages, a new model strategy should be developed in order to enable the model to create such large topology changes. The way of growth of L_0 is probably insufficient for such growth. There are several conceptual possibilities how to solve this model deficiency but it is impossible to explain details and which one is the best one prior to their testing.

It is evident that there is a permanent competition between the model accuracy and the computational load imposed by the model. The truth is that one goes against the other. Hence, the model should be carefully balanced from this point of view.

It has to be mentioned that the model is open to insert local volume forces and/or local change of the Young modulus according to the cell types. We have to stress that all already known biological knowledge [1, 32] enables to build fairly complicated models which could have properties close to the observed ones. The work presented here should be understood as the one possible model of the whole bunch of such computational models. Author of this contribution strongly believes that such bottom-to-top models have the potential to capture the essential properties of biological tissues undergoing morphological development.

13.8 Conclusions

This chapter has two main parts. In the first one, the general program of the research dealing with modelling of morphological growth realized by mechanical interaction of mesenchyme and epithelium under conduction of gene regulatory network using diffusion of signalling chemicals are presented. Special attention is focussed to a relatively detailed explanation of all important processes operating in living cells and tissues which are important for any successive model of morphological growth.

In the second part, research results coming from a partial realization of this program are presented. The results generated by the mechanical part of the model describing morphological development of tissues—i.e. by mechanical interaction of mesenchyme and pseudo-epithelium—which is defined and consequently tested in this contribution are presented. Mechanical influence of epithelium is simulated by use of external forces acting at the top layer of nodes of the whole block of nodes connected by fibres—contrary to living cells where this force is produced by living cell themselves. Tissue located below applied external forces is deformed and shaped into an invagination within this tissue—where depth depends on the size of applied force. Surrounding tissue parts are due to influence of fibres interconnecting neighbouring nodes elevated compared to their initial positions.

The model is prepared to take into account localized mechanical influence of epithelium and stimulated proliferation of mesenchyme where both are generating mechanical pressure on mesenchymal-epithelial complex. This should be realized by incorporation of diffusion of signalling chemicals and a gene regulatory network. It is shown that a tissue composed from living cells can be simulated by a set of nodes mutually interconnected by deformable fibres.

Acknowledgements

This work is dedicated to Jaroslava. Supported by the Czech Ministry of Education, Youth and Sports under the grant number MSM 4977751303.

References

[1] Alberts B, Johnson A, Lewis J, Raff M, Roberts K, Walter P (2002) Molecular biology of the cell. (4th ed.) Garland Science (Taylor & Francis Group), New York
[2] Kroc J (2002) LNCS 2329:773–782
[3] Toffoli T, Margolus N (1987) Cellular Automata Theory. MIT Press, Cambridge
[4] Ilachinski (2001) A Cellular Automata: A Discrete Universe. World Scientific Publishing Co. Pte. Ltd., New Jersey London Singapore, Hong Kong
[5] Resnick M (2006) StarLogo - programmable environment for exploring decentralized systems flocks, traffic jams, termite and ant colonies. Technical report, MIT, http://education.mit.edu/starlogo
[6] Toffoli T (1984) Physica 10D:117–127
[7] Vichniac GY (1984) Physica 10D:96–116
[8] Wolfram S (2002) A New Kind of Science. Wolfram Media Inc., Champaign
[9] Ingber DE (1998) Scientific American 278:48–57
[10] Ingber DE, Heidemann SR, Lamoreux P, Buxbaum RE (2000) J. Appl. Physiol. 89:1663–1670
[11] Lamoreux P, Heidemann SR, Buxbaum RE (2000) J. Appl. Physiol. 89:1670–1674
[12] Ingber DE (2000) J. Appl. Physiol. 89:1674–1677
[13] Ingber DE, Heidemann SR, Lamoreux P, Buxbaum RE (2000) J. Appl. Physiol. 89:1677–1678
[14] Hajela P, Kim B (2001) Struct. Multidisc. Optim. 23:24–33
[15] Gurdal Z, Tatting B (2000) Cellular automata for design of truss structures with linear and nonlinear response. In: 8th AIAA/USAF/NASA/ISSMO Symposium on Multidisciplinary Analysis and Optimization, American Institute for Aeronautics and Astronautics, Long Beach, CA
[16] Kita E, Toyoda T (2000) Struct. Multidisc. Optim. 19:64–73
[17] Slazar-Ciudad I, Jernvall J, Newman SA (2003) Development 120: 2027–2037

[18] Chaturvedi R, Huang C, Kazmierczak B, Schneider T, Izaguirre JA, Glimm T, Hentschel HGE, Glazier JA, Newman SA, Alber MS (2005) J.R. Soc. Interface 2: 237–253
[19] Glazier JA, Graner F (1993) Phys. Rev. E 47:2128–2154
[20] Zeng W, Thomas GL, Newman SA, Glazier JA (2003) A novel mechanism for mesenchymal condensation during limb chondrogenesis in vitro. In: Mathematical modelling and computating in biology and medicine. Fifth Conference of the European Society of Mathematical and Theoretical Biology
[21] Thesleff I (2003) Journal of Cell Science 116:1647–1648
[22] Jernvall J, Thesleff I (2000) Mech. Dev. 92:19–29
[23] Salazar-Ciudad I, Jernawall I (2002) Proc. Nat. Acad. Sci. USA 99:8116–8120
[24] Thesleff I, Mikkola M (2002) Int. Rev. Cytol. 217: 93–135
[25] Buttler PM (1956) Biol. Rev. 31: 30–70
[26] Jernvall J, Aberg T, Kettunen P, Keranen S, Thesleff I (1998) Development 125: 161–169
[27] Jernvall J, Kettunen P, Karavanova I, Martin LB, Thesleff I (1994) Int. J. Dev. Biol. 38:463–469
[28] Kettunen P, Laurikkala J, Itaranta P, Vainio S, Itoh N, Thesleff I (2000) Dev. Dyn. 219:322–332
[29] Pilot F, Lecuit T (2005) Compartmentalized morphogenesis in epithelia: From cell to tissue shape. Developmental Dynamics 232:685–694
[30] Hay ED (2005) The mesenchymal cell, its role in the embryo, and the remarkable signaling mechanisms that create it. Developmental Dynamics 233:706–720
[31] Ball EMA, Risbridger GP (2001) Activins as regulators of branching morphogenesis. Developmental Biology 238:1–12
[32] Heidemann SR, Wirtz D (2004) Towards a regional approach to cell mechanics. TRENDS in Cell Biology 14:160–166
[33] Kroc J (2006) Model of mechanical interaction of mesenchyme and epithelium in living tissues. Lecture Notes in Computer Science 3994:847–854
[34] Kroc J (2007) Modelling of morphological development of tooth using simple regulatory network: Mechanical model of mesenchyme. Mathematics and Computers in Simulation, in print
[35] Kroc J (2004) Diffusion Controlled Cellular Automaton Performing Mesh Partitioning. Lecture Notes in Computer Science 3305:131–140

14

Artificial Chemistry and Molecular Darwinian Evolution of DNA/RNA-Like Systems I - Typogenetics and Chemostat

Marian Bobrik, Vladimir Kvasnicka, and Jiri Pospichal

Institute of Applied Informatics, Faculty of Informatics and Information Technologies, Slovak Technical University, 84216 Bratislava, Slovakia bobrik@cauldron.sk, kvasnicka@fiit.stuba.sk, pospichal@fiit.stuba.sk

Summary: Two simplified models of Darwinian evolution at the molecular level are studied by applying the methods of artificial chemistry. *First*, a metaphor of a chemical reactor (chemostat) is considered. It contains molecules that are represented by binary strings, the strings being capable of replication with a probability proportional to their fitness. Moreover, the process of replication is not fully precise, sporadic mutations may produce new offspring strings, which are slightly different from their parent templates. In the framework of this approach we postulate a folding of binary strings into a secondary 2D structure. The proposed chemostat method offers a detailed view of mechanisms of the molecular Darwinian evolution, in particular of the meaning and importance of neutral mutations. *Second*, a simplified formal system Typogenetics, introduced by Hofstadter, is discussed. Concepts of replicators and hypercycles, defined within Typogenetics, belong to the basic entities in current perception of artificial life. A metaphor of chemical reactions is applied to study an emergence of replicators and hypercycles.

Key words: Artificial life; Artificial chemistry; Fitness landscape; Eigen theory of replicators; Molecular Darwinian evolution; Neutral mutations; Neutral evolution; Typogenetics; strand; replicator; hypercycle; evolutionary method.

14.1 Introduction

Darwinian evolution belongs to standard subjects of interest of *Artificial Life* [1, 37]. In particular, the main stimulus was observed at the end of the eighties, when evolutionary algorithms suddenly emerged as a new paradigm of computer science based on the metaphor of Darwinian evolution. This paradigm may be traced back to 1932 when Sewall Wright [41] has postulated an *adaptive landscape* (nowadays called the *fitness landscape or fitness surface*) and characterized Darwinian evolution as an adaptive process (nowadays we say an optimization process), where the genotype of population is adapted in such a way that it reaches a local (even global) maximum on the fitness surface. Forty years later, this ingenious idea was used by John Holland [24] as a metaphor for creation of *genetic algorithms*, which may be now interpreted as an abstraction of Darwinian evolution in the form of universal optimization algorithm [15] (see Dennett's seminal book [7]).

In this chapter we present simple computational models of Darwinian evolution, which may reflect some of its most elementary aspects appearing on biomacromolecular level (e.g. see experiments of Spiegelman [37] from the end of the sixties). These "molecular" models of Darwinian evolution can offer a detailed quantitative view of many of its basic concepts and notions, e.g. the role of neutral mutations may be studied as an auxiliary device to overcome local valleys of fitness surface in the course of the adaptation process. Artificial chemistry plays a very important role in the present study [2–6, 8–10, 16, 21, 27, 28], which may be considered as a subfield of artificial life based on the metaphor of chemical reactor (in our forthcoming discussions called the chemostat).

The chemostat is composed of "molecules" that are represented by abstract objects (e.g. by strings composed of symbols, trees, formulae constructed within algebra, etc.), which are transformed stochastically into other feasible objects by "chemical reactions". The probability of these transformations is strictly determined by the structure of incoming objects, resulting - outgoing objects are returned to the chemostat. Kinetics of the processes running in the chemostat is well described by Eigen's replicator differential equations [11–14], which were constructed on the basis of the well-known physico-chemical law of mass action. The main objects of artificial chemistry are (*i*) to study formal systems that are based on the chemical metaphor and that are potentially able to perform parallel computation, and (*ii*) to generate formal autocatalytic chemical systems (molecules are represented by structured objects) for purposes of "*in silico*" simulations of an emergence of living systems.

The purpose of this chapter about Typogenetics and of the following chapter about programmable folding is not to provide a tool for computer science by harnessing models of real chemical (biological) processes to construct artificial processes for computation. In this aim, the presented approach is different from a typical application of otherwise closely related evolutionary algorithms. We focus the other way round, i.e., we use computational models to provide an insight into processes on the edge between biology and chemistry connected with emergence of self-replicating systems. Since quantum chemical models are too complicated to provide an answer to dynamic processes in biology involving thousands of atoms, we use computational models, which employ very basic rules. The presented models are closely related in this effort to artificial life models. Presented models are not yet developed to the extent, that they could provide exact solutions for problems in real biological processes. No models concerning self-replication achieved yet such an advanced stage. However, this is the final goal of these kinds of models.

Newman and Engelhardt [33] have shown that many aspects of the molecular Darwinian evolution *in silico* may be studied by making use of a fitness surface based on a generalization of Kauffman's *NK* [26] rugged function with tunable degree of neutrality. They demonstrated that almost all basic results obtained by Peter Schuster's Vienna group [16–20, 34–36], based on a realistic physico-chemical model of RNA molecules and their folding, may be simply and immediately obtained by this simple model of fitness surface. In the present communication we use our previous results with binary strings [27, 28] in place of "molecules" that fill an artificial-chemistry chemostat. Each binary string is evaluated by a planar secondary structure called folding. The secondary structure of binary strings specifies their fitness function, which is directly related to the probability of a replication process of strings. The folding of binary strings – genotypes - is considered as a phenotype that specifies the fitness of the genotype. This simple triad ***genotype – phenotype – fitness*** is fundamental for our computer simulation of the molecular Darwinian evolution, such that the evolution is interpreted through changes of string phenotypes.

A Typogenetics is a formal system initially devised by Hofstadter in his famous book *Dialogues with Gödel, Escher, Bach: An Eternal Golden Braid* [23] (cf. refs. [36, 40, 41]). In Typogenetics a string (called the strand) codes a sequence of elementary operations so that their sequential application to the strand transforms this strand (parent) onto another strand (offspring). Typogenetics was discussed by Hofstadter in connection with his attempt to explain or classify a "tangled hierarchy" of DNA considered as a replicative system. In particular, a DNA strand contains, among other things, instructions prescribing a production of enzymes that are capable of different types of operations acting on the strand itself. A part of information contained in sequences of bases of DNA strands prescribes a synthesis of enzymes that are capable to make a copy of the DNA strand itself.

Typogenetics as presented by Hofstadter [23] was not formulated in a very precise and exact way, many concepts and notions were presented only in a "fuzzy" verbal form and the reader was left to improvisation and to ad-hoc additional specification of many notions of Typogenetics. Morris [31] was the first who seriously attempted to formulate the Typogenetics in a precise manner and presented many illustrative examples and explanations that substantially facilitated an understanding of Typogenetics. Varetto [38] has published an article where he demonstrated that Typogenetics is a proper formal environment for a systematic constructive enumeration of strands that can autoreplicate. Recently, Varetto [39] published another paper where Typogenetics was applied to a generation of the so-called tanglecycles that are a simplified version of hypercycles [11–14] of Eigen and Schuster.

We present a simplified version of Typogenetics that will be still capable to form a proper environment for Artificial Life studies of replicators and hypercycles, both entities that belong to basic concepts of modern efforts [2–6, 8–10, 16, 21, 27, 28] to simulate life *in-silico*. Simplification of our version of Typogenetics consists mainly in trimming the instruction set, where all instructions that introduce or delete bases in strands were omitted. It is demonstrated that a construction of replicators and hypercycles belongs to very complicated combinatorial problems and therefore an effort of their systematic constructive enumeration is hopeless. This is the main reason why we turned our attention to evolutionary methods of spontaneous emergence of replicators and hypercycles.

One of the objectives of this chapter is to demonstrate an effectiveness of a simple version of evolutionary algorithm to create replicators and hypercycles in a way closely related to Darwinian evolution. The used approach is expanded to include hypercycles, which are composed of coupled systems of replicators with a cyclic kinetic structure, where a replication of its ith constituent is catalyzed by an enzyme produced by the previous (i-1)th constituent. Hypercycles are considered in recent efforts of artificial life [34] as a proper formal tool suitable for specific explanation of a phenomenon called the increase of complexity. We show that evolutionary algorithms are capable of inducing an emergence of hypercycles from a population initialized by random strands. More complicated hypercycles (composed of three or four replicators) represent for evolutionary algorithms very hard combinatorial problems. This is the main reason why we turned our attention to a sequential step-by-step method of their construction, a given hypercycle is evolutionary enlarged to a larger hypercycle by adding one additional replicator.

The last part of this communication is dedicated to devising an artificial chemistry system which aims to extend modeling of binary string replicators, so, that it is more close to behavior of real biomacromolecules, by using secondary 2D structure (folding) to specify a "code" of its replication mechanism. That is, a phenotype of binary strings is not specified only by their folding but also by a "computer program" that should be performed by a replicator in its replication process. In other words, the code hidden in the secondary structure – folding specifies an ability of a given replicator to be replicated. Thanks to these enlarged possibilities of simple binary strings that are able to create a secondary 2D structure, we may create a sophisticated system of artificial chemistry, which is closely related to RNA molecules, where their properties are not determined immediately by a sequence of tokens but by their secondary structure. Such a system offers very effective possibility to study an evolution of biomacromolecules by principles that are closely related to real living systems.

14.2 Eigen Theory of Molecular Replicators

Manfred Eigen published in the early seventies a seminal paper entitled "*Self organization of matter and the evolution of biological macromolecules*" [11], where he postulated a hypothetical chemical system composed of the so-called replicators. This system mimics Darwinian evolution even on an abiotic level. Later, Eigen and Schuster [12–14] discussed the proposed model as a possible abiotic mechanism for increasing complexity on a border of abiotic and biotic systems.

Let us consider biomacromolecules (called *replicators*) $X_1, X_2, ..., X_n$, which are capable of the following chemical reactions:

$$X_i \xrightarrow{k_i} X_i + X_i \quad (i = 1, 2, ..., n) \tag{14.1}$$

$$X_i \xrightarrow{\phi} \emptyset \quad (i = 1, 2, ..., n) \tag{14.2}$$

The reaction (14.1) means that a molecule X_i is replicated onto itself with a rate constant k_i, whereas the reaction (14.2) means that X_i becomes extinct with a rate parameter ϕ (this parameter is called the *"dilution flux"* and will be specified further). Applying the mass-action law of chemical kinetics, we get the following system of differential equations

$$\dot{x}_i = x_i (k_i - \phi) \quad (i = 1, 2, ..., n) \tag{14.3}$$

The dilution flux ϕ is a free parameter and it will be determined in such a way, that the following condition is satisfied: a sum of time derivatives of concentrations $\dot{x}$'s is vanishing, $\sum \dot{x}_i = 0$, we get

$$\dot{x}_i = x_i \left(k_i - \sum_{j=1}^{n} k_j x_j \right) \quad (i = 1, 2, ..., n) \tag{14.4}$$

where the condition $\sum x_i = 1$ is used without a loss of generality of our considerations. Its analytical solution is as follows

$$x_i(t) = \frac{x_i(0) e^{k_i t}}{\sum_{j=1}^{n} x_j(0) e^{k_j t}} \tag{14.5}$$

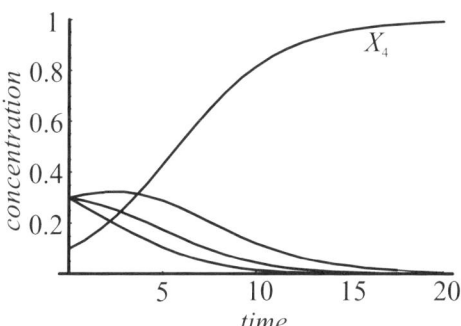

Fig. 14.1. A plot of relative concentrations of four component system with rate constants $k_1=1$, $k_2=2$, $k_3=3$, and $k_4=4$. We see that only molecules X_4 survive in the end.

This solution has an asymptotic property, where only one type of molecules (with the maximum rate constant k_{max}) survives while others become extinct

$$\lim_{t \to \infty} x_i(t) = \begin{cases} 1 & (\text{for } k_i = k_{max} = \max\{k_1, ..., k_n\}) \\ 0 & (\text{otherwise}) \end{cases} \tag{14.6}$$

Loosely speaking, each type of molecules may be considered as a type of species with a fitness specified by the rate constant k. Only those molecules - species "survive" in a chemostat that are best fitted, i.e. that have the highest rate constant k_{max}, and all other molecules with smaller rate constants become extinct (see Fig. 14.1). The condition of invariability of the sum of concentrations (i.e. $\sum x_i = 1$) thus introduces a "selection pressure" to replicated molecules.

The proposed model may be simply generalized [11] in such a way that mutations are introduced into process of replications. The system (14.3), (14.4) is modified as follows

$$\dot{x}_i = x_i (k_{ii} - \phi) + \sum_{\substack{j=1 \\ (j \neq i)}}^{n} k_{ji} x_j \quad (i = 1, 2, ..., n) \tag{14.7}$$

where k_{ij} is a rate constant assigned to a modified reaction (14.1)

$$X_i \xrightarrow{k_{ij}} X_i + X_j \quad (i, j = 1, 2, ..., n) \tag{14.8}$$

There is postulated that a rate constant matrix $\boldsymbol{K} = (k_{ij})$ has dominant diagonal elements, i.e. nondiagonal elements are much smaller than diagonal ones. This requirement directly follows from an assumption that imperfect replications in Eq. (14.8) are very rare, the product X_j is considered as a weak mutation of autoreplicated X_i, $X_j = O_{mut}(X_i)$. The dilution flux ϕ from (14.7) is determined by the condition that the sum of time derivatives of concentrations is vanishing, $\sum \dot{x}_i = 0$. We get

$$\phi = \sum_{i,j=1}^{n} k_{ji} x_j \tag{14.9}$$

Analytical solution of (14.7) with dilution flux specified by (14.9) is [25]

$$x_i(t) \approx \frac{\sum_{j=1}^{n} q_{ij} x_i(0) e^{\lambda_i t}}{\sum_{m,j=1}^{n} q_{mj} x_j(0) e^{\lambda_j t}} \tag{14.10}$$

where $\boldsymbol{Q} = (q_{ij})$ is a nonsingular matrix that diagonalizes the rate matrix $\boldsymbol{K}$, $\boldsymbol{Q}^{-1} \boldsymbol{K} \boldsymbol{Q} = \Lambda = \mathrm{diag}(\lambda_1, \lambda_2, ..., \lambda_n)$. Since we have postulated that nondiagonal elements of $\boldsymbol{K}$ are much smaller than its diagonal elements, its eigenvalues λ's are very close to diagonal elements, $\lambda_i \doteq k_{ii}$, and the transformation matrix $\boldsymbol{Q}$ is closely related to a unit matrix, $q_{ij} \doteq \delta_{ij}$ (a Kronecker's delta symbol). This means that introduction of weak mutations does not change dramatically general properties of the above simple replicator system without mutations. In particular, the final asymptotic state (for $t \to \infty$) will be composed almost entirely of molecules with the highest rate constant k_{max} (see Fig. 14.2). These molecules are weakly accompanied by other replicators with rate constants k's slightly smaller than k_{max}.

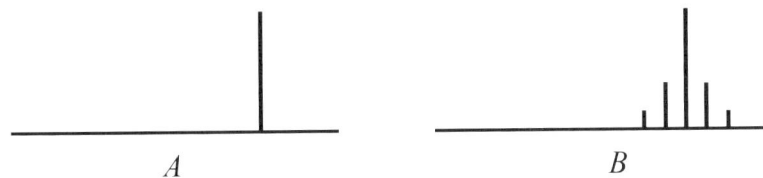

Fig. 14.2. A difference between resulting asymptotic states, (A) Replication process is without mutations (i.e. replication process is exact), whereas (B) is a replication process with mutation (asymptotic state is composed of a pure population of one replicator – winner, which is accompanied by a cohort of tightly related replicators).

14.2.1 Replicators and Molecular Darwinian Evolution

Eigen's system of replicators with mutations (i.e. with imperfect replications) presented in the previous section can be simply used for description of the *molecular Darwinian evolution*. Let us consider a hypothetical reaction system composed of a sequence of n replicators $X_1, X_2, X_3, ..., X_n$. They are endowed with a property that X_i may produce by imperfect replication the juxtaposed replicators $X_{i\pm1}$ (see Fig. 14.3, diagram A). If an initial concentration of X_1 is $x_1(0)=1$, then in the course of evolution there exist concentration waves that are consecutively assigned $X_2, X_3, ..., X_n$ (see Fig. 14.3, diagram B). This fact may be simply interpreted as a manifestation of the molecular Darwinian evolution, where fitness of single "species" are specified by diagonal rate constants k_{ii}. The evolution process was started by a population composed entirely of X_1. Since its replication is imperfect, it may occasionally produce (specified by the rate constant k_{12}) the next replicator X_2 with a greater fitness (rate constant k_{22}) than its predecessor X_1 ($k_{11} < k_{22}$). This means that in the course of the forthcoming evolution, "species" X_2 will survive (i.e. its concentration will rise almost to unity while the concentration of X_1 will decline to a very small value). This process is repeated for the replicator X_2 considered now as an initial replicator (it plays the same role as the replicator X_1 in the previous stage). Since the replication of X_2 is imperfect, "species" X_3 is produced with a low probability. However, since X_3 has a greater fitness than its predecessor X_2 ($k_{33} > k_{22}$), this new "species" X_3 will survive. This process is finished when the last replicator X_n has appeared initially as a consequence of imperfect replication of X_{n-1} and then its concentration increases to unity by its autoreplication.

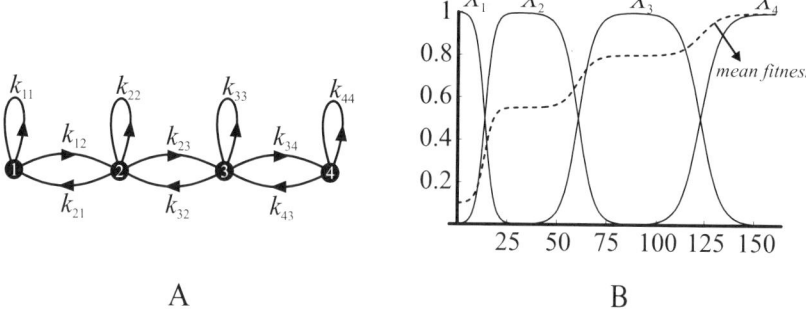

Fig. 14.3. Diagram (A) represents a four-replicator system, where a replicator X_i produces by imperfect replications juxtaposed replicators X_{i-1} and X_{i+1}. Edges of the diagram are evaluated by rate constants, their numerical values are specified by matrix $\mathbf{K}$ (see Eq. (14.11)), where diagonal elements are well separated and much greater than nondiagonal ones. Edges corresponding to zero elements are omitted. Diagram (B) displays plots of replicator concentration profiles that form a sequence of concentration waves. This diagram also contains a plot of mean fitness specified by $\bar{k} = k_{11}x_1 + \ldots + k_{44}x_4$, which forms a typical nondecreasing "stair" function.

An assumption of good separability of concentration waves gives a strong condition for rate constants concerning the replicator X_i in particular: we may say that for a particular replicator the sum of "outgoing" rate constants must be much smaller than the sum of "incoming" rate constants. In other words, loosely speaking, *the "probability" of creation of a particular replicator from its juxtaposed replicators by their imprecise replications must be much greater than the "probability" of destroying the respective replicator by its imprecise replication.*

The above simple considerations are numerically verified for a simple four-replicator system with rate constants specified by the following matrix of rate coefficients

$$\mathbf{K} = \begin{pmatrix} 0.1 & 10^{-3} & 0 & 0 \\ 10^{-7} & 0.55 & 10^{-7} & 0 \\ 0 & 10^{-11} & 0.8 & 10^{-11} \\ 0 & 0 & 10^{-7} & 1.0 \end{pmatrix} \quad (14.11)$$

This matrix satisfies both the above postulated conditions: (i) Its diagonal matrix elements are much greater than its nondiagonal ones, and (ii) the nondiagonal rate constants satisfy inequalities derived in [28]. This means that we may expect a Darwinian behavior of the replicator system. This expectation nicely coincides with our numerical results displayed in Fig. 14.3, diagram B, where concentration profiles of single replicators are shown, which form a sequence of concentration waves typical of Darwinian evolution. Summarizing the present section, we may say that ***Eigen's phenomenological theory of replicators forms a proper theoretical framework for numerical studies of the molecular Darwinian evolutionary theory*** (i.e. applied to biomolecules capable of replication process like RNA or DNA).

14.2.2 Artificial Chemistry and a Metaphor of Chemostat

Let us consider a *chemostat* (chemical reactor) [8, 16, 21] composed of formal objects called the molecules. It is postulated that the chemostat is not spatially structured (in chemistry it is said that the reactor is well stirred). Molecules are represented by formal structured objects (e.g. token strings, rooted trees, λ-expressions, etc.). An interaction between molecules is able to transform information, which is stored in the composition of the molecules. Therefore a chemical reaction (causing changes in the internal structure of reacting molecules) can be considered as an act of information processing. The capacity of the information processing depends on the complexity of molecules and chemical reactions between them.

General ideas of the chemostat approach will be explained by an example of chemostat as a binary function optimizer that resembles many features of the molecular Darwinian evolution emphasized in the previous section (see Fig. 14.4). Let us consider a binary function

$$f : \{0,1\}^n \to [0,1] \quad (14.12)$$

This function $f(\mathbf{g})$ maps binary strings $\mathbf{g} = (g_1, g_2, ..., g_n) \in \{0,1\}^n$ of length n onto real numbers from the closed interval [0,1]. We look for an optimal solution

$$\mathbf{g}_{opt} = \arg \max_{\mathbf{g} \in \{0,1\}^n} f(\mathbf{g}) \quad (14.13)$$

Since the cardinality of the set $\{0,1\}^n$ of solutions is equal to 2^n, a CPU time necessary for solution of the above optimization problem grows exponentially

$$t_{CPU} \approx 2^n \quad (14.14)$$

This means that the solution of the binary optimization problem (14.13) may in general belong to a class of hard numerical NP-complete problems. This is the main reason why the optimization problems (14.13) are solved by the so-called evolutionary algorithms [12–14, 21], which represent very efficient numerical heuristic of solving binary optimization problems. The purpose of this subsection is to demonstrate that a metaphor of replicator provides an efficient stochastic optimization algorithm.

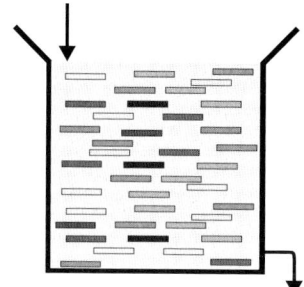

Fig. 14.4. The chemostat contains a homogeneous "solution" (mixture) of molecules, a few molecules are fully randomly selected (with a probability determined by their concentrations). Then these molecules undergo a chemical reaction that consists of a transformation of some of them. The produced molecules are returned to the chemostat in such a way that they may eliminate some other molecules.

```
P:=randomly generated chemostat of molecules g;
epoch:=0;
for epoch:=1 to epoch_max do
begin select randomly a molecule g;
  if random<f(g) then
  begin g':=O_mut(g);
    product g' substitutes in chemostat a randomly selected molecule;
  end
end;
```

Algorithm 1. A pseudo Pascal implementation of chemostat optimization. The algorithm is initialized by a chemostat composed of randomly generated molecules (binary strings of the fixed length). A copy of a randomly selected molecule **g** is transformed with a probability equal to its functional value $f(\mathbf{g})$ by a mutation operator onto a new molecule **g**'. The mutation operator causes an actual change only very rarely. This new mutated molecule substitutes a randomly selected molecule. Value *random* stands for a random number from the uniform distribution over the interval [0, 1].

Let a chemostat be composed of molecules that are realized by binary strings $\mathbf{g} = (g_1, g_2, ..., g_n) \in \{0,1\}^n$. An imperfect duplication is considered (cf. Eq. (14.8))

$$\mathbf{g} \xrightarrow{f(\mathbf{g})} \mathbf{g} + \mathbf{g}' \qquad (14.15)$$

where the formed molecule $\mathbf{g}'$ substitutes a randomly selected molecule from the chemostat. A term $f(\mathbf{g})$ assigned to the chemical reaction is interpreted as the probability (rate constant) of the occurrence of reaction (14.15). In evolutionary algorithms a selection pressure in population of solutions (chromosomes) is created by a reproduction process based on chromosome fitness. Chromosomes with a greater fitness have the greater chance to take part in a reproduction process (a measure of quality of chromosomes); on the other hand, chromosomes with a small fitness are rarely used in the reproduction process. This simple manifestation of Darwin's natural selection ensures a gradual evolution of the whole population. In the present approach the mentioned principle of fitness selection of molecules is preserved, but it is now combined with an additional selection pressure due to the constancy of number of molecules in the chemostat. A molecule incoming to the reaction is randomly selected from the chemostat. After evaluation of the quality of the selected molecule it is then stochastically decided whether the reaction is performed or not (see Algorithm 1) and, moreover, the resulting molecule substitutes another randomly selected molecule. Finally, we specify the product $\mathbf{g}'$ from the right-hand side of (14.15) as mutation [24] of an incoming molecule $\mathbf{g}$

$$\mathbf{g}' = O_{\text{mut}}(\mathbf{g}) \qquad (14.16)$$

where O_{mut} is a stochastic mutation operator that changes single bits with a probability P_{mut}. A pseudo Pascal code for the replicator algorithm is presented in Algorithm 1.

As an illustrative example we will study the chemostat approach specified for a simple unimodal function determined over binary strings of length 4. Let us postulate that a chemostat is formed by a multiset composed of binary strings of length 4

$$\{...., (1100), ...\} \subset \{0, 1\}^4 \qquad (14.17)$$

Each binary vector α is evaluated by a rational number from the closed interval $\langle 0, 1 \rangle$

$$\text{real}(\mathbf{g}) = \frac{1}{2^4 - 1} \text{int}(\mathbf{g}) \qquad (14.18)$$

where int(g) is the integer represented g. A rate constant k assigned to the binary string is specified as follows

$$k(\mathbf{g}) = f(\text{real}(\mathbf{g})) = \frac{1}{2}(1 - \sin(2\pi \cdot \text{real}(\mathbf{g}))) \qquad (14.19)$$

with an optimum $\mathbf{g}_{opt}$=(1011), where real($\mathbf{g}_{opt}$)=11/15 and f(11/15)=0.9973.

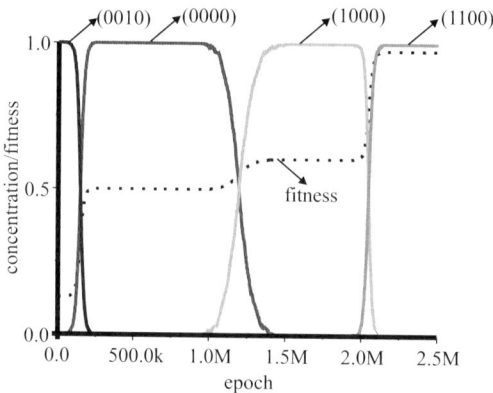

Fig. 14.5. Plot of frequencies of appearance of some dominant binary strings of length 4. At the beginning of the process, the chemostat was composed entirely of strings (0010). After 2.5×10^6 time steps, the most dominant final solution is $\mathbf{g}_{fin}$ =(1100), where real($\mathbf{g}_{opt}$)=12/15 and f (12/15)=0.9755. This final solution is juxtaposed in rational number evaluation to the optimal solution $\mathbf{g}_{opt}$ =(1011), where real($\mathbf{g}_{opt}$)=11/15 and f (11/15)=0.9973, but the Hamming distance d of binary strings (1100) and (1011) is great, d =3 (in theory of GA this effect is called the Hamming cliff). This relatively great size of the Hamming distance is the main reason why the algorithm is unable to achieve the global solution (1011).

The chemostat is composed of 1000 binary strings and the mutation operator O_{mut} is specified by a 1-bit probability $P_{mut}=10^{-5}$. The obtained numerical results are displayed in Fig. 14.5. We see that those binary strings are spontaneously emerging in the chemostat, which correspond to a suboptimal solution with a rational numerical value closely related to real($\mathbf{g}_{opt}$)=0.80. Main results of this section may be summarized as follows: (1) *A metaphor of Eigen's replicators offers an effective stochastic optimization algorithm, where a proof of its convergence to a global solution immediately follows from the existence of a unique asymptotically stable solution with the greatest rate constant*, and (2) *if the probability of mutations is a very small number, then the obtained results are very similar to those obtained by Eigen's replicator equations with mutations* (see Fig. 14.5).

14.2.3 Summary

We have demonstrated that a chemical metaphor (based on Eigen's replicators) may be applied in design of the so-called replicator algorithm. This algorithm resembles in many features standard evolutionary algorithms, but the most important feature of the present metaphor is its introduction of unexpected new possibilities how to look at the optimisation procedure from a different perspective. In particular, since the proposed algorithm is based on a chemical metaphor, an application of a standard "chemical kinetics" offers new ways how to use its already established chemical formalism in analysis of optimisation process.

Other important aspect of artificial chemistry may be "in silico" performance of hypothetical chemical processes that could not be realized by the standard "in vitro" chemistry. Recently, many chemical processes running on the border of abiotic and biotic systems are simulated by "in silico" techniques. This approach represents a substantial part of the current artificial life area of computer science. In particular, Eigen and Schuster's [11–14] replicators and hypercycles are easily modeled by chemostats. This possibility will be extensively discussed in the forthcoming part of this communication.

14.3 Hofstadter's Theory of DNA-Like Molecules, Typogenetics

Typogenetics is a formal artificial-chemistry system initially devised by Douglas Hofstadter in his famous book *Dialogues with Gödel, Escher, Bach: An Eternal Golden Braid* [23] (cf. refs. [31, 38, 39]). Typogenetics replaces DNA molecules by strings (called the strands), defining a DNA molecule as a sequence of four kinds of letters, when each letter codes a basis (chemical group forming building block of DNA). The really significant simplification consists in definition of parts of DNA sequences which code elementary operations acting in turn on the DNA sequence itself. In reality a part of the DNA substrings code the instructions prescribing a production of enzymes. Each enzyme codes a different type of operation acting on DNA. These enzymes then use the DNA which coded them as a plan to create a copy of this DNA or a copy of another molecule (another strand in the Typogenetics formalism). While in the real life these substrings used for definition of enzymes are very large, in Typogenetics these codes of "enzymes" or "elementary operations" are smaller by orders of magnitude. Typogenetics is using the sequence of elementary operations coded by a strand to transform this strand (parent) onto another strand (offspring). Typogenetics was discussed by Hofstadter in connection with his attempt to explain or classify a "tangled hierarchy" of DNA considered as a replicative system.

Typogenetics as presented by Hofstadter [23] was not formulated in a very precise and exact way, many concepts and notions were presented only in a "fuzzy" verbal form and the reader was left to an improvisation and an ad-hoc additional specification of many notions of Typogenetics. Morris [31] was the first one who seriously attempted to formulate the Typogenetics in a precise manner and presented many illustrative examples and explanations that substantially facilitated an understanding of Typogenetics. More than ten years ago Varetto [38] has published an article where he demonstrated that Typogenetics is a proper formal environment for a systematic constructive enumeration of strands that are capable of autoreplication. Varetto [39] published also another paper where Typogenetics was applied to a generation of the so-called tanglecycles that are simplified versions of hypercycles [11–14] of Eigen and Schuster.

We introduce a simplified version of Typogenetics that will be still capable to form a proper environment for Artificial Life studies of replicators and hypercycles, both entities that belong to basic concepts of modern efforts [2–6, 8–10, 16, 21, 27, 28] to simulate life *in-silico*. Simplification of our version of Typogenetics consists mainly in trimming of an instruction set, where all instructions that introduce or delete bases in strands were omitted. It is demonstrated that a construction of replicators and hypercycles belongs to very complicated combinatorial problems and therefore an effort to generate them by a systematic constructive enumeration is hopeless. This is the main reason why we turned our attention to evolutionary methods of spontaneous emergence of replicators and hypercycles. One of objectives of the present chapter is to demonstrate an effectiveness of a simple version of evolutionary algorithm to create replicators and hypercycles in a way closely related to Darwinian evolution.

Strands are determined as strings composed of four symbols A, C, G, and T. Then a DNA is specified as a double strand composed of a strand and its complementary strand. A simple way how to assign an enzyme to an arbitrary strand is demonstrated. The enzyme is composed of a sequence of elementary instructions and the so-called binding site. In our simplified Typogenetics we retain only those instructions that do not change the length of strands, which excludes for example instructions for insertion or deletion of bases. An action of enzyme upon the strand is strongly deterministic, it is applied to the binding site which first appears when going on the strand from the left to the right. Replicators are determined as double strands with such a property that each of both replicator strands is replicated by application of an enzyme. Firstly the double strands are separated. Then each strand produces an enzyme, which is in turn applied to the same strand and produces its complementary DNA copy. The enzyme is produced from the code by a prescription "start from the left, translate a couple of entries into an instruction and move to the right", creating from neighboring couples of strand entries a sequence of "instructions". This sequence of "instructions", which is a sort of metacode of an enzyme, is in this formalism equated with an enzyme. Instructions of such an enzyme usually do not make the copy of its "parental" strand by a straightforward "start from the left, copy and move to the right". They work more like a Turing machine on a tape (a metaphor from computer science), where the instructions can move the enzyme to the left or to the right on the strand. Such a copying process can create the copy e.g. with starting from the middle and jumping back and forth to the left and right, adding entries to the copy of a strand from both sides in turn. The copy can even be created in nonadjacent parts with the conjunctive entries copied at the end. This specification of replicators represents, in fact, a hard constraint, so that their construction is nontrivial combinatorial problem. Fortunately, it can be effectively solved by making use of evolutionary methods. Hypercycles composed of double strands are studied in Section 14.3.3. The notion of hypercycles [11–14] is a generalization of replicators such that a hypercycle is a cyclic kinetic structure, where a replication of its ith constituent is catalyzed by an enzyme produced by the previous (i-1)th constituent. Hypercycles are considered in recent efforts of artificial life [34] as a proper formal tool suitable for specific explanation of a phenomenon called the increase of complexity. We show that evolutionary algorithms are capable of inducing an emergence of hypercycles from a population initialized by random strands. More complicated hypercycles (composed of three or four replicators) represent for evolutionary algorithms very hard combinatorial problems. This is the main reason why we turned our attention to a sequential step-by-step method of their construction, where a given hypercycle is evolutionary enlarged to a larger hypercycle by adding one additional replicator.

14.3.1 Basic Principles of Typogenetics

Let us consider a set $B=\{A, C, G, T\}$, where elements – bases are called the adenine, cytosine, guanine, and thymine, respectively. These four elements are further classified as purines (A and G) and pyrimidines (C and T), i.e. $B = B_{pur} \cup B_{pyr}$. Moreover, bases are alternatively called *complementary*, A is complementary to T and C is complementary to G. In other words, we say that A is paired with T and C is paired with G (and vice versa). In Typogenetics the basic entity is the so-called *strand S* determined as a string composed of four different bases

$$S = X_1 X_2 ... X_n \in B^* = B \cup B^2 \cup B^3 \cup ... \quad (14.20)$$

This strand is composed of n bases $X_1, X_2, \ldots, X_n \in B$, where the natural number n specifies its *length*, $|S| = n$. Examples of strands are CCA, TTGGACTTG, ..., their lengths are 3 and 9, respectively.

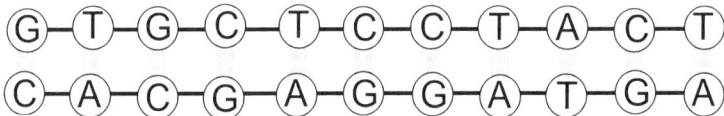

Fig. 14.6. An illustrative example of DNA composed of two complementary strands S (lower strand) and R (upper strand). Shaded areas represent interactions between complementary bases (realized by two or three hydrogen bonds).

A *complementary strand* $\bar{S}$ with respect to the strand $S = X_1 X_2 ... X_n$ is determined by $\bar{S} = \bar{X}_1 \bar{X}_2 ... \bar{X}_n$, where $\bar{A} = T$, $\bar{C} = G$, $\bar{G} = C$, and $\bar{T} = A$ are complementary bases [1]. For illustration let us consider the above mentioned two strands S_1=CCA, S_2=TTGGACTTG, their complementary forms are $\bar{S}_1 = GGT$ and $\bar{S}_2 = AACCTGAAC$, respectively. A *double strand* called the *DNA* is specified by two strands S (lower strand) and R (upper strand) that are complementary, $R = \bar{S}$ (see Fig. 14.6)

$$A = \begin{pmatrix} R \\ S \end{pmatrix} = \begin{pmatrix} \bar{S} \\ S \end{pmatrix} \quad (14.21)$$

where a base X_i is paired with Y_i of $R = Y_1 Y_2 ... Y_n \in B$ (and vice versa), for $i=1,2,\ldots,n$.

---
[1] In the real DNA content, the complimentary strand of AACCT is not TTGGA, as presented in the chapter, but AGGTT. Meaning, besides complimentary nucleotides exchange, the directionality need to be changed as well.

In order to simplify our forthcoming considerations, let us enlarge the set B by a symbol that corresponds to an empty position on the strands, this additional symbol is represented by a hash symbol (#). If a strand contains at least one hash, then the strand is called the *quasistrand* (e.g. S=AACG##CCT). Formally, the above notion is simply realized when the set B is enlarged to $\tilde{B} = B \cup \{\#\}$, then quasistrands are determined as strings of

$$\tilde{B}^* = (B \cup \{\#\})^* = \{A, AA, ..., A\#C, ..., CCGT, ..., GGT\#\#T, ...\} \quad (14.22)$$

A *distance* between two (quasi)strands $S = X_1 X_2 ... X_n \in \tilde{B}$ and $R = Y_1 Y_2 ... Y_n \in \tilde{B}$ (of the same length) is determined as follows

$$d(S,R) = 1 - \frac{1}{n} \sum_{i=1}^{n} \delta(X_i, Y_i) \quad (14.23)$$

$$\delta(X,Y) = \begin{cases} 1 & (\text{if } X = Y \text{ and } X, Y \in B) \\ 0 & (\text{otherwise}) \end{cases} \quad (14.24)$$

where a unit increment corresponds to a situation when both bases are identical and not equal to hash symbols. For illustration, let us consider two strands S =CGTT###AAT and R =TGT###AAAG, according to (14.23),(14.24), the distance between them is

$$d(S,R) = 1 - \frac{1}{10}(0+1+1+0+0+0+0+1+1+0) = 1 - \frac{4}{10} = \frac{3}{5}$$

A zero distance between two strands S and R means that they are identical and do not contain hash symbols.

14.3.2 An Expression of Strands by Enzymes

The purpose of this Section is to specify one of the most important concepts of Typogenetics, an expression of a strand by a sequence of instructions, that is called euphemistically the *enzyme*. Let us consider a set

$$B^2 = \{AA, AC, AG, ..., TT\} \quad (14.25)$$

composed of sixteen base pairs (doublets). Each strand $S = X_1 X_2 ... X_n \in B^*$ can be expressed by making use of doublets of (14.25) as follows

$$\begin{array}{ll} S = D_1 D_2 ... D_p & (\text{for } n = 2p) \\ S = D_1 D_2 ... D_p X_{2p+1} & (\text{for } n = 2p+1) \end{array} \quad (14.26)$$

where the first (second) possibility is applicable if the length of S is even (odd). Let us consider two mappings

$$instruction : B^2 \rightarrow \{mvr, mvl, cop, off, rpy, ...\} \quad (14.27)$$

$$\text{inclination} : B^2 \to \{s,l,r\} \tag{14.28}$$

where the first mapping *instruction* assigns to each strand a sequence of instructions that will be sequentially performed over the strand when an enzyme (specified by the strand and the second mapping *inclination*) is applied. Details of these mappings will be specified later. If doublets of a strand are mapped by (14.27), (14.28) (see Table 14.1), we arrive at the so-called *primary structure of the enzyme* that is specified by a sequence of instructions

$$\text{instruction}(S) = \text{instr}(D_1) - \text{instr}(D_2) - \ldots - \text{instr}(D_p) \tag{14.29}$$

A *tertiary structure* (2D) of the enzyme is determined by the mapping *inclination*, it offers the following sequence of inclinations assigned to doublets (see Table 14.1)

$$\text{inclination}(S) = \text{inclin}(D_1) - \text{inclin}(D_2) - \ldots - \text{inclin}(D_p) \tag{14.30}$$

Table 14.1. Specification of mappings *instruction* and *inclination*

No.	Doublet	Instruct.	Inclin.	No.	Doublet	Instruct.	Inclin.
1	AA	*mvr*	*l*	9	GA	*rpy*	*s*
2	AC	*mvl*	*s*	10	GC	*rpu*	*r*
3	AG	*mvr*	*s*	11	GG	*lpy*	*r*
4	AT	*mvl*	*r*	12	GT	*lpu*	*l*
5	CA	*mvr*	*s*	13	TA	*rpy*	*r*
6	CC	*mvl*	*s*	14	TC	*rpu*	*l*
7	CG	*cop*	*r*	15	TG	*lpy*	*l*
8	CT	*off*	*l*	16	TT	*lpu*	*l*

Table 14.2. Description of single instructions from Table 14.2.

No.	Instruction	Description
1	*cop*	Enzyme turns on copy mode, until turned off, enzyme produces complementary bases
2	*off*	Enzyme turns off copy mode
3	*mvr*	Enzyme moves one base to the right
4	*mvl*	Enzyme moves one base to the left
5	*rpy*	Enzyme finds nearest pyrimidine to the right
6	*rpu*	Enzyme finds nearest purine to the right
7	*lpy*	Enzyme finds nearest pyrimidine to the left
8	*lpu*	Enzyme finds nearest purine to the left

Both sequences (14.29),(14.30) that are assigned to a strand specify a transformation of the original (parent) strand onto a derived (offspring) strand. Loosely speaking, this transformation is considered as an application of the corresponding enzyme specified by sequences (14.29),(14.30), where the enzyme is visualized as a robot arm operating on the given strand, carrying out the commands that are coded by a sequence (14.29), which is unambiguously determined by mapping (14.27) based on the strand doublets (see also Table 14.1. Single instructions are specified by Table 14.2.

What remains to be determined is a starting position on the strand, where a sequence of enzyme actions is initialized. Such a position is called the *binding site* and it is represented by a base. An application of enzyme is then started on the first base (going from the left to the right) on the strand. If the strand does not contain such a base we say that the given enzyme is inapplicable to the strand. The binding site X is specified by the sequence of inclinations (14.30) such that going successively from left to right, we construct recurrently a sequence of arrows oriented to the right, left, up, or down. This process is initialized by the first position such that it is automatically set to arrow $\Rightarrow$, see Fig. 14.7, so that the first inclination is not enacted. When the sequence of inclinations is constructed or analyzed, we get the direction of the last arrow. The binding site is unambiguously determined by the first inclination symbol and by the last arrow (see Table 14.3)

$$X = f(\text{first inclination symbol}, \text{last arrow}) \tag{14.31}$$

This formula simply determines the binding site on the strand, e.g. according to Table 14.3, a sequence of arrows presented by diagram E in Fig. 14.7 determines the binding site X=A. It means that a corresponding enzyme is initially applied to a base A (going first from the left on a strand). Many different enzymes can have the same binding site. Formally, the whole procedure of construction of an enzyme assigned to a strand S is expressed by

$$enzyme(S) = (instruction(S), X) \tag{14.32}$$

where its first component corresponds to an instruction sequence (14.29) and the second component specifies a binding site. This relatively complicated way of determination of the binding site was introduced by Morris [31]. Original Hofstadter's approach [23] is much simpler, the binding site is specified only by the last arrow in the 2D enzyme structure, i.e. the type of the last arrow directly specifies a binding site.

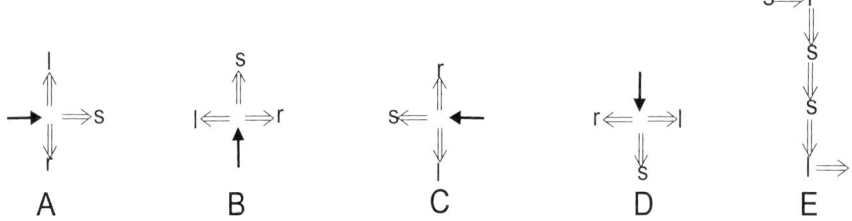

Fig. 14.7. An outline of four different cases of local properties of inclinations (A to D), where an initial arrow is specified by a black bold arrow. For instance, the first diagram A represents three possible folds (directions of double arrow) created from the bold arrow (oriented from the left to the right) if inclinations *s*, *l*, and *r* are applied. Diagram E corresponds to a 2D structure produced by an inclination sequence *s - r - s - s - l*.

Table 14.3. Different possibilities for binding site determination for three types of inclination. *s* straight *r* right *l* left

No.	1st inclin.	Last arrow	Binding	No.	1st inclin.	Last arrow	Binding
1	*s*	⇒	A	7	*l*	⇐	G
2	*s*	⇑	C	8	*l*	⇑	T
3	*s*	⇓	G	9	*r*	⇑	A
4	*s*	⇐	T	10	*r*	⇐	C
5	*l*	⇓	A	11	*r*	⇒	G
6	*l*	⇒	C	12	*r*	⇓	T

For a given strand S and its *enzyme*(S) we may introduce the so-called replication process consisting in an application of the *enzyme*(S) to the strand S. This replication process is formally composed of the following two steps:

Step 1. Construction of an enzyme composed of a sequence of instructions (amino acids)

$$instruction(S) = instr(D_1) - instr(D_2) - ... - instr(D_p) \quad (14.33)$$

and a binding site X, i.e.

$$enzyme(S) = (instruction(S), X) \quad (14.34)$$

Step 2. Enzyme *enzyme*(S) is applied to the strand S so that its application is initialized at the base X incoming first from the left and then instructions are step-by-step performed over the strand.

This simple process of transformation of the (*parent*) strand S onto another quasistrand (in general, it may contain also hash symbols) R is called the *replication*

$$replication(S) = R \tag{14.35}$$

A strand R (*offspring*) is created in the course of replication as a result of the replication process if in some replication stage the enzyme was switched to *on* mode. In general, this strand R may be composed of a number of empty hash symbols that appear in the resulting strand when its length is smaller than a length of the parent strand S. If the result of replication is not a continuous strand, a strand R is defined as the first continuous part of the result of replication. Diagrammatic representation of the above two-step transformation (replication) is outlined in Fig. 14.8.

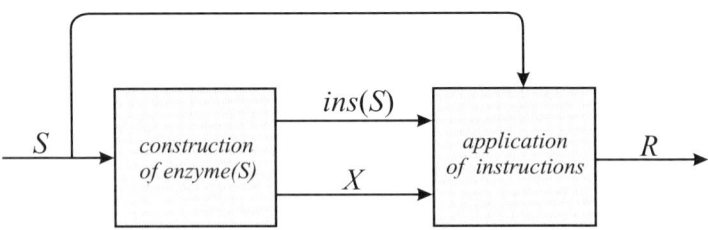

Fig. 14.8. A schematic outline of a replication process of a strand S. At the first stage an enzyme *enzyme(S)* is constructed, then, at the second stage this enzyme is applied to the strand S by a set of instructions *ins(S)*, starting at a binding site X. Loosely speaking, we may say, that each strand contains a necessary information for its replication process.

Finally, we will discuss how to apply an enzyme *enzyme(S)* to a strand S. Let us postulate that the enzyme is specified by $enzyme(S) = (instruction(S), X)$, where X specifies a binding site on the strand S. Two different situation should be distinguished:

1. If $X \notin S$, then the enzyme is inapplicable to the strand.
2. If $X \in S$, then the enzyme is applied to the first appearance (from the left) of the base X. Enzyme instructions (amino acids) are sequentially stepbystep applied to the strand S.

14.3.3 Replicators

One of the central notions of artificial (or algorithmic) chemistry [1–6, 9, 11–15, 17, 19–22, 24–28], are *replicators*, initially introduced in the beginning of seventies by Eigen and Schuster [11–14] as hypothetical biomacromolecules that are endowed with standard "mass-law" kinetics and that are capable of replication catalyzed by themselves. These authors demonstrated that in this "abiotic" level there is already possible to observe phenomena closely resembling Darwinian evolution based on the surviving of best fitted individuals (i.e. best adapted biomacromolecules). A double strand

$$A = \begin{pmatrix} R \\ S \end{pmatrix} \quad (14.36)$$

is called the *replicator* if the replication process applied to both its parts results in

$$replication(S) = R, replication(R) = S \quad (14.37)$$

in a composed form

$$replication(replication(S)) = S \quad (14.38)$$

i.e. the strand S is replicated to R, and the strand R is replicated to S. In typogenetic environment we always manipulate single strands, the above presented definition should be considered as a two-step process: in the first step the strand S is replicated to an offspring R, and then R is replicated to the next offspring identical with the parent strand S, see Fig. 14.9. The requirement, that each of replicator's complementary strands is replicated exactly onto the other one, is very restrictive.

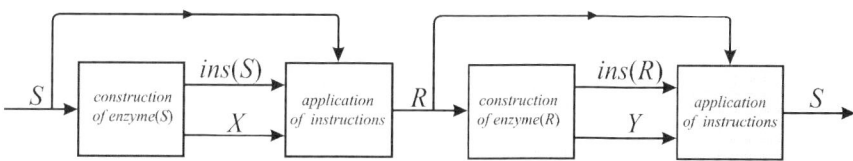

Fig. 14.9. A schematic outline of an replication process of a strand S, it may be considered as a double application of a scheme presented in Fig. 14.8. If the strand S is an replicator, then an output from two replications is again the same strand S.

For an application of evolutionary methods [15, 22, 24] to construction of replicators we need a quantitative measure of a fact whether a strand is replicator or not. We introduce the so-called *fitness* of strands that achieves the maximum value if the strand is an replicator. Let us have a strand S, its fitness will reflect its ability to be an replicator. In particular, let $R = \bar{S}$ be a complementary strand to the original strand S, applying to these two strands independent replication processes we get

$$replication(S) = R', replication(R) = S' \quad (14.39)$$

Then a fitness of S is determined as follows

$$fitness(S) = \frac{1}{2}\left(2 - d\left(S, \bar{R}'\right) - d\left(R, \bar{S}'\right)\right) \quad (14.40)$$

with values ranged by

$$0 \leqslant fitness(S) \leqslant 1 \quad (14.41)$$

Its maximum value ($fitness_{max}=1$) is achieved for $S = \bar{R}'$ and $R = \bar{S}'$ (i.e. strands S, R' and R, S' are complementary). This means that the maximum fitness value is achieved for strands that are replicators.

A mutation represents a very important innovation method in evolutionary algorithms. In particular, going from one evolutionary epoch to the next epoch, individuals of a population are reproduced with small random errors. If this reproduction process were always without spontaneously appearing errors, then the evolution would not contain "variations" that are a necessary presumption of the Darwinian evolution.

Let us consider a strand $S = X_1X_2...X_n$, this strand is transformed onto another strand $T = Y_1Y_2...Y_n$, (where Y's are bases or empty symbols) applying a stochastic mutation operator O_{mut}

$$T = O_{mut}(S) \tag{14.42}$$

This operator is realized in such a way that going successively from the left to the right each element (base) with a small probability P_{mut} is either changed (mutated) to another base, or deleted from the strand, or enlarged from the right by a new randomly selected base

$$O_{mut}(AACGTTA) = \begin{cases} \underline{T}ACGTTA & \text{(mutation)} \\ AA\blacktriangle GTTA & \text{(deletion)} \\ AACG\underline{A}TTA & \text{(insertion)} \\ AACGTTA & \text{(exact copy)} \end{cases} \tag{14.43}$$

where the first three particular cases (mutation, deletion, and insertion) are realized with the same probability.

Evolution of strands towards an emergence of replicators in a population (composed of strands that are considered as objects of Darwinian evolution) is simulated by a simple evolutionary algorithm. Individuals in a population are represented by single strands, and in a reproduction process a mutation operator is applied to a randomly selected parent – strand, creating one offspring. A strand is quasirandomly selected for a reproduction process, a probability of this selection is proportional to the strand fitness. The reproduction process consists of a simple copy process, where a strand is simply reproduced with a possibility of appearance of stochastic mutations (specified by the probability P_{mut}). When a new population composed of offspring from the reproduction process achieves the same number of individuals as the original population, then the old population is replaced by the new population.

The above formal definition of the replicator is relatively complicated, it requires a two-step process to verify whether a strand is a replicator. Varetto [38] studied a systematic constructive way for the construction of replicators, which is applicable for shorter strands or for strands with the same repeated "motif". In order to demonstrate the full capacity of Typogenetics for AL studies, a simple evolutionary algorithm is applied to achieve an evolutionary spontaneous emergence of replicators. The basic parameters of the algorithm were set as follows: size of population $N=1000$, minimum and maximum lengths of strands $l_{min}=15$ and $l_{max}=30$. The probability P_{mut} was varied during the course of evolution, at the beginning of evolution its value is maximum $P_{mut}^{(max)}$ and then it decreases to a minimum value $P_{mut}^{(min)}$. A current value of probability for an evolutionary epoch t is determined by

$$P_{mut} = P_{mut}^{(max)} - \left(P_{mut}^{(max)} - P_{mut}^{(min)}\right) \frac{t}{t_{max}} \qquad (14.44)$$

where t_{max} is the length of evolution (maximum number of epochs). In our calculations we set $P_{mut}^{(max)} = 0.01$ and $P_{mut}^{(min)} = 0.001$.

A proper method how to visualize evolution is a plot of distance between the temporarily best strand $S_{best}^{(t)}$ (specified for the evolutionary epoch t) and the best strand resulting from the whole evolution $S_{best}^{(all)}$. Since the strands $S_{best}^{(t)}$ and $S_{best}^{(all)}$ may be, in general, of different length, the distance specified in Section 14.3.1 (see eqs. (14.23),(14.24)) is not applicable for this consideration. It means that we have to determine a notion of distance in a more general way than that one mentioned in the previous part of this report. Let us consider two strands $S = X_1 X_2 \ldots X_n$ and $R = Y_1 Y_2 \ldots Y_m$, their lengths are $|S| = n$ and $|R| = m$, respectively. Let $p = \min\{m,n\}$ be a minimum distance of strands S and R, then an alternative distance between them is determined by

$$D(S,R) = |S| + |R| - 2 \sum_{i=1}^{p} \delta(X_i, Y_i) \qquad (14.45)$$

where δ is an analogue of Kronecker's delta already defined by ((14.24). A positive value of this new distance reflects a measure of difference between strands S and R, its vanishing value corresponds to a fact that both strands are identical. A plot of $D\left(S_{best}^{(t)}, S_{best}^{(all)}\right)$ visualizes evolution of temporarily best strands to the resulting best strand that may be considered as a result of the evolutionary emergence of replicators.

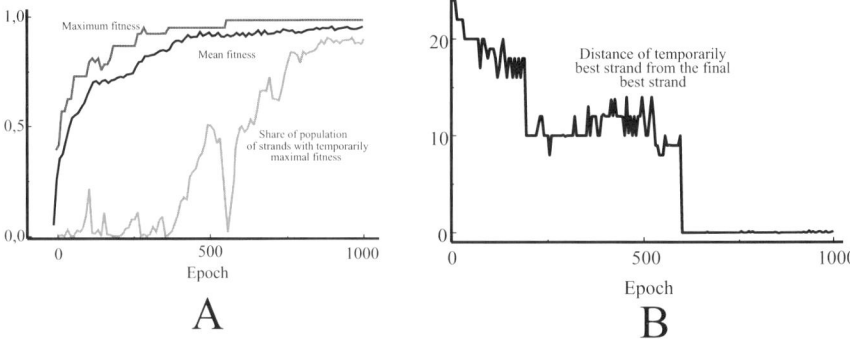

Fig. 14.10. Two different plots that characterize evolutionary emergence of replicators. Diagram A shows plots of maximum fitness, mean fitness, and a share of population of temporarily best strand. Diagram B shows plot of distance $D\left(S_{best}^{(t)}, S_{best}^{(all)}\right)$, where $S_{best}^{(t)}$ is a temporarily best strand (for an epoch t) and $S_{best}^{(all)}$ is the best strand (a replicator) produced by the evolution of population. The distance D is determined by (14.45). The displayed plot indicates that distance D "monotonously" decreases (with some small fluctuations due to a random genetic drift in the population) to zero value, which indicates a spontaneous emergence of a replicator ($S_{best}^{(all)}$) at the end of evolution.

Typical resulting plots are shown in Fig. 14.10. The first diagram A corresponds to plots of maximum and mean fitness and a frequency of appearance of temporarily best strand. A mixture of different strands appeared at the beginning of evolution. As the population was more evolved (say starting from 500 epochs), where a final solution (a replicator) was already created, its share of population almost monotonously increased to 100%. The second diagram B corresponds to a plot of a distance D between temporarily best strand and the best final strand (replicator) produced by the evolution of population. We see that the distance decreases with small fluctuations so that starting from the half of evolution this distance is vanishing, i.e. the correct strand (or strands) has emerged from the evolution.

The following set of observation from our numerical results can be formulated (cf. ref. [28]):

1. *There are no dramatic changes in the composition of best strands throughout the whole population period. Rather, we see that evolution of replicators is very opportunistic, it contains only small changes in compositions of strands such that the whole evolution is inherently directed to an emergence of replicators.*
2. *Moreover, there exist long evolutionary periods in which the maximum fitness is kept fixed and small changes appeared in composition of strands. Such evolutionary periods are called the neutral periods, in which evolution "gathers" an information for changes that lead to a substantial increase of quality of strands towards their ability to be replicators.*

14.3.4 Hypercycles

According to Eigen and Schuster [11–14], a *hypercycle* is a kinetic composition of replicators, where a replication of A_i is catalyzed by enzymes produced by the previous replicator A_{i-1}

$$A_i + E_{i-1} \rightarrow 2A_i + E_{i-1} \quad (for\, i=1,2,...,n) \tag{14.46}$$

where E_{i-1} is an enzyme produced by the previous replicator A_{i-1}, and $A_0 = A_n, E_0 = E_n$.

Hypercycles may be considered as multilevel hierarchical catalytic kinetic systems. They represent an important concept of the current mental image of an abiotic period of molecular evolution. Replicators, which emerged in the first stage of this evolution, may be integrated into higher level kinetic systems that represent units relatively independent from other replicators or hypercycles. Moreover, hypercycles represent an uncomplicated example of an increase of complexity [34], with a well described mathematical model and a simple computer implementation [12–14].

Let us consider a sequence of replicators $S_1, S_2, \ldots, S_n$, that are mutually related in such a way that a replication of S_i is catalyzed by an enzyme $enzyme(S_{i-1})$ produced by the previous strand S_{i-1} (a previous strand with respect to S_1 is a strand S_n). Applying a metaphor of chemical reactions, a hypercycle can be represented as a sequence of the following reactions

$$S_i \xrightarrow{enzyme(S_{i-1})} S_i + \bar{S}_i \quad and \quad \bar{S}_i \xrightarrow{enzyme(\bar{S}_{i-1})} \bar{S}_i + S_i \tag{14.47}$$

for $i=1,2,\ldots,n$. We see that their precise determination is highly restrictive and may give rise to very serious doubts whether hypercycles can exist and be constructed (e.g. within Typogenetics).

Varetto [39] has introduced the so-called tanglecycles as an alternative to our hypercycles that were specified in a way *closely related to their original meaning* proposed by Eigen and Schuster [11–14]. In particular, in a specification of tanglecycles there is suppressed an autoreplication character of strands, Varetto only required that there exists a replication of a strand S_i onto another strand S_{i+1} and this process is catalyzed by an enzyme of S_{i-1} strand (he does not specify properties of complementary strands taking part in the tanglecycle)

$$S_i \xrightarrow{enzyme(S_{i-1})} S_i + S_{i+1} \quad (i = 1, 2, ..., n) \tag{14.48}$$

where $S_0 = S_n$ and $S_{n+1} = S_1$. The main difference between hypercycles and tanglecycles consists in the fact that the strands in hypercycles, unlike the tanglecycles, are coupled only through enzymatic catalysis, while in tanglecycles inside a "replication" of S_i there is created the forthcoming strand S_{i+1}. The present version of our Typogenetics machinery is not applicable to a study of tanglecycles, since a replication product S_{i+1} of a strands S_i (see eq. (14.48)) should be a complementary strand to S_i, i.e. we could not expect that by applying a sequence of reactions (14.48) for $n \geq 3$ we get at its end a product identical with the initial strand S_1.

A population P is composed of hypercycles (or hopefully future hypercycles) that are composed of the same number n of strands. Each hypercycle of the population is evaluated by a fitness that reflects an ability of all its components to replicate themselves. Hypercycles are selected quasirandomly (with a probability proportional to their fitness) for reproduction with a possibility of stochastic mutations (controlled by a probability P_{mut}). The design of the evolutionary algorithm is the same as for the evolution of single replicators.

The fitness of a hypercycle is determined as follows: Let us consider a hypercycle and its complementary form

$$\mathbf{x} = (S_1, S_2, ..., S_n) \quad \text{and} \quad \bar{\mathbf{x}} = (\bar{S}_1, \bar{S}_2, ..., \bar{S}_n) \quad (14.49)$$

$$S_i \xrightarrow{e(S_{i-1})} S_i + R_i \quad \text{and} \quad \bar{S}_i \xrightarrow{e(\bar{S}_{i-1})} \bar{S}_i + R'_i \quad (14.50)$$

Each ith component (S_i and $\bar{S}_i$) is evaluated by a "local" fitness

$$fitness_i = \frac{1}{2} \left(2 - d(S_i, \bar{R}_i) - d(\bar{S}_i, \bar{R}'_i) \right) \quad (14.51)$$

A fitness of the hypercycle x is determined as a *minimum* of local fitness of its constituents

$$fitness(\mathbf{x}) = \min_i fitness_i \quad (14.52)$$

Loosely speaking, a fitness of a hypercycle is determined by a local fitness values of its weakest replicator (a chain is as strong as its weakest link). A Darwinian evolution of strands towards an emergence of hypercycles in a population is simulated by a simple evolutionary algorithm used for an evolution of replicators (see Fig. 14.11).

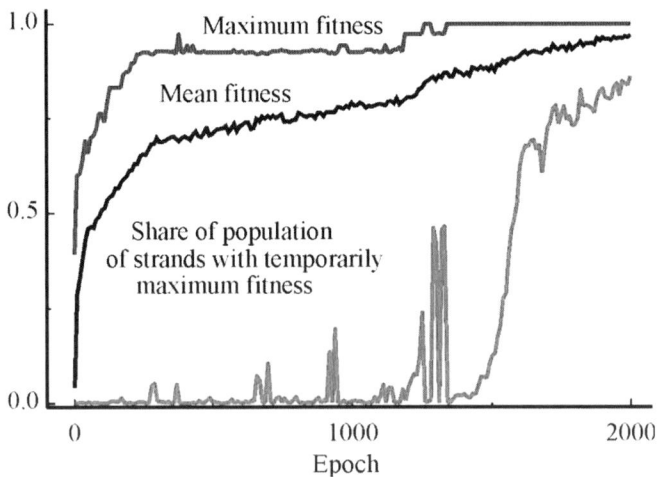

Fig. 14.11. Three different plots that characterize evolutionary emergence of hypercycles composed of two replicators (2-hypercycle).

The basic parameters of the present evolutionary algorithm that was used for an emergence of hypercycles are set as follows: size of population $N=2000$, mutation probability $P_{mut}=0.001$, minimum and maximum lengths of strands $l_{min}=15$ and $l_{max}=30$, and the evolution of population is watched two thousands epochs (i.e. $t_{max}=2000$). The evolutionary approach produced 2-hypercycles; if the same approach was used for higher hypercycles, then we never succeeded in their emergence. Main conclusions from computer simulations of evolutionary emergence of hypercycles are following:

1. *An evolutionary emergence of hypercycles composed of more than two replicators is a very improbable evolutionary event. In other words, it represents for evolutionary algorithms a very difficult combinatorial tasks.*
2. *More complex hypercycles may be constructed by evolution from simpler hypercycles such that they are enlarged by another replicator with evolutionarily optimized composition.*

14.3.5 Summary

It seems, according to our results, that Typogenetics offers new analogies and formal tools for computer scientists active in artificial life. A central "dogma" of the typogenetics is that strands have twofold role: *First* they are replicators, and *second*, they code an information about the way of their replication. Formally, Typogenetics may be considered as a molecular automaton (cf. ref. [39]) that on its input reads strands and on its output it replicates strands. To make such an automaton more interesting, we may endow strands with additional properties enabling them to behave in some specific manner. In the present simple approach, strands have infinite resources for their replications. If we introduce a limited space of resources, then we get an additional selective pressure (a struggle for raw materials) with respect to a selection entirely based on strand fitness that reflect their capability of replication. An introduction of a "geographical" distributions of strands in a population might be very important, which was already clear from the evolutionary construction of hypercycles. In that case the population could not be considered as a homogeneous one in a well-stirred vessel. A replication function of strands usually requires only a fraction of the enzyme that is coded in the strand; it is then possible, in general, to code additional strand or enzyme properties that may give rise to an emergence of new properties and hierarchically organized structures. Summarizing, Typogenetics represents a very rich and flexible formal tool, closely related to basic concepts of molecular biology, that opens new possibilities and horizons for artificial life activities and efforts.

14.4 Folding of RNA-Like Molecules that are Represented by Binary Strings

In an analogy with RNA molecules which are endowed with the so-called folding [35] (secondary structure), we will study a similar property specified also for binary strings (see Fig. 14.12). The folding of a binary string may be specified by a list of matched pairs $i-j$ (for $i<j$) and unmatched singles k

$$\text{fold}(\mathbf{g}) = \{i_1-j_1, i_2-j_2, ..., i_r-j_r; k_1, k_2, ..., k_q\} \quad (14.53)$$

where the pairs are restricted by the following three conditions: (1) For any pair $i-j$ holds

$$j-i \geqslant 2 \quad (14.54)$$

(2) For any two pairs $i-j$ and $k-l$ (restricted by $i \leqslant k$) holds either

$$i = k \Leftrightarrow j = l \quad (14.55)$$

$$k < j \Rightarrow i < k < l < j \quad (14.56)$$

The first condition (14.54) means that a minimum length of the so-called *hairpin* in the produced folding is two (see the right-hand part of secondary structure in Fig. 14.12). The second condition (14.55) means that each string entry can take part in no more than one matched pair. Finally, the third condition (14.56) implies that the so-called pseudoknots are forbidden (i.e. each folding may be represented by a planar graph; the appearance of pseudoknots in folding could cause its non-planarity). Moreover, the folding of $\mathbf{g}$ is defined such that it contains a maximum number of matched pairs; this condition reflects a physical meaning of folding as a most stable secondary structure. The last two conditions (14.55), (14.56) are very important for application of dynamic programming technique for construction of folding.

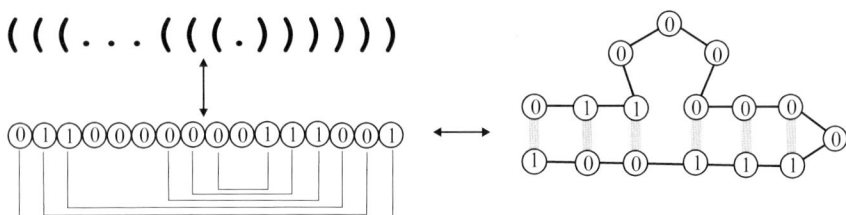

Fig. 14.12. A binary string (a linear graph with vertices assigned to binary entries that are connected by edges) may be folded into a two-dimensional structure (called the secondary structure) in such a way that complementary binary pairs are matched together. A bracket representation of folding is presented in the upper part of the drawing, where dot symbols correspond to noninteracting string entries and brackets '(' and ')' correspond to a pair of matched complementary entries.

The folding $fold(\mathbf{g})$ of binary string $\mathbf{g}$ may be alternatively expressed by a bracket formalism (see Fig. 14.12). This means that each folding of the binary string may be expressed by a string composed of three symbols $\{(,),.\}$, formally $fold(\mathbf{g}) \in \{(,),.\}^n$.

Of course, actual forms of these strings are strongly restricted such that all three conditions (14.54), (14.55), (14.56) should be satisfied. The simplest way to ensure the correctness of bracket representation is to postulate that bracket strings are formulae of a simple context–free grammar $\langle V_N, V_T, S, R \rangle$ where $V_N = \{S\}$ is a set of nonterminal symbols, $V_T = \{(,),.\}$ is a set of terminal symbols, S is a starting nonterminal symbol, and R is a rule set composed of the following three rules

$$S \to (S)|SS|. \qquad (14.57)$$

A feasible folding $fold(g)$ which satisfies all three restrictions (14.54), (14.55), (14.56) is interpreted as a formula composed entirely of terminal symbols that belongs to the language L generated by the grammar (14.57), i.e. $fold(g) \in L$. An illustrative example of grammar production looks as follows

$$S \to \underline{SS} \to (\underline{S})S \to ((\underline{S}))S \to ((\underline{SS}))S \to ((.\underline{S}))S$$
$$\to ((..))\underline{S} \to ((..))\underline{SS} \to ((..))\underline{SSS} \to ((..))S(\underline{S})S$$
$$\to ((..))S(\underline{SS})S \to ((..))S(.\underline{S})S \to ((..))\underline{S}(..)S$$
$$\to ((..)).(..)\underline{S} \to ((..)).(..).$$

```
for i:=1 to n do S[i,i]:='.';
for i:=1 to n-1 do S[i,i+1]:='..';
for d:=2 to n-1 do
 for i:=1 to n-d do
 begin
  j:=d+i;
  S[i,j]:=max{i≤k≤j-1,S[i,k]⊕S[k+1,j]};
 end;
folding:=S[1,n];
```

Algorithm 2. A dynamic-programming scheme for the calculation of folding of a binary string of length n. The resulting folding is coded in the bracket representation and is stored at the string entry $S_{1,n}$.

We use a simple dynamic-programming technique for the construction of folding of binary strings. In general, it can be used as an alternative to backtrack searching methods (these have an exponentially increasing CPU time, when a respective system may be decomposed into smaller subsystems such that the used evaluation of system is always additive with respect to its subparts (then an exponential time complexity e^n is reduced to a cubic complexity n^3). Let S_{ij} be a substring of bracket representation assigned to a folding between i and j (including) binary entries. These entries are initialized as follows

$$S_{ii} = '.' \quad \text{and} \quad S_{i,i+1} = '..' \qquad (14.58)$$

The forthcoming entries S_{ij}, for $j - i \geq 2$, are recurrently constructed by

$$S_{i,j} = \max_{i \leq k \leq j-1} S_{ik} \oplus S_{k+1,j} \qquad (14.59)$$

where $\oplus$ is the symbol of concatenation of "substrings" S_{ik} and $S_{k+1,j}$ which were already constructed in the previous stages of the algorithm (see Algorithm 2). Moreover, if S_{ik} ($S_{k+1,j}$) contains in the leftmost (rightmost) position dot symbol '.' and ith and jth binary entries are complementary, then the respective dot symbols are substituted by (and) symbols. Symbol "max" in (14.59) means that we select that index k, which produces maximum pairing in S_{ij}. The resulting folding in the form of bracket representation is stored at entry S_{1n}.

Table 14.4. All possible genotypes represented by binary string (for $n=7$), the respective phenotypes and fitness.

No.	Genotype	Phenotype	Fitness[a]
1	(0000000)(1111111)	....	1
2	(0000001)(0000100)(1111011)(1111110)	....(.)	1
3	(0000010)(1111101)	...(.).	0
4	(0000011)(0001001)(0001101)(0010010)(0010110)(0011000) (0011100)(0100011)(0100111)(0101001)(0110010)(0110110) (0111000)(0111100)(1000011)(1000111)(1001001)(1001101) (1010110)(1011000)(1011100)(1100011)(1100111)(1101001) (1101101)(1110010)(1110110)(1111100)	..(.))	0
5	(0000101)(0010001)(0101100)(0101110)(0110000)(0111010) (1000101)(1001111)(1010001)(1010011)(1101110)(1111010)	.((.).)	3
6	(0000110)(0011010)(1100101)(1111001)	.((.)).	5
7	(0000111)(0001111)(0010011)(0011011)(0100101)(0101101) (0110001)(0111001)(1000110)(1001110)(1010010)(1011010) (1100100)(1101100)(1110000)(1111000)	(((.)))	7
8	(0001000)(1110111)	...(..)	0
9	(0001010)(1110101)	((.).).	0
10	(0001011)(0001100)(0001110)(0011001)(0011110)(0100001) (0100100)(0100110)(0110011)(0110100)(1001011)(1001100) (1011001)(1011011)(1011110)(1100001)(1100110)(1110001) (1110011)(1110100)	.(.)(.)	0
11	(0010000)(1101111)	..(...)	1
12	(0010100)(0111011)(0111110)(1000001)1000100)(1101011)	(.).(.)	1
13	(0010101)(0101010)(1010101)(1101010)	.((..))	1
14	(0010111)(0011101)(0100010)(0101000)(1010111)(1011101) (1100010)(1101000)	.(.(.))	0
15	(0011111)(1100000)	((.)..)	2
16	(0100000)(1011111)	.(....)	1
17	(0101011)(1010100)	(..)(.)	0
18	(0101111)(1010000)	(.(.).)	5
19	(0110101)(0110111)(1001000)(1001010)	(.)(..)	0
20	(0111101)(1000010)	(..(.))	2
21	(0111111)(1000000)	(.....)	3

[a]Fitness is calculated as a graph-theory based similarity measure between the respective phenotype and the so-called required phenotype represented by $p_{req}=(((.)))$, see eqs. (14.60).

The main problem in actual implementation of this algorithm for construction of folding of binary strings consists in the fact that although it constructs a folding with maximum matchings, it offers as a result only one result of many possible. Therefore, the algorithm should be considered as a test-bed for development of phenotype of genotypes and also as an integral part of evaluation of genotypes by fitness.

The notion of folding allows us to introduce a triad of fundamental concepts from evolutionary biology, in particular *genotype*, *phenotype*, and *fitness*. The genotype $\mathbf{g}$ is represented by a binary string of length n, $\mathbf{g} = (g_1 g_2 ... g_n) \in \{0,1\}^n$, the phenotype $p(\mathbf{g})$ corresponds to a folding of $\mathbf{g}$; formally, it may be expressed by the bracket notation, $p(\mathbf{g}) = \text{fold}(\mathbf{g}) \in \{(,),.\}^n$. Finally, the fitness, a numerical attribute of $\mathbf{g}$, is specified by making use of the respective phenotype. For our forthcoming considerations the fitness will be specified as a similarity between a phenotype $p(\mathbf{g})$ and an ad-hoc *required phenotype* p_{req}

$$\text{fitness}(\mathbf{g}) = s\left(p(\mathbf{g}), p_{req}\right) \tag{14.60}$$

This means that maximum fitness equal to n is achieved when a similarity between the respective phenotype $p(\mathbf{g})$ and the required phenotype p_{req} is maximum (n) (i.e., $p(\mathbf{g})=p_{req}$). On the other hand, if $s(p(\mathbf{g}), p_{req}) < n \Leftrightarrow p(\mathbf{g}) \neq p_{req}$, then the fitness is smaller than n; in a limit case, when the foldings are fully dissimilar (i.e. $s(p(\mathbf{g}), p_{req})=0$), the fitness of $\mathbf{g}$ is vanishing, fitness($\mathbf{g}$)=0. The notion of similarity will be specified in the forthcoming section. Table 14.4. contains illustrative results, where genotypes represented by all possible binary strings of length $n=7$ are evaluated by phenotype foldings and fitness. We see that many different binary strings are evaluated by the same folding, and similarly, many different foldings are evaluated by the same fitness. This simple observation immediately implies that mappings of genotypes onto phenotypes and phenotypes onto fitness are of the many-to-one type, i.e. there exist a huge redundancy in both mappings (see Fig. 14.13). A single binary string could be theoretically evaluated by more foldings than one, but the mapping produced by an application of the Algorithm 2 is the first one, which was found with a particular maximum number of matched pairs.

An interrelationship between the elements of this triad "genotype-phenotype-fitness" is formally expressed as a sequence of two mappings (see Fig. 14.13)

$$G \xrightarrow{p} P \xrightarrow{\text{fitness}} [0, \infty) \tag{14.61}$$

This means that the basic entity is the genotype: it is initially mapped onto the phenotype, and then the phenotype is mapped onto the fitness. An abbreviated form of this composite mapping is as follows

$$G \xrightarrow{f=\text{fitness} \circ p} [0, \infty) \tag{14.62}$$

This new mapping immediately maps the genotype strings onto fitness without the necessity to consider explicitly an intermediate called the phenotype. In this connection one may ask why there is worthwhile to introduce the phenotype as a mediator between the genotype and the fitness. Of course, such a question is fully acceptable from the pure mathematical point of view, but it must be noted that the concept of phenotype is a very effective and fruitful heuristic for interpretation of the Darwinian evolutionary theory. In particular, a given form of phenotype is usually considered as an evolutionary goal, and therefore we may say that the Darwinian evolution is represented mainly as a sequence of phenotypes which are progressively closer to the evolutionary phenotype goal.

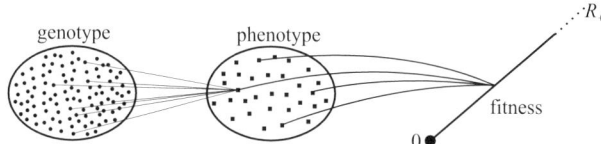

Fig. 14.13. Schematic outline of the composite mapping (14.62). Both respective mappings are of the many-to-one type, i.e. many gene strings are mapped onto one phenotype string, and similarly, many phenotype strings are mapped onto one value of fitness. This means that there exists a huge redundancy of the genotype coding, many different genes (strings) may be evaluated by one value of fitness. This property of the huge redundancy of genotype coding is of considerable importance for the existence of neutral stases in the Darwinian evolutionary theory.

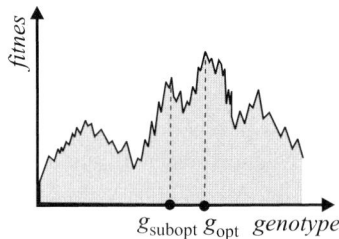

Fig. 14.14. Fitness landscape (or more precisely, fitness surface) was initially introduced into theory of the Darwinian evolution in 1932 by Sewall Wright [41], who characterized the Darwinian process as an optimization process over the fitness landscape specified by a composite mapping f (14.62). The resulting population genotype corresponds to a point – optimal genotype g_{opt} – with a maximum fitness. Loosely speaking, the Darwinian evolution should have tools to find a way from a suboptimal solution g_{subopt} to optimal solution g_{opt}.

Sewall Wright in 1932 [41] introduced one of the most fundamental concepts of the Darwinian evolution called the *fitness surface* (see Fig. 14.14). Moreover, by making use of this concept he characterized the Darwinian evolution as an optimization process, where the evolved population seeks a global maximum (or another solution closely related to this global one)

$$g_{opt} = \arg \max \; f(g) \qquad (14.63)$$

This complex optimization combinatorial problem will be solved by methods of artificial chemistry based on the metaphor of Eigen's replicators. It will be demonstrated that the "chemostat" formalism offers an effective tool for optimization of problems of the form (14.63), i.e. "replicator" methods of artificial chemistry are very well suitable to mimic the molecular Darwinian evolution.

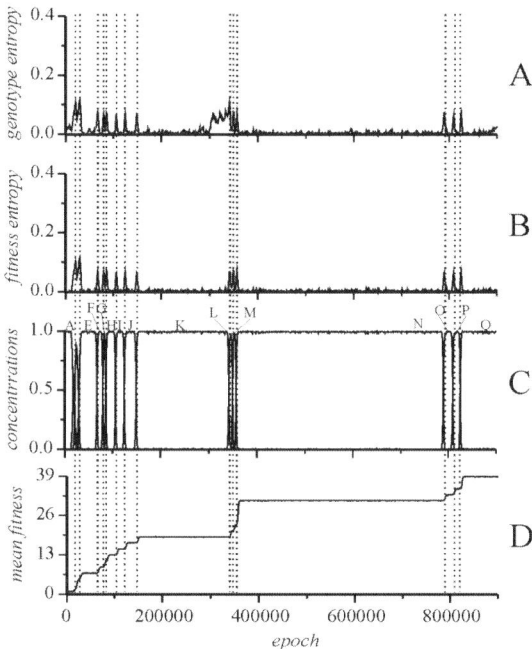

Fig. 14.15. Plots of (A) genotype entropy, (B) fitness entropy, (C) concentrations of strings with respective fitness, and (D) mean fitness. Mean fitness is a nondecreasing plot with two relatively long neutral stases. Its stairs are well indicated by fitness and genotype entropies. The plot of genotype entropy (A) at the end of the first neutral stasis indicates a substantial increase in genotype entropy whereas the fitness entropy is simultaneously almost vanishing. From this observation we may conclude that there exists huge appearance of "neutral mutants" that have the capability of producing by 1-bit mutations a new string with a higher fitness. Plot (C) displays relative concentrations of strings with given fitness. Each concentration profile is identified with labels of phenotypes in Fig. 14.16.

To summarize the main results of this section, *we have observed that in our scenario both mappings of genotype onto phenotype as well as phenotype onto fitness are of strongly stochastic nature with huge redundancy (both mappings are of the many-to-one type). General properties of these mappings may be specified only by making use of computersimulation tools, i.e. instead of exact "deterministic" description of properties of mappings, we generate histograms of appearances of their different entities and then we deduce from them some general properties of statistical validity.*

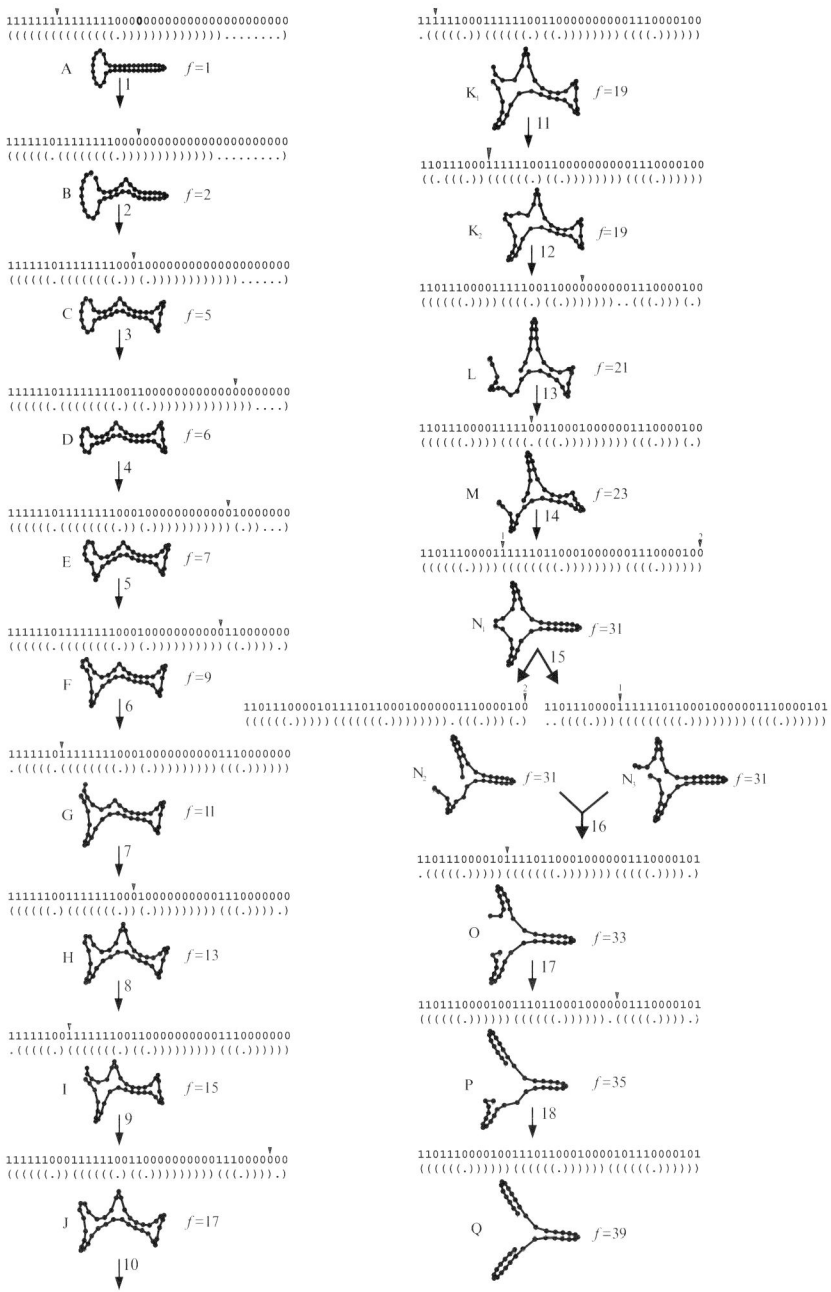

Fig. 14.16. A trajectory T (g_{ini}, p_{req}), where the initial genotype is specified by (14.4.1) and the required phenotype is outlined by diagram Q (see (14.4.1)).

14.4.1 Chemostat Simulation of Molecular Darwinian Evolution

The chemostat approach outlined in the first part of this communication will be used as an algorithmic framework for simulation of the molecular Darwinian evolution. An initial composition of chemostat is made by identical strings of length 39

g_{ini}=111111111111111000000000000000000000000

The required phenotype is specified by

p_{req}=((((((.))))))((((((.))))))((((((.))))))

Its secondary propeller-like structure is composed of three shafts (see secondary structure Q in Fig. 14.16). This phenotype will serve as a goal phenotype, all fitness calculations of binary strings being realized with respect to the required phenotype. This means that we expect a genotype with folding fully specified by the required phenotype p_{req} to emerge in the chemostat. The mutation operator O_{mut} (14.16) is specified by a probability of 1-bit mutation P_{mut}=0.0001. The used probability of 1-bit mutation is sufficiently small to ensure that the produced trajectory is composed of adjacent strings (with unit Hamming distance) in the respective genotype graph (see Fig. 14.16). Further important parameter, the size of chemostat (number of strings), is equal to 500. The length of trajectory in Fig. 14.16 is 18, in all transient states the used mutations are of the 1bit type (between respective strings there is unit Hamming distance). There exist two cases of neutral mutations, in particular transitions 11 and 15. These transitions are different, the former corresponding to a sequence of neutral mutations, whereas the latter to a "parallel" appearance of two neutral mutations (i.e. the trajectory is split into two paths which are connected in the next step.

The composition of chemostat is characterized by two different types of entropies that are determined as follows: Let $w(x)$ be the probability that the chemostat string is evaluated by entity x (fitness or genotype). Then

$$S_X = -\sum_x w(x) \ln[w(x)] \qquad (14.64)$$

These entropic parameters are very sensitive to composition changes of the chemostat. For a homogenous chemostat (composed of the same strings), both entropies are vanishing. A *fitness entropy* $S_{fitness}$ may serve as a proper indicator of intermediate transient states where a new genotype with a higher fitness substitutes an older genotype with lower fitness. This moment of transition can be detected from a fast temporary increase of the fitness entropy $S_{fitness}$ from its usual zero value. The genotype entropy is capable of detecting such transient stages where fitness remains unchanged, but the genotype composition of chemostat is temporarily changed due to the existence of the neutral mutation. This means that the genotype entropy is capable of detecting very rare events when fitness remains invariant but there appear temporarily different neutral genotypes. Both entropies have nonnegative values; it is possible to assess their maximum values as follows. At most time stages the chemostat composition is homogeneous, then S_x=0. A deviation from this homogeneity is usually realized as a two-component system (e.g. two different types of the genotype or phenotype, with respective concentrations α and 1-α). Then the entropy is specified by $S_x = -\alpha \cdot \ln\alpha - (1-\alpha) \cdot \ln(1-\alpha)$, for $0 < \alpha < 1$. Its maximum value is achieved for $\alpha=1/2$, $S_x(1/2) = \ln 2 \approx 0.7$. This usually means that great positive values of the respective entropy indicate that the chemostat is composed of two components with roughly equal concentrations.

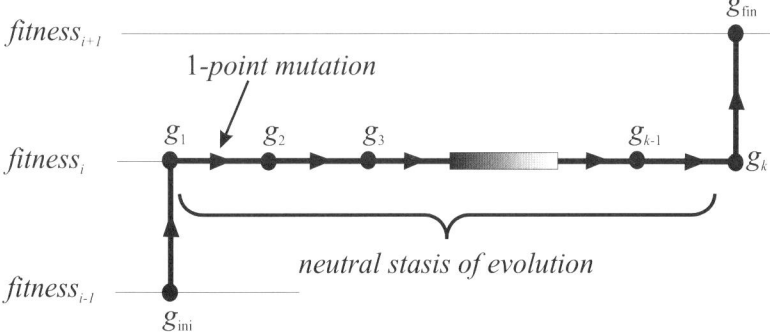

Fig. 14.17. Schematic outline of neutral stasis between "jumps" from the neutral graph with *fitness*$_i$ into another neutral graph with *fitness*$_{i+1}$. At the first neutral stage, hill-climbing forms a sequence of actual solutions within a cluster. The first solution in this sequence corresponds to a result from the previous "jump" and the last solution enables a "jump" to the forthcoming neutral graph *fitness*$_{i+1}$. Then the neutral stasis is repeated until a proper solution is found, which can be used for the next "jump" to further neutral graph.

Numerical results of our computer simulation of the molecular Darwinian evolution are displayed in Figs. 14.15 and 14.16. We see that the produced plot of the chemostat mean fitness (diagram D in Fig. 14.15) is a nondecreasing step function, with a few relatively long neutral stases. Diagrams A and B correspond to a genotype and fitness entropy, respectively, where these plots unambiguously indicate that at the end of the first neutral stasis (about 300 000 epochs) a considerable deviation from genotype homogeneity exists, i.e. in this evolutionary stage the chemostat is likely composed of two different genotypes with the same fitness. This deviation from the chemostat homogeneity can be considered as a necessary preliminary stage before an evolutionary transition to a next stage with higher fitness. The same situations can be found also in the previous stages of evolution, in particular for phenotype transitions A →B and E →F. Diagram C represents concentration profiles of different genotypes with respective fitness; we see these profiles to nicely agree with the Eigen's theory prediction of their form (see Fig. 14.3, diagram B). In particular, they form a sequence of well separated profiles. The dotted vertical auxiliary lines mark evolutionary transitions well indicated by entropies. Fig. 14.16. shows a sequence of phenotypes that appeared for single evolutionary stages (see Fig. 14.15). We got 17 different genotypes that are evaluated by different phenotypes (secondary folding structures). Their similarity to the required phenotype (14.4.1) specifies directly their fitness.

We see that neutral mutation plays an important role for the molecular Darwinian evolution to be able to escape local maxima on fitness hypersurface (see Figs. 14.17 and 14.18). In many cases, when a respective string g is not adjacent in the genotype graph $\hat{G}$ to another string g' with higher fitness (i.e. a transition $g \to g'$ causes an evolutionary jump), it is useful to stochastically look for another string $\tilde{g}$ in the neighborhood of g which has the same fitness, but for which an evolutionary jump $\tilde{g} \to g'$ with an increase of fitness, fitness $(g') >$ fitness $(\tilde{g})$, already exists.

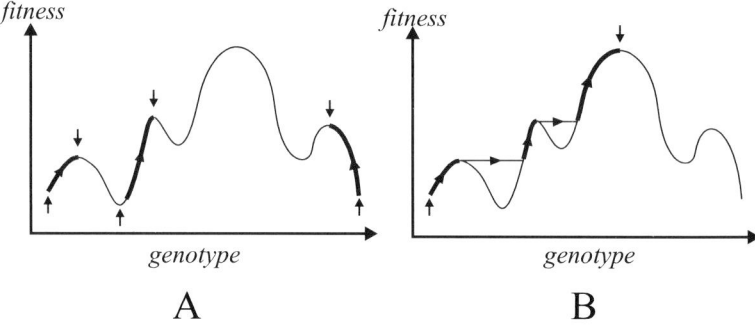

Fig. 14.18. (A) Schematic illustrative plot of the molecular Darwinian evolution when neutral mutations do not exist. An evolutionary adaptation ends at the nearest local maximum (in this case we may say that the Darwinian evolution is a local optimizer, population fitness is "scrambled" on fitness hypersurface to nearest maxima). On the other hand, (B) when neutral mutations are considered (fitness hypersurface is composed of many "plateaus" with constant value of fitness), a local character of Darwinian adaptation may be abridged by neutral "plateaus", which allow to overcome valleys with lower fitness. This means that the molecular Darwinian evolution has a good chance to achieve a global maximum on fitness hypersurface in the course of adaptation process. (After Schuster [35])

14.4.2 Summary

The main purpose of this Section was to study a simple model of molecular evolution based on binary strings and their folding into a secondary structures. Binary strings are evaluated by fitness that reflects a graph-theory based similarity measure between the respective folding and the required folding considered as an evolutionary goal. Binary strings – genotypes are able to replicate with the probability proportional to their fitness. The replication process, is not entirely perfect, there exists a very small probability of mutations that produce binary strings slightly different from their parent templates. The dynamics of the replication is fully specified by Eigen's kinetic differential equations that form sound phenomenological basis of theory of molecular replications with mutations.

Eigen's theory of replicators forms a sound phenomenological foundation of the molecular Darwinian evolution. Its differential-equation solutions which are specified by a proper selection of the required rate constants offer concentration very similar to those experimentally observed [37] (see Figs. 14.3 and 14.5). The Darwinian evolution is an interplay between Monodian [30] *chance and necessity*, between stochastic and deterministic processes. The Darwinian evolution is composed of parts that are fully deterministic, which are fully predictable (e.g. genotype – phenotype mapping), but integral parts of evolution involve also processes of a strong stochastic character that could not be well predicted, we can speak only about their basic statistic characteristics (e.g. mutations).

Sewall Wright's idea [41] of *fitness hypersurface* (adaptive or fitness landscape) is of a great heuristic importance and can be considered as one of the greatest achievements of the theory of Darwinian evolution. Then, after this concept, the Darwinian evolution may be interpreted as a kind of an ***evolutionary algorithm*** [15, 22, 24, 29] for solution of complicated (obviously NP-complete) combinatorial optimization problems. The used model provides a simple mechanism for an explanation of *neutral mutations* and their importance for the Darwinian evolution (see Figs. 14.17 and 14.18). The existence of neutral mutations on the fitness surface is of great importance for overcoming evolutionary traps of local maxima. The Darwinian evolution is divided into long-term neutral stases, where mean fitness of population remains unchanged, but the composition of population strings slowly stochastically wanders towards strings with the possibility of 1-point mutational jumps to strings with greater fitness.

Time orientation of the Darwinian evolution is unambiguous. This is manifested, for example, by the existence of nondecreasing population mean fitness plot. Fitter strings have an evolutionary advantage with respect to other string, they are reproduced more frequently than strings with smaller fitness. In other words, we can say that the Darwinian evolution is a progressive change of mean population genotype such that the corresponding mean fitness is nondecreasing during the whole evolution.

Two different time scales [35] may be distinguished in the Darwinian evolution, in particular adaptive stages and neutral stages. An ***adaptive stage*** corresponds to a sudden change of mean fitness (see Fig. 14.15), where two different phenotypes coexist; old phenotype has a smaller fitness than a new phenotype. Since the probability of replication of strings is proportional to their fitness, strings corresponding to the new phenotype have a greater chance to be reproduced than the old ones. New strings with a greater fitness win in the course of several evolutionary steps; consequently, an adaptive stage, when a string species is substituted by another string species, seems to an external observer as an extremely short evolutionary stage. On the other hand, a ***neutral stage*** of the Darwinian evolution consists in a long-term stasis, where the appearance of neutral mutations stochastically prepares a sudden emergence of the next adaptive stage.

Evolutionary properties of the presented chemostat model are nicely specified by two types of entropies that are introduced for specification of changes in the chemostat composition. The *fitness entropy* reflects composition changes of binary strings with respect to their fitness, i.e. the so-called neutral mutations do not affect this type of entropy. On the other hand, the ***genotype entropy*** is very sensitive to each composition change in the chemostat; consequently, it is affected by neutral mutations. Therefore, their simultaneous observation in the course of evolution allows us to simply distinguish between nonneutral and neutral mutations on the evolutionary trajectories.

What are the ***limits of the present model***? The used forms of genotype and its mapping onto phenotype are extremely simple, they do not reflect more complex organisms other than viruses, bacteriophages, and some prokaryotic bacteria. For complex organism, the model of genotype (and its mapping onto phenotype) must be much more complex, it should take into account such concepts as variable length, hierarchical structure, other mutations than 1-point ones, etc. An important problem of the recent theory of Darwinian evolution is a lack of a theoretical model explaining the emergence of the so-called "*interlocking complexities*" [32] together with a catalytic repertoire of RNA. The present model is unable to explain this problem even on an elementary level. Recent efforts in Artificial Life are concentrated in the areas that might be of importance for elaboration of a more general theory of the Darwinian evolution than the one presented here. In particular, modular aspects of the genotype are recently very intensively studied [40] and the problem of symbiosis is modeled [40]. Both problems require a much more complex genotype than the linear strings of symbols with constant lengths which are studied here.

References

[1] Adami C (1998) Introduction to Artificial Life. Springer, New York
[2] Banatre J-P, Le Metayer D (1990) The Gamma Model and its Discipline of Programming. Sci of Progr 15: 55-77
[3] Banzhaf W (1993) Self-replicating sequences of binary numbers – I. Foundations, Self-replicating sequences of binary numbers – II. Strings of length N=4. Biological Cybernetics 69: 269-281
[4] Banzhaf W (1994) Self-organization in a system of binary strings. In: Brooks R, Maes P (eds) Artificial Life IV. MIT Press, Cambridge, MA, pp 109-119
[5] Banzhaf W, Dittrich P, Eller B (1999) Topological Interactions in a Binary String System. Physica D 125: 85-104
[6] Berry G, Boudol G (1992) The Chemical Abstract Machine. Theoret Comp Sci 96: 217-248
[7] Dennett DC (1995) Darwin's Dangerous Idea - Evolution and the Meaning of Life. Penguin Press, London
[8] Dittrich P (1999) Artificial Chemistries. Tutorial held at ECAL'99, 13-17 September 1999, Lausanne, Switzerland
[9] Dittrich P, Banzhaf W (1998) Self-Evolution in a Constructive Binary String System. Artificial Life 4: 203-220.
[10] Dittrich P, Ziegler J, Banzhaf W (2001) Artificial Chemistries A Review. Artificial Life 7: 225-275

[11] Eigen M (1971) Self-organization of matter and the evolution of biological macromolecules. Naturwissenschaften 58: 465-523
[12] Eigen M, Schuster P (1977) The Hypercycles: A Principle of Natural Evolution. Part A: Emergence of the Hypercycle. Naturwissenschaften 64: 541-565
[13] Eigen M, Schuster P (1978) The Hypercycles: A Principle of Natural Evolution. Part B: The Abstract Hypercycle. Naturwissenschaften 65: 7-41
[14] Eigen M, Schuster P (1978) The Hypercycles: A Principle of Natural Evolution. Part C: The Realistic Hypercycle. Naturwissenschaften 65: 341-369
[15] Fogel DB (1995) Evolutionary Computation. Towards a New Philosophy of Machine Intelligence. IEEE Press, Piscataway, NJ
[16] Fontana W (1991) Algorithmic Chemistry. In: Langton CG (ed) Artificial Life II. Addison Wesley, Reading, MA, pp 159-210
[17] Fontana W, Schnabl W, Schuster P (1989) Physical aspects of evolutionary optimization and adaptation. Phys Rev A 40: 3301:3321
[18] Fontana W, Schuster P (1987) A computer model of evolutionary optimization. Biophys Chem 26: 123-147
[19] Fontana W, Schuster P (1998) Continuity in evolution. On the nature of transitions. Science 280: 1451-1455
[20] Fontana W, Wagner G, Buss L (1994) Beyond digital naturalism. Artificial Life 1: 211-227.
[21] Gillespie DT (1977) Exact Stochastic Simulation of Coupled Chemical Reactions. J Phys Chem 81: 2340-2361
[22] Goldberg DE (1989) Genetic Algorithms in Search, Optimization, and Machine Learning. Addison-Wesley, Reading, MA
[23] Hofstadter D (1979) Dialogues with Gödel, Escher, Bach: An Eternal Golden Braid. Basic Books, Inc, New York, Chapters XVI and XVII
[24] Holland JH (1975) Adaptation in Natural and Artificial Systems. University of Michigan Press, Ann Arbor
[25] Jones BL, Enns RH, Rangnekar SS (1976) On the theory of selection of coupled macromolecular systems. Bull Math Biol 38: 15-28
[26] Kauffman SA (1993) The Origins of Order: Self-Organization and Selection in Evolution. Oxford University Press, New York
[27] Kvasnicka V (2000) An evolutionary model of symbiosis. In: Sincak P, Vascak J (eds) Quo Vadis Computational Intelligence? Physica-Verlag, Heidelberg, pp 293-304
[28] Kvasnicka V, Pospichal J (2003) Artificial Chemistry and Molecular Darwinian Evolution In Silico. Collection of Czechoslovak Chemical Communications 68: 139-177
[29] Mitchell M (1996) An Introduction to Genetic Algorithms. MIT Press, Cambridge, MA.
[30] Monod J (1971) Chance and Necessity. An Essay on the Natural Philosophy of Modern Biology. Vintage, New York
[31] Morris HC (1989) Typogenetics: A logic for artificial life. In: Langton CG (ed) Artificial Life. Addison-Wesley, Reading, MA, pp 369-395

[32] Muller HJ (1939) Reversibility in evolution considered from the standpoint of genetics. Biological Reviews of the Cambridge Philosophical Society 14: 261-280
[33] Newman MEJ, Engelhardt R (1998) Effects of neutral selection on the evolution of molecular species. Proc R Soc London, Ser B, 265: 1333-1338
[34] Schuster P (1996) How does complexity arise in evolution. Complexity 2: 22-30
[35] Schuster P (2002) Molecular insight into evolution of phenotypes. In: Crutchfield JP, Schuster P (eds) Evolutionary Dynamics - Exploring the Interplay of Accident, Selection, Neutrality, and Function. Oxford University Press, Oxford UK (see many Vienna group's citations therein)
[36] Schuster P, Fontana W (1999) Chance and Necessity in Evolution: Lessons from RNA. Physica D, 133: 427-452
[37] Spiegelman S (1971) An Approach to the Experimental Analysis of Precellular Evolution. Q Rev Biophys 4: 213-253
[38] Varetto L (1993) Typogenetics: An artificial genetic system. J Theor Biology 160: 185-205
[39] Varetto L (1998) Studying artificial life with a molecular automaton. J Theor Biology 193: 257-285
[40] Watson RA (2006) Compositional Evolution. The Impact of Sex, Symbiosis, and Modularity on the Gradualist Framework of Evolution. The MIT Press, Cambridge, MA
[41] Wright S (1932) The Roles of Mutations, Inbreeding, Crossbreeding and Selection in Evolution. In: Jones DF (ed) Proceedings of The Sixth International Congress of Genetics, Vol I, pp 356-366. Available at the Internet address http://www.blackwellpublishing.com/ridley/classictexts/wright.pdf.

15

Artificial Chemistry and Molecular Darwinian Evolution of DNA/RNA-Like Systems II – Programmable folding

Marian Bobrik, Vladimir Kvasnicka, and Jiri Pospichal

Institute of Applied Informatics, Faculty of Informatics and Information Technologies, Slovak Technical University, 84216 Bratislava, Slovakia bobrik@cauldron.sk, kvasnicka@fiit.stuba.sk, pospichal@fiit.stuba.sk

Summary: Third simplified model of Darwinian evolution at the molecular level, following the two studied in our previous approach, is studied by applying the methods of artificial chemistry. An artificial-life application is designed as a modification of the metaphor of chemical reactor (chemostat), where the secondary structure of binary strings (RNA-like molecules) specifies instructions for replication of binary strings. It means that a molecular phenotype is interpreted as a computer program for an artificial-life system. Properties of such a system unambiguously demonstrate its capability to model quick evolutionary emergence of replicators – programs that are able of quick and complete replication.

Key words: Artificial life; Artificial chemistry; Fitness landscape; Eigen theory of replicators; Molecular Darwinian evolution; Neutral mutations; Neutral evolution; Typogenetics; strand; replicator; hypercycle; evolutionary method.

15.1 Programmable Folding of RNA-Like Molecules

Typogenetics [12] was the first attempt to create an artificial chemistry system intended to incorporate knowledge of the molecular biology of its time. In the following decades, numerous artificial life systems modeling replication of virtual organisms followed, even surpassed capabilities of typogenetics, which, though capable of reproducing interesting behavior, like self-replicators or hypercycles, is likely not computationally universal [25]. In a generic sense, a replicator can be anything capable of self-replication. Here it means either RNA molecule, or a string - an artificial model of RNA molecule. This string retains basic properties of RNA, which are self-replication capability and mapping of the string at secondary (two-dimensional) structure. Hypercycle is a possible scenario for the origin of self-replicating molecular systems. These systems contain replicating cycles with catalytic feedback loops wherein molecule A begets molecule B which begets molecule C which begets molecule A and so on. "Organisms" in these systems are analogous in their conduct to the so-called "replicator-first" scenarios of origin of life on Earth, since, at least in the beginning, their whole activity consists in production of their copies. The first replicator on Earth is presumed to be RNA, and for its catalytic properties, which are fundamental for replication, its spatial structure is essential. However, no secondary structure is assumed in the virtual organisms of artificial life systems. Their behavior is determined directly by a sequence of symbols, i.e. [1, 14, 18, 22, 24]. A digital organism is typically represented by a sequence of instructions – program, which is then carried out step by step; that feature of digital organism is then more similar to data-processing in classical computer than to functioning of biological systems.

There exist other models simulating evolution and behavior, which are based on computation of secondary structure, but these models do not belong to "classical" systems of artificial life, where computationally universal programs replicate. No system, both computationally universal and at the same time functioning at least roughly analogically to RNA, was designed yet, even though a system in this direction is discussed in [26] or [9].

To fill this gap we designed a system, which decodes genotype into phenotype using a secondary structure. The secondary structure is then interpreted as a program in a system of artificial life. The design of such a phenotype uses a property of secondary structure of RNA, that it can be represented by a root tree in terms of graph theory. This tree can be then used in a tree representation of a program similarly to a representation of programs in evolutionary automatic programming technique called genetic programming. In this way it is possible to create a system of artificial chemistry, in which a sequence of symbols in a chain–molecule does not determine its behavior directly. Instead, similarly to RNA, where a sequence of bases determines its behavior indirectly through its spatial structure, the resulting behavior of the sequence in artificial chemistry is also determined by its secondary structure, which is then interpreted as a program, after inserting some additional information from the chain.

The resulting system thus combines the most suitable properties of conventional artificial life systems, that is, genetic programming and RNA. It allows us to study behavior and evolution of programs working on principles closer to real life forms, than previously existing artificial life systems.

15.2 Source of the Instruction Set

Simple, but efficient system of operators for program tree nodes is derived from an "esoteric" programming language called *brainf..k*. [19], see Table 15.1. Its variant was used in [13], and shown the ability of **"digital abiogenesis" – emergence of a self-replicator among randomly generated programs**. To study this ability, a further reduced system, in which only data processing instructions were preserved, was implemented here. Other instructions were replaced by the instruction N, *nop*, and interaction between programs was completely omitted. This system was then used to test density of self-replicators among all possible programs (maximum program length was limited to 512 instructions due to original system restrictions, so, there are $2^{2048} \doteq 3 \times 10^{616}$ different programs).

It is quite easy to design a self-replicator directly from instruction set. It is only five instruction long program: [<}V**,** which is also the shortest possible replicator. Density of self-replicators among all programs can be measured simply by generating large number of random programs, and determine whether they produce their copies as their output or not. However, for modeling "digital abiogenesis" it is not strictly necessary that a program produces exactly its own copy. It is enough that at least one in the chain of program $P_0 \to P_1 \to .... \to P_n$ will produce one of its progenitors $P_0 \to P_1 \to ... \to P_n \to P_{n+1} \to P_{n+m} \to P_n$, forming a hypercycle like in previous chapter. There has to be also limit for the number of executed instructions, because large portion of the programs ends up in an infinite loop, and, because brainf..k is Turing-complete, there is no way to tell, whether a program will finish or not. So, to obtain a lower bound estimate while keeping computational requirements acceptable, only programs which produced its output after less than 10^4 instructions, and which after one "bootstrapping" run yielded one-step replicator $P_0 \to P_1 \to P_1$ were counted. Even with these restrictions, in 10^7 programs tested, as many as 1 in 62500 programs were self-replicators. This high replicator density means that in a modern computer it is literally a matter of a few seconds, until the first replicator appears among randomly generated programs. All found replicators fall into two categories.

Table 15.1. Instruction set of the simplified brainf..ck based alife

Code	Instruction	Pascal equivalent
0	0	Exit;
1	∨	p := p + 1;
2	∧	p := p - 1;
3	+	a := a + 1;
4	-	a := a - 1;
5	<	a := memory[p];
6	>	memory[p] := a;
7	{	a := io_buffer[p];
8	}	io_buffer[p] := a;
9	[	while a <> 0 do begin
A	]	end;
B	N	
C	X	tmp := memory[pc]; memory[pc] := a; a := tmp; pc := pc + 1;
D	N	
E	N	
F	Z	a := 0; p := 0;

** At the beginning a = F; p = pc = 0; io_bufer, memory are filled with 0.

Typical replicators, whose function is equivalent to above mentioned minimal replicator copy all instructions from the beginning of memory until they encounter some terminating character which in 90% was '0', occasionally 'F', or '1'. They are significantly longer than the minimal replicator (19.25 instructions on average), because most of their instructions do not perform any useful function. The remaining instructions are equivalent to instructions of minimal replicator, except for occasional doubling part of the replication loop before or after the loop (see Fig. 15.1).

Atypical replicators are significantly rarer, only 1 in 22 replicators is atypical, hence the name. While typical replicators copy memory only until they encounter a terminating character, atypical replicator copies the whole memory almost regardless of its content. This functionality was achieved by only two instructions more than the minimal replicator which test whether the next position in io_buffer contains a specific character other than '0', see Fig. 15.2.

15 Artificial Chemistry and DNA/RNA-Like Systems   341

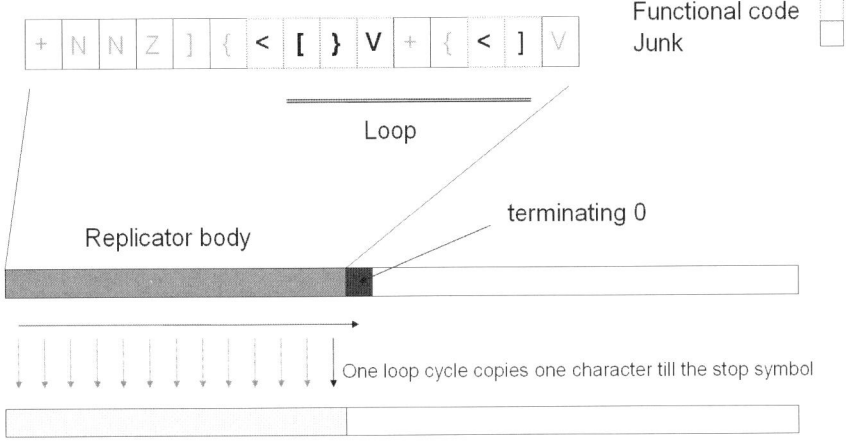

Fig. 15.1. Typical replicator and its function

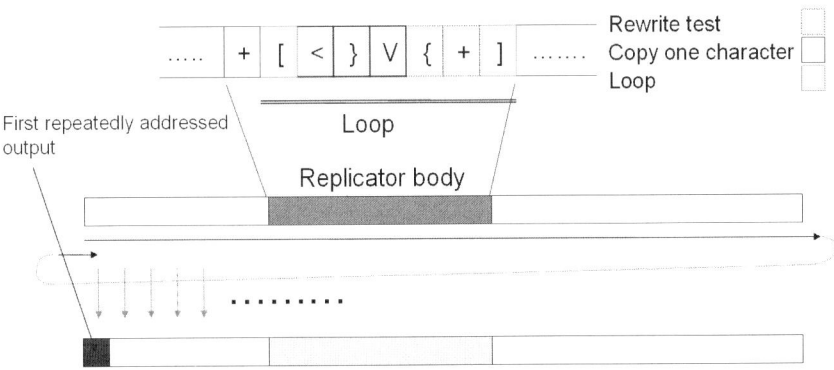

Fig. 15.2. Atypical replicator function

The io_buffer is initialized to '0', so, if it contains anything other, it means that the whole memory has been copied, and the position is being addressed the second time. The replicator however does not test for *any* value different from '0', it looks only for occurence of one specific value (with two instructions it can check only 'v' or 'F'), Thus it copies the part of memory until the first occurence of the tested character twice. So, the "cost" of this sophistication is, that it requires at least two more instructions in the right place, and needs more instructions to copy itself.

In both cases the high chance (compared to traditional programming languages) of a random program to be self-replicator could be attributed to three factors. The first was the small number of instructions necessary for a replicator. The second was large amount of instruction combinations that mutually cancel their effect, like '+-', '∧∨' '∧+∧ − ∨∨', and instructions that overwrite and thus cancel results of previous instructions. Example of such behavior provides a sequence '++{-<' in which the last instruction overwrites A register, and thus eliminates results of all previous instructions. The third factor is that the '0' instruction uniformly distributed through the memory caused the executed part to be relatively short – the average position of first occurrence of '0' which then terminates the program execution in the 16th instruction. Because of this, most random programs were behaviorally identical variants of a relatively few short programs, one of them being the replicator. This caused the high probability of its occurrence.

15.3 Architecture of Programmable RNA System

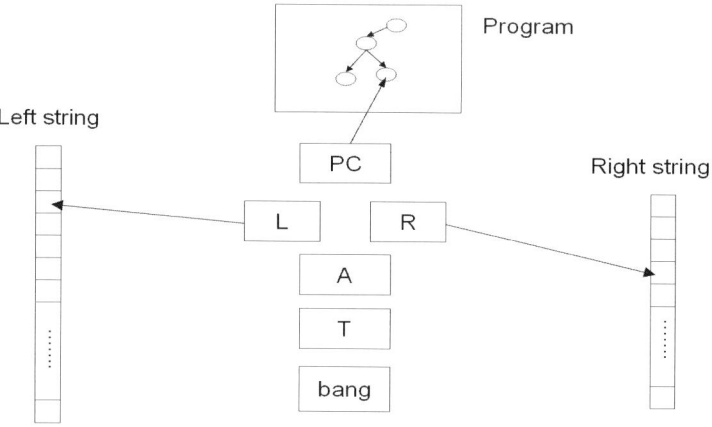

Fig. 15.3. Virtual machine architecture. Program is in the form of a program-tree, the register **PC** points to currently executed command. Two symmetric memories *Left string* and *Right string* are addressed through **L** and **R** registers, **A** register serves as the main target and/or operand for most commands, the complementary register **T** is used only for two-operand commands. The **bang** register is set by an attempt to move **L** or **R** register past memory boundary in either direction, and cleared by successfully executing a *grab* command.

To create a system that combines encoding of a program by secondary structure, and the universality of common instruction-based a-life systems, it would suffice just to assign instructions from previous section to nodes of tree representation of secondary structure.

However, such system would lack two important properties of biomacromolecules. Firstly, interaction with other molecules and secondly, that a real world RNA replicating enzyme always copies other molecules, not directly itself. The original architecture, which contained only output buffer and a directly accessible program memory had thus to be modified. Program memory (its primary structure) is not longer directly accessible, but there are two symmetrical buffers, which the program can use, and read input sequences into them through special commands (react with adjacent molecules, in analogy), or put their content to output (release molecules, in analogy), see Fig. 15.3.

Two more registers were added. The T register, which serves as a complement register to A (for example, loop exit condition may be $A = T$) and the *bang* register, which indicates that one of previous instructions tried to move R or L pointer past memory end or beginning. Another difference is that memory structure is not cyclical – moving pointer past one end does not result into returning it to the other end. It is also impossible to overwrite a location in memory directly, but, on the other hand, it can be manipulated like a string, which can be read, characters can be inserted into it, or deleted. Overwriting can thus be achieved by deleting a character from the string and inserting another one.

Unlike systems, where the sequence of symbols directly represents the program, the primary structure of the currently used strand has to be processed in three steps. First, the secondary structure is computed through dynamic programming as mentioned in previous chapter. It is then converted to a tree representation then, which, together with additional information from the primary structure for special commands, will be then interpreted as the actual program (see Fig. 15.4).

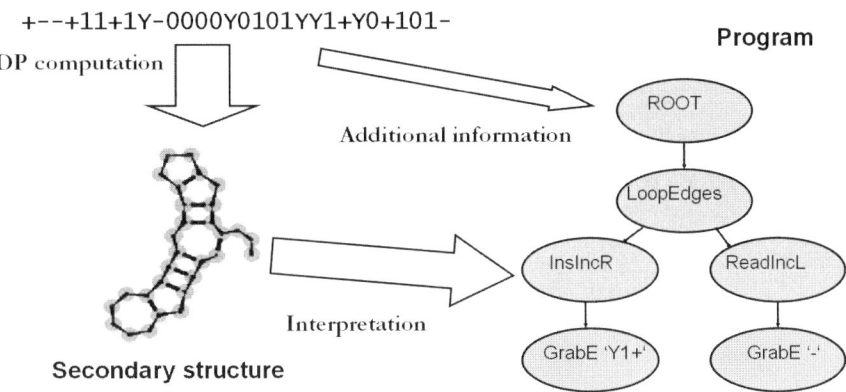

Fig. 15.4. Primary structure => program translation. The program is then executed with both memories empty, L and R registers 0, bang register set to 'false', PC register pointing to initial external loop node ROOT, and A register set to the first symbol of the primary sequence, T register to the last symbol.

For computing the secondary structure, the usual dynamic programming procedure is used [8], resp. [11], with following simple formula for the energy of the molecule

$$V_{ij} = \max \begin{pmatrix} Pair(i,j) + Hp(j-i-1), \\ Vlp(j-i-1) + \max(i < m < j, V_{im} + V_{mj}), \\ Pair(i,j) + V_{i+1,j-1} \end{pmatrix} \quad (15.1)$$

if $i < j$; $V_{ij} = 0$ if $i = j$; and $V_{ij} = -\infty$ for $i > j$, where V_{ij} is the decrease of free energy of substring from ith symbol to jth, in folded state, and $Pair(i,j)$ is pairing energy of ith and jth symbol, $Hp(x)$ is the value of hairpin of length x, $Vlp(x)$ is the value of loop of length x.

This formula is largely simplified in comparison with real RNA secondary structure computation. Only linear approximation for loop and energy is used, and effects like base stacking or dangling ends are omitted. This reduces similarity to real RNA, but this is a necessary compromise with computational power requirements, because of the huge number of strings to be evaluated.

The secondary structure computed by DP is then converted to tree representation, and this is interpreted as a program. The program "language" consists of 46 commands, which are assigned to various secondary structure shapes (see Fig. 15.5 and Table 15.2 and Table 15.3).

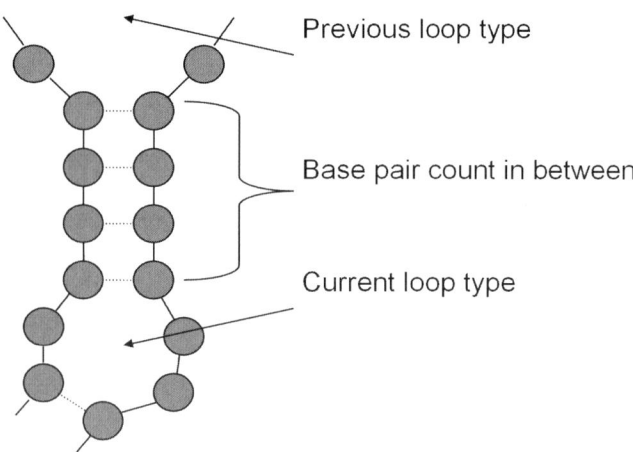

Fig. 15.5. Instruction encoding. Instruction is determined by three parameters. Type of the loop, number of base pairs between current node/loop, and previous loop, and the type of previous loop. Not all instructions are determined by all three parameters

The loop type is determined by the following rules: There are three types of a loop:

All external loops are of the type *Eloop*, Multiloops are *Mloop* and hairpins are *Hairpin*. Types assigned to inner loops and bulges a are described in Table 15.2. (For the classification of RNA secondatry structure shapes, like *Hairpin*, or *Bulge*, see [8])

Table 15.2. Loop types for command determination, LenL and LenR are unpaired base counts in the loop in the direction of reading

Loop type	Condition
BulgeL1	(LenL + 2) / 3 > LenR
BulgeR1	(LenR + 2) / 3 > LenL
BulgeL2	(LenL + 1) * 2 /3 > LenR
BulgeR2	(LenR + 1) * 2 /3 > LenL
Iloop1	(LenR + LenL) mod 4 >= 2
Iloop2	((LenR + LenL) mod 4 < 2

Table 15.3. Commands. Data manipulation instructions in the first part of the table, and flow control instructions below, depend only on current loop type, and base pair number. Special instructions type depend on the previous loop type, and base pair number, and the symbol sequence forming the hairpin loop forms the operand.

	Base pairs between this and previous loop				
Type	1	2	3	4	5
BulgeL1	incL	readIncL	insIncL	delIncL	cutIncL
BulgeR1	incR	readIncR	insIncR	delIncR	cutIncR
BulgeL2	decL	readDecL	insDecL	delDecL	cutDecL
BulgeR2	decR	readDecR	insDecR	delDecR	cutDecR
ILoop1	incA	incT	xchgAT	AtoT	sumAT
ILoop2	decA	decT	ligate	TtoA	sumTA
Mloop	Base pairs between this and previous loop				
	1	2	3	4	
command	loopEdges	loopEdgesM	loopIncA	loopDecA	
	5	6	7		
command	loopIncT	LoopDecT	loopNop		
Hairpin	Previous loop type				
	Eloop	Mloop	BulgeL1	BulgeR1	
command	SetT	SetT	GrabEL	GrabER	
	BulgeL2	BulgeR2	ILoop1	ILoop2	
command	GrabBL	GrabBR	SetA	SetA	

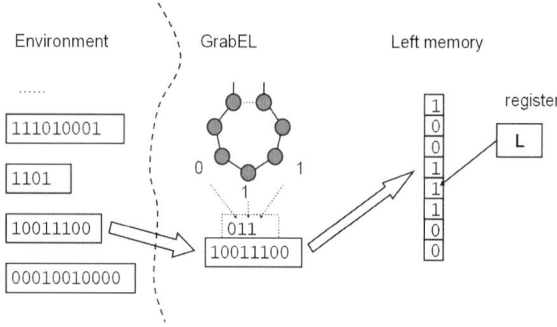

Fig. 15.6. Command grab captures a molecule from the environment, seeking only those which contain subsequence matching the content of their hairpin loop without the first and last base. If none is found, or the memory is already filled with an other string, the command returns as unsuccessful.

Typical operations of commands are shown in Fig. 15.6 and Fig. 15.7. Another main difference from the instruction set in previous section is that pointer movement is joined to memory operation. For example, command *readIncL* reads one symbol from a memory location pointed by L register into A, and subsequently increments L by 1. The reason for this change was to compensate for the increased complexity by simplifying the most often used operations.

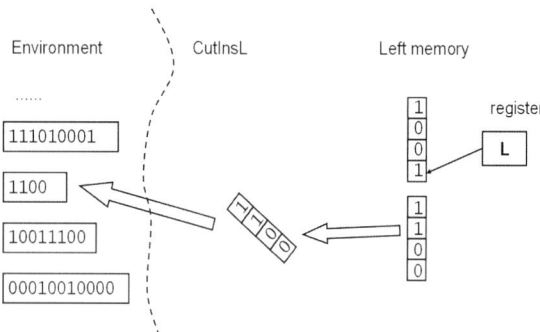

Fig. 15.7. Command cut releases part of the string to environment. Which part stays and which part is released is determined by the Inc/Dec modificator. Inc means that the upper part is released, dec that the lower part is.

15.4 Comparison with the Instruction Based System

To compare "digital abiogenesis" capability with the original instruction-based system in section 15.2, the same test the of density of replicators is performed in the new system. Using the following virtual RNA grammar { 0,1,+,-,Y }, energies of base pairs $E(0\bullet1) = 15$, $E(+\bullet-) = 5$, where $E(x\bullet y)$ denotes the energy decrease for pair $x - y$. Energy per unpaired base in of hairpin Len $> 2 = -1$, otherwise $-\infty$, with following variants given in the Table 15.4.

Table 15.4. Self-replicator density in various encoding variants

Variant	replicators/ 10^7 strings	Avg. len
no change	144	52.5
more than 6 base loops count as *Mloop*	95	50.4
$E(+\bullet Y) = -1, E(-\bullet Y) = -1$	277	61.4
$E(+\bullet Y) = 0.5, E(-\bullet Y) = 0.5, E(+\bullet 0) = 0.25, E(-\bullet 1) = 0.25$	324	58.8

Finding an replicator manually is not as easy as in the reference system, but it is still possible to find out that the shortest self-replicator is 24 symbols long, one of the many strings, which are equivalent to it is "0++Y+Y+Y—0000YYY1Y1111", translating to a program in Fig. 15.8, which can capture and copy itself, and any string beginning with the sequence "0+".

The replicator search is similar but the addition of the environment interaction. The interaction was simplified by supplying a *grab* command with a template for copying if it demanded the appropriate sequence, or an arbitrary string less than 5 symbols, which are considered to be ubiquitous in the 'prebiotic soup'. The program run is limited by a 10^4 instruction limit, and if the program releases two strings identical to the template, it is counted as a self-replicator, though technically it replicates other strings, rather than directly itself. As the Table 15.4 shows, even if the minimal replicator length increased nearly fivefold, and the average replicator length 2.5 to 3 times, and the rules of the sequence => function mapping were more complex, replicator density in the worst variant is only 40% smaller, and in the best it even increased by 50%. So, the instruction "transplant" from a conventionaly determined program to a program determined by the secondary structure can be considered successful.

ROOT :
    LoopEdges :
        ReadIncL
            GrabEL 'textbf+'
            InsIncR
        GrabER 'textbfY'

Fig. 15.8. Translated minimal replicator. At first, the program goes inside the *LoopEdges* loop, because the *bang* register is not set. Unsuccessfully attempts to read, by now empty, *Left* string. The *GrabEL* '+' command then captures a string containing a '+', and sets the L pointer to it. *InsIncR* then inserts to *Right* the symbol contained in A, which at the beginning is initialized to '0'. *GrabER* is thus always unsuccessful. In the next cycle of LoopEdges, the symbol at which L points is read into A by *ReadIncL* , and inserted at the end of R by *InsIncR* , moving both registers to the next symbol. The cycle repeats until the last symbol is read. Then, because of the bang register set, the *LoopEdges* loop ends, and with it the whole program. Both left and right strings are then released.

15.5 Replicator Evolution by Artificial Selection

As an in silico analog to attempts to evolve in vitro a self-replicator from real RNA, i.e. [17], the experiment described by Fig. 15.9 was created.

At the beginning of the simulation, the chemostat is empty, and slowly fills with random influx strings, and after reaching maximum capacity, for each new string, one random string is deleted, so population size remains constant. Pairs of strings are chosen at random and tested for fitness, and with probability proportional to the fourth power of their fitness are duplicated with a small (p = 0.01/ per symbol) chance of point mutation - change, insertion or deletion.

Fitness is evaluated by test of the string replicator capability, in which one of the string pair, $S_{passive}$, served as the replicated one, and the other, S_{active}, as the replicating one. Similarly to the previous search for a replicator in random strings, the *grab* command returns $S_{passive}$ if there is a match, the demanded sequence, if it is shorter than 5 characters, and 0 otherwise. S_{out} are strings released as a result of the reaction. The fitness is then defined as

- *Fit = 0*, if the program did not execute *grab* command on $S_{passive}$ (such program is considered inert)
- *Fit = 0*, if S_{out} is empty (the program destroyed its input)
- If the minimal difference between a string in S_{out} to $S_{passive}$, D_{min} is not zero, *Fit = 0.5 / (1 + D_{min})*, because the program damaged the original string
- if $D_{min} = 0$ and S_{out} has only one member, *Fit = 0.5* (the program neither copied, nor damaged the string)
- if $D_{min} = 0$, and S_{out} has at least two members, then *Fit = 0.5 * (1 + 1 / (1 + D_{min2}))*, where D_{min2} is the second smallest difference between a string in S_{out} and $S_{passive}$ (the imperfect replicator)

- if $D_{min} = 0$, $D_{min2} = 0$, then $Fit = 1$ (the final replicator)

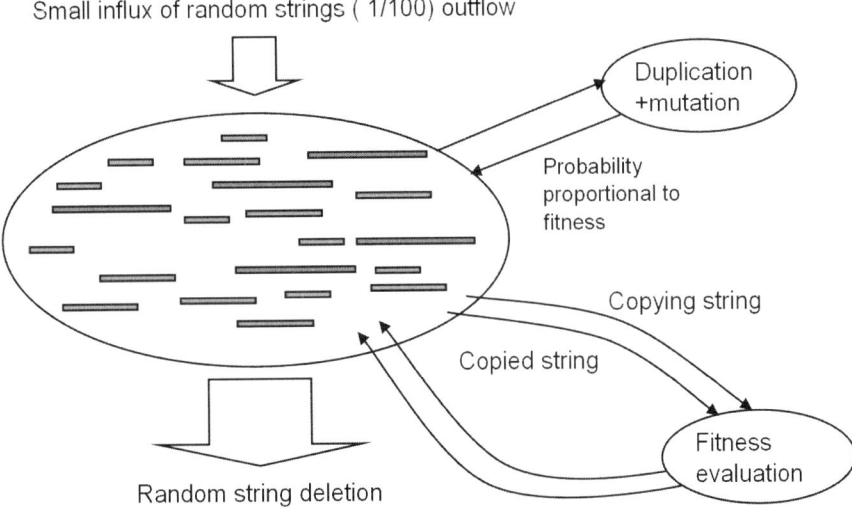

Fig. 15.9. Replicator evolution scheme. Strands are rewarded by fitness only for copying accurately, and being copied accurately.

Total fitness of a string is defined then as

$$Fitness = \sqrt{\frac{\sum Fit_{active} \sum Fit_{passive}}{Cnt_{active} Cnt_{passive}}} \qquad (15.2)$$

where Fit_{active} is fitness in replication test where the string was S_{active}, $Fit_{passive}$ is fitness in replication test where the string was $S_{passive}$, Cnt_{active} the number of tests, where the string was S_{active}, $Cnt_{passive}$ the number of tests, where the string was $S_{passive}$, The aim of this fitness function is that a string to be considered successful should both copy other strings accurately, and be easily copied by all other strings. A string that is good at copying other strings but itself can not be copied, is as useless, as a string which can not copy at all.

15.5.1 The behavior of the System

Following Fig. 15.10 and Fig. 15.11 show a typical behavior of the system. The simulation after roughly 500000 steps always ends in a state where most of the chemostat consists of self-replicators, and the rest are various mutants with significantly decreased fitness; their share of population keeps constant because of rather high mutation rate. Clearly visible is the initial stasis when during 200000 steps the best strand could only capture other strand without modification.

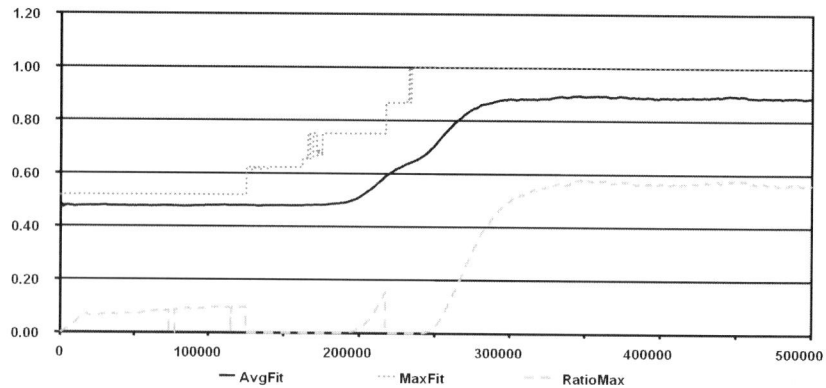

Fig. 15.10. Average and maximum fitness and concentration of the replicators with maximum fitness

Rapid evolution occurred after 220000 steps, when improved strands first arose, and were relatively quickly displaced by even better ones until after 280000 the first 100% replicator appeared, displaced other strands, and remained the dominant molecule until the end of the simulation.

Fig. 15.12 shows all ancestor sequences of the final replicator, from the initial random string, at the beginning of the simulation, to one of its ancestors with fitness

= 1 at the end of the simulation. Only 6 mutations separate the replicator from the initially completely passive molecule, 5 symbol changes, and one deletion. Three times the point mutation induced a major change in the secondary structure (strand 1 to 2, 3 to 4, and 4 to 5), twice a local modification occurred (between 2 and 3, and 5 and 6), the last mutation (6 to 7) was neutral. This means, that both radical rearrangements of the secondary structure, and changes that correspond to local code changes only, even though they happen through a complicated primary to secondary structure mapping, played a role in the evolution of the replicator.

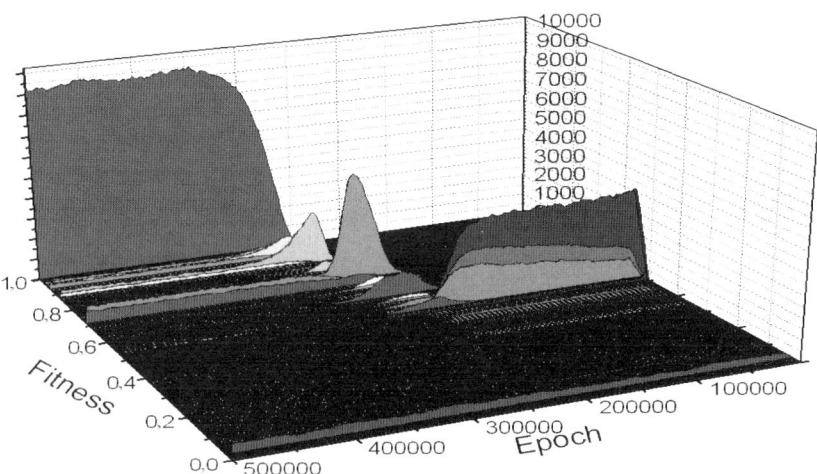

Fig. 15.11. Distribution of fitness during the evolution. Initial population of inert strings on the right is replaced in a brief period of rapid evolutionary 'experimentation' by the final replicator.

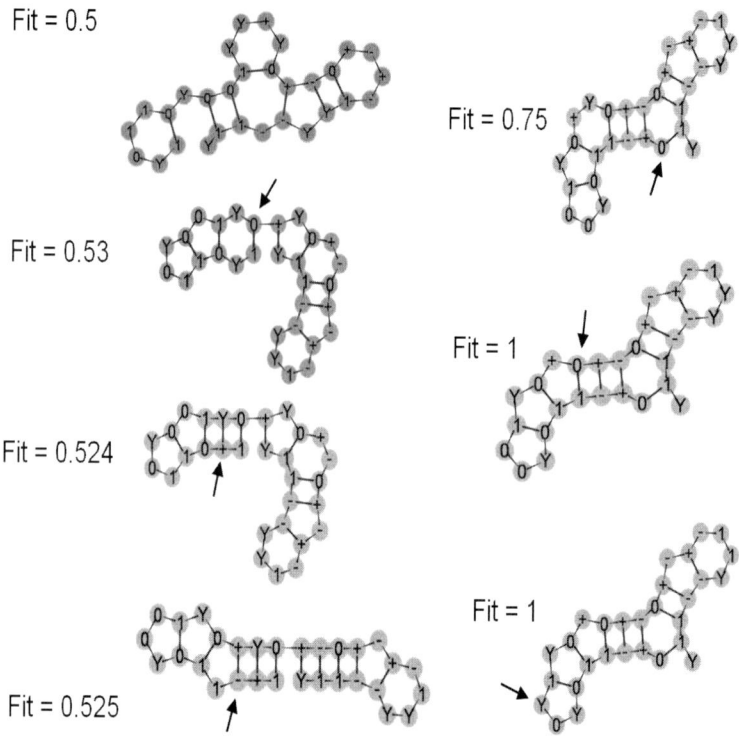

Fig. 15.12. The evolution of the replicator. An arrow marks mutations.

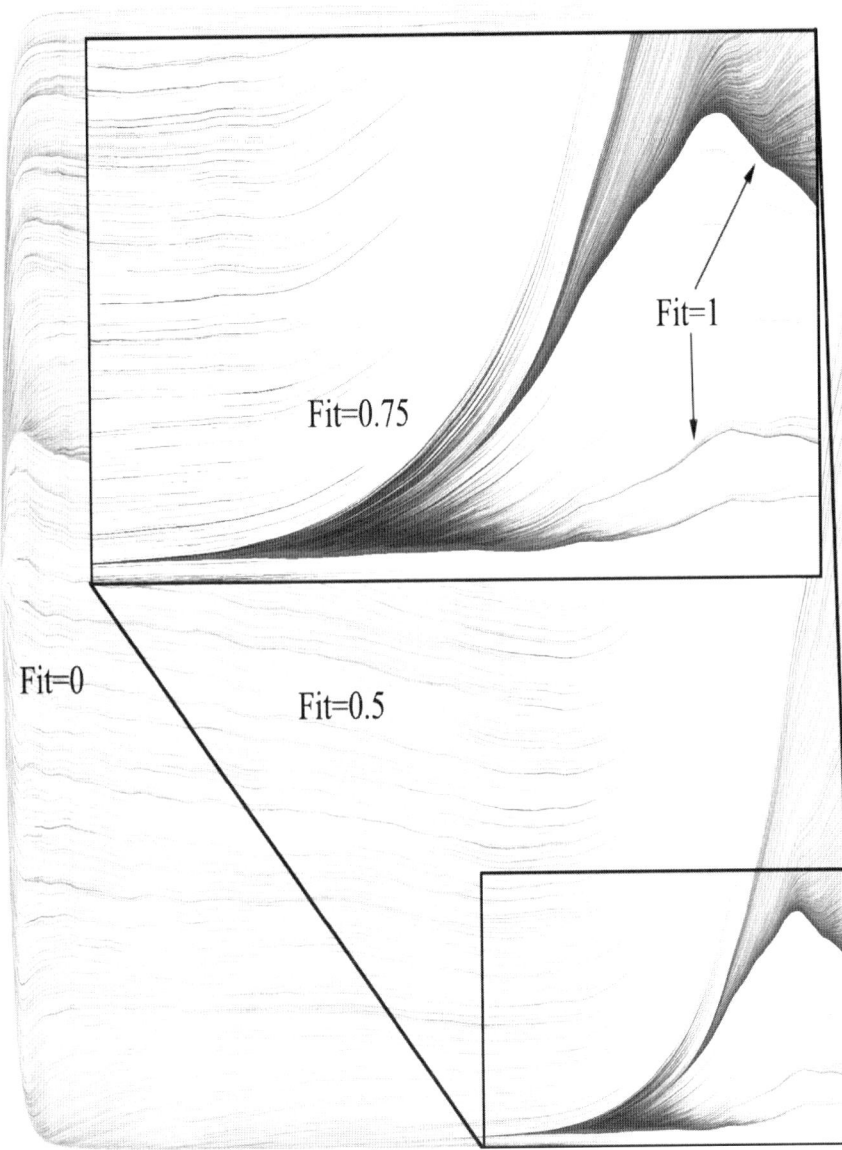

Fig. 15.13. Genealogy tree of the chemostat population. Most strands belong to one of four groups; inert strands with Fit = 0 are marked yellow, and were common only at the beginning. Passive strands that dominated the chemostat during the static phase with Fit = 0.5, are red. Imperfect replicators which originate from one ancestor, and expand exponentially until their successor emerges, with Fit = 0.75 are blue. Finally, replicators capable of perfect copying, which dominate the chemostat at the end, with Fit = 1, are colored green.

An alternative to a representation of the evolution in the chemostat shown as a fitness plot changing in time, like in Fig. 15.10, is to directly visualize the entire history of the chemostat in a form of a genealogy tree of all strands, which is shown in Fig. 15.13. In this form, details of the evolution are far better visible. Initial filling of the chemostat, disappearance of unsuitable random strands, a phase of neutral evolution, appearance of the first imperfect replicator, its spread and decline of the original population. Details, which would be hidden in other representations, become visible – both imperfect replicators, and their successor appeared long before their biggest expansion, and during their decline, one of the imperfect replicators gave rise to a new, separate lineage of full replicators. (the smaller, separate fit = 1 line).

15.5.2 String Splitting

A common function which ribozymes perform in vivo is cleaving other RNA at a specific place. To check, how strong the intended analogy between the real RNA, and this system is, the chemostat can be modified so, that the fitness is dependent on the capability of the strand to split an input sequence correctly. The input string S_{in} consists of a "-+-" tag and random sequence of '0' and '1' 7 to 33 characters long. Approximately in the middle is an 'Y' symbol, which marks the desired cleavage site. The input string should be cut in two S_{lo} and S_{hi} just before it, see Fig. 15.15.

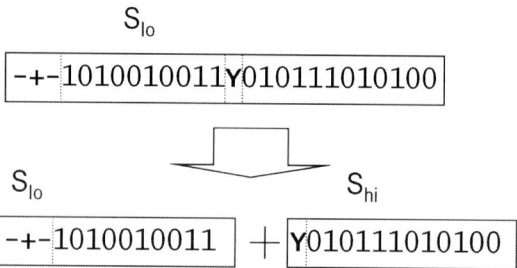

Fig. 15.14. A string splitting example. The string marked by initial tag "-+-" should be cut into two pieces in the place marked by "Y"

The fitness Fit is then defined as

- Fit = 0, if the program did not execute *grab* command on S_{in}, or performed it more than once
- Fit = 0, if the program did not produce any output
- If it produced only one output, Fit = 0.5 / (1+D_{lo} + D_{hi}), where D_{lo}, resp. D_{hi} is difference between it and S_{lo}, resp. S_{hi}.
- If it produced two outputs, Fit = 1 / (1+D_{lo} + D_{him}), where D_{lom}, resp. D_{him} is the difference of the closest output to S_{lo}, resp. S_{hi}.

- If it produced more than two outputs, $Fit=0.9/(1+D_{lom}+D_{him})$, where D_{lom}, resp. D_{him} is the difference of the closest output to S_{lo}, resp. S_{hi}.

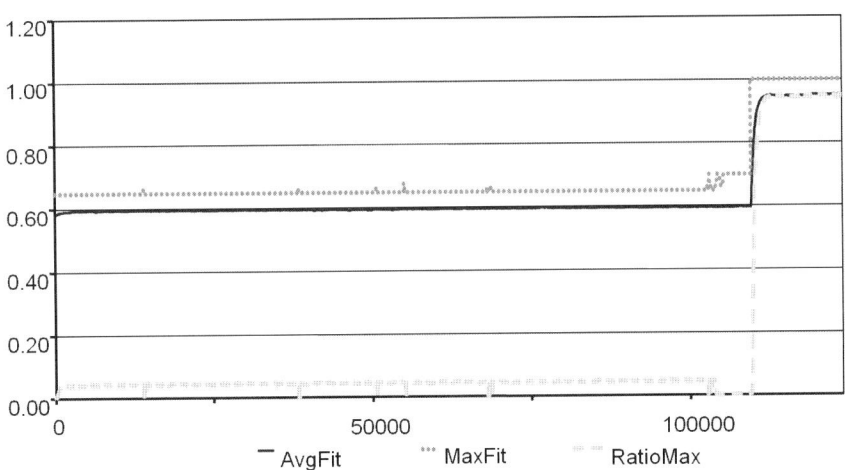

Fig. 15.15. Average and maximum fitness and concentration of the programs with maximum fitness.

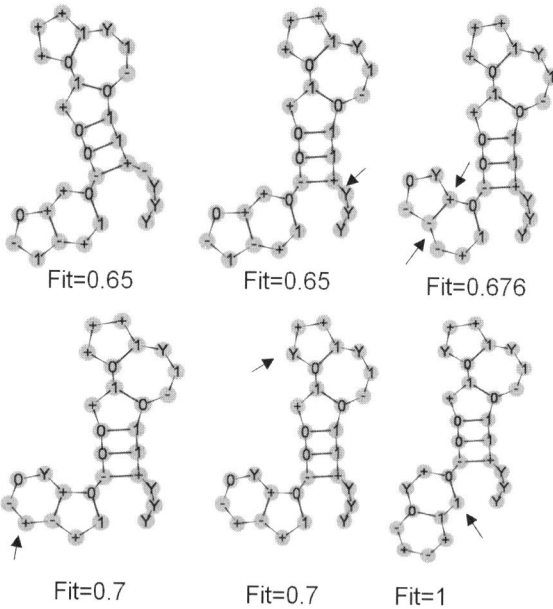

Fig. 15.16. Distribution of fitness during evolution. The transition from initial imperfect program, to final is almost instantaneous.

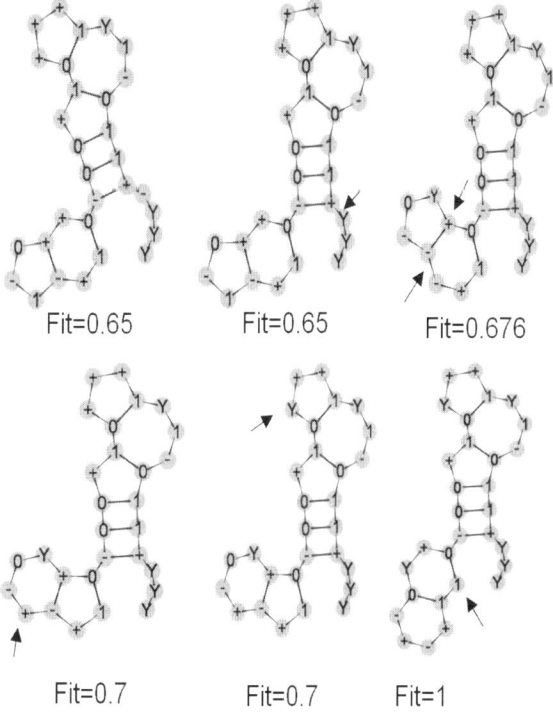

Fig. 15.17. The evolution of the string-spliting program. An arrow marks mutations.

The results of a typical execution of the program are shown in Fig. 15.15, Fig. 15.16, Fig. 15.17 and Fig. 15.18. As it is visible from the shorter time until the programs with fitness 1 take over the replicator, the strand suitable for this task is substantially simpler to evolve than a replicator is. Even among the first strands, there were some with fitness 0.65, and after half the time it took to evolve a replicator, the first strand with fit = 0.7 appeared, quickly evolving into the final program.

Fig. 15.17 shows, that only four non-neutral mutations were required to transform an original random string into a functional sequence splitting program, and no radical change of the secondary structure was needed. Although this behavior was not originally planed or expected, similarly to the real RNA, accurate cutting of other molecules is an easier task than duplicating them.

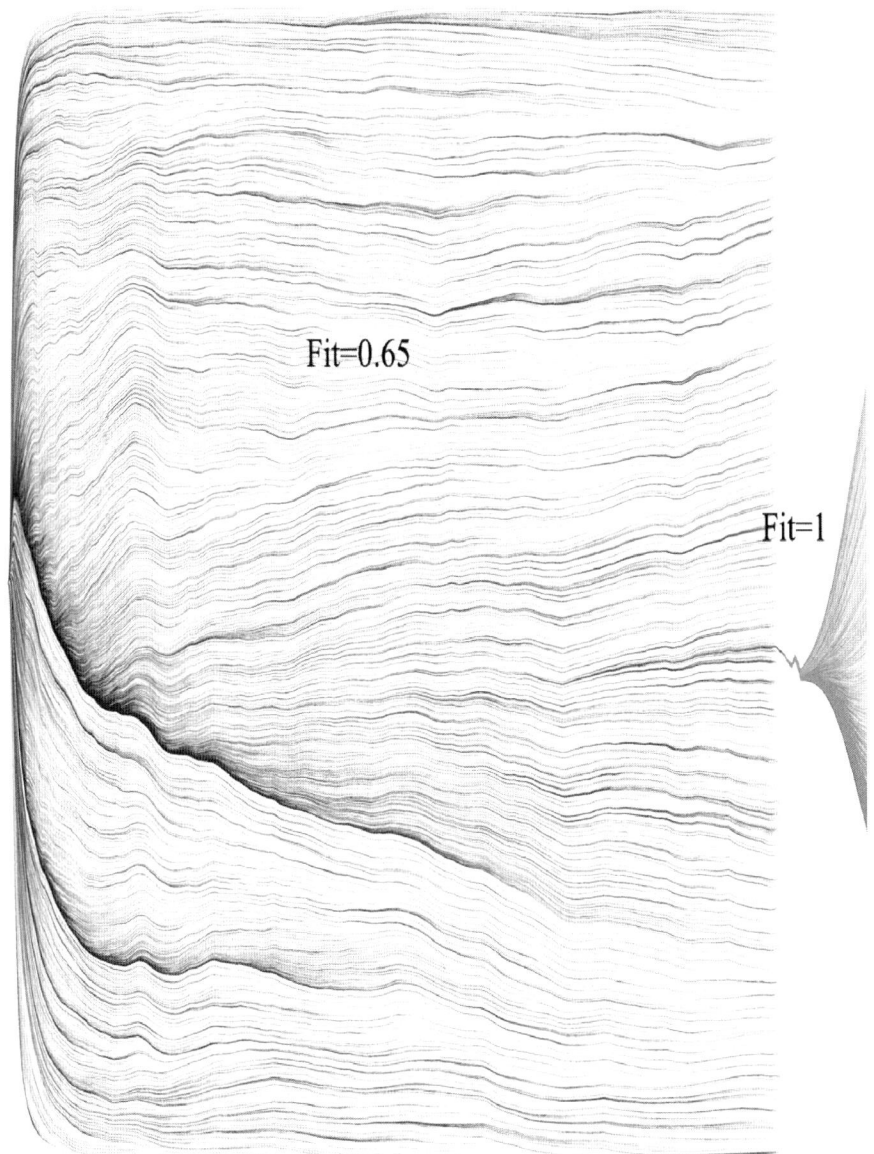

Fig. 15.18. The genealogy tree of the chemostat population. Fit = 0.65 violet, Fit = 1 green.

15.6 The Chemostat

The strands in the previously described cases had one shortcoming as models of replicators. These strands did not replicate by themselves; they were duplicated according to their fitness, which was correctly maximum in the case of a true replicator, but which also reached non-zero values in the case, when the replicator produced at the output other strand than itself. This last property would not be feasible, if the replication were wholly in competence of replicators themselves, i.e. the contents of the chemostat would depend, save the influx and outflux, only on the kinds of produced and used strands during their mutual interactions, see Fig. 15.19.

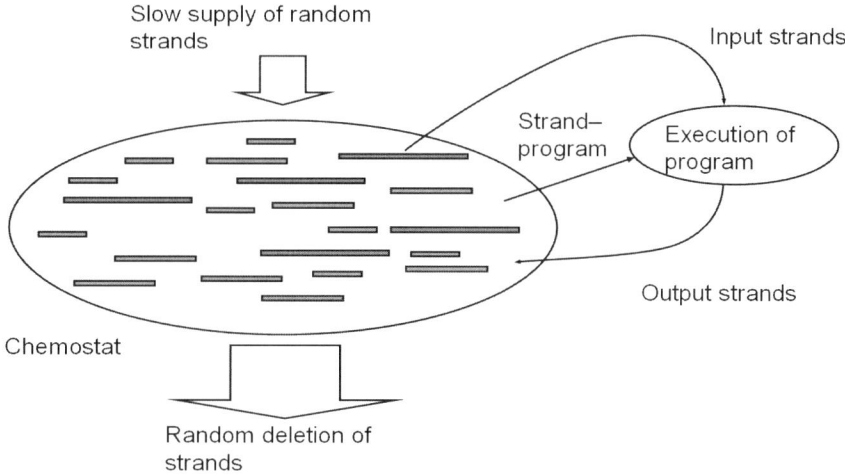

Fig. 15.19. Chemostat without external fitness. The only source of new strings, besides the input are reactions between strands.

In the case of "real" self–replication of molecules inside the chemostat, the result of the imperfect replicator would be an increase of concentration values of other strands, not of the imperfect replicator. The fitness of the imperfect replicator would be thus zero, the same as the fitness of an inert strand. The exception would be of course in a situation, when the products of the strand would be in the next reactions transformed onto the original strand, thus creating a hypercycle. However, also in this case the single steps - reactions of hypercycle must produce each strand, from which the hypercycle is composed, otherwise the whole cyclic reaction network would stop.

The emergence of a true replicator by a gradual selection of incorrect, but progressively improving replicators is therefore not feasible. The first replicator, whether it is one molecule, or a hypercycle, must appear in the chemostat complete right away, without flaws. Since the replicators in our system are represented among randomly generated strands in a relatively high proportion (about one in 30 000), the outright appearance of replicator should not be a major hindrance.

15.6.1 Perfectly Mixed Chemostat

A more serious issue than a random appearance of replicator is the fact, that the system was designed in such a way, that a replicator can never make a copy of itself directly, but it can only copy another molecule. If this molecule, which is copied, is identical to the replicator copying it, the result of the reaction are three identical molecules–products from the initial two molecules–reactants. However, if the other molecule, which is copied, is different from the replicator, the replicator makes a copy of this other molecule, not a copy of itself. It is true, that the functionality of the command Grab ensures, that only those strands–molecules will be duplicated, that contain the corresponding substring. However, there still exist a great number of strands–molecules that can free-ride replication, while the majority of these strands does not help the replicator to create its copy. These strands–molecules therefore act as parasites.

In the case, that the system will be simplified to contain only two kinds of substances, replicators R, and parasites P, the dynamics of the chemostat without spatial structure can be approximated by equations

$$\dot{R} = R(R(1-R-P) - Outf) + In_R \quad \dot{P} = P(R(1-R-P) - Outf) + In_P \quad (15.3)$$

where R is the concentration of the replicator, P is the concentration of the parasite, $Outf$ is the outflux from the chemostat and In_R, resp. In_P is the influx of the random strands, which are either replicators or parasites. The inequality $Outf > In_R + In_P$ holds, since some of the strands are inert and $In_P > In_R$. Any equilibrium state in chemostat must satisfy the following condition

$$\frac{R}{P} \approx \frac{In_R}{In_P} \quad (15.4)$$

From the formula follows that in a chemostat without a spatial structure, which is allowed to evolve into an equilibrium, the replicators will not appear more often than among randomly generated strands.

15.6.2 Chemostat with Spatial Structure

In [4] the authors suggested to solve the problem of parasites (i.e. free–riders on replication) by taking into account also the spatial distribution of molecules in a chemostat. This should provide an advantage for replicators, since when only local interactions are allowed, the number of parasites interacting with a replicator will decrease. This also means, that areas with locally highest concentration of replicators tend to expand into the neighborhood at the expense of the areas with lower concentration. The result is a dynamic equilibrium, which allows the replicator to keep high concentration in chemostat despite the presence of parasites, similarly to [26].

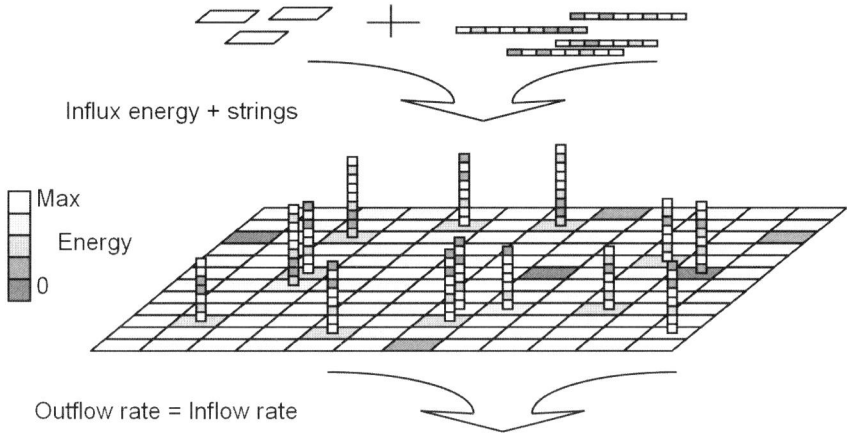

Fig. 15.20. Unstirred chemostat without external fitness. The spatial structure is a 2D grid, each cell can have at most one strand in it, and has an 'energy' – property representing the nutrient concentration in it, which is depleted by strand reactions. The influx and outflow are realized by overwriting cells at random by new energy and content.

The spatial structure used here is a 2D grid with a toroidal topology, where each square can be either empty, or occupied by exactly one replicator–strand. Each square has also one integer value – energy, which determines, how many instructions can carry out a program placed on the square, see Fig. 15.20. The neighborhood is defined by supremum metric, with neighborhood size 1, resp. 2, which means 8, resp. 24 squares in the neighborhood.

One step of the simulation means, that one of the following operations is carried out

Influx: a random square is chosen. If it is already occupied by a strand, this will be deleted, the energy of the square will be set to *MAX* value, and with a probability *Pin* it will be occupied by a random string, which will be also copied to a random neighboring square, otherwise the square will be left empty[1].

Mutation: a random square is chosen. If it is already occupied by a strand, this strand will undergo a small random change, and the energy of the square will increase by a small value *Emut*.

Diffusion: a random square will be chosen, and its content will be swapped with a content of another randomly chosen square from its neighborhood.

---

[1] Any replication needs at least two molecules close enough for mutual interaction. Without providing another, neighboring, molecule by the Influx operation, the replication would start only if at least two suitable molecules would happen to be neighbors, which is unlikely, and thus the period of initial "static" state without a replicator would be extremely prolonged. Without provision of the second molecule by the Influx operation the replicator emerged in average after 2.4×10^7 Influx operations, which decreased to 1.7×10^4 Influx operations when 2 neighboring molecules were deposited.

Execution: a random square will be chosen, and if it contains a string, it will be interpreted as a program.

The execution of the program is identical to the previous experiments, except for the instructions *Grab* and *Release* which work only within the neighborhood of the square with the active strand: If *Grab* finds among neighboring strands a strand, which contains the corresponding sequence, this strand will be processed by the currently active program, and the square of the processed string will be marked as empty. If the active program carries out the instruction *Release*, the newly created string will be deposited onto a randomly chosen square from the neighborhood. However, *Release* takes into account priorities of the states of the neighboring squares. Random selection is restricted only to the squares with the highest priorities from the neighborhood:

- The highest priority, A, have squares emptied by the instruction Grab. Without this rule the strands would through their interaction artificially increase diffusion.
- The priority B is assigned to empty squares with a non-zero energy; this rule decreases the destructivity of the strand for its neighborhood.
- The priority C is assigned to occupied squares with a non-zero energy. If the new strand is placed onto an already occupied square, the old strand is deleted.
- The lowest priority D is given to squares with zero energy level.

During the run of the program defined by the strand, the energy from its square is consumed. A small amount of energy is consumed even before the initialization of the program, the aim of this rule is to shorten a lifespan of inert strands in comparison with active ones. Then each instruction consumes one unit of energy, and when the energy level reaches zero, the run of the program is terminated, similarly to a regular termination of the program. One of the four operations mentioned above is chosen randomly at each step, with probabilities $Pin = 0.05$, $Pmut = Pdif = 0.01$; the size of the grid was in all experiments equal 128 x 128 squares.

15.6.3 Replicator Spatial Structures

The behavior of the system is characterized by two phases and a sudden switch between them. After the initialization, a variably long phase of stasis follows, when the chemostat does not contain any molecule, which would be able to influence more substantially the reactions in the chemostat. This phase in average takes 230 000 operations, which for the fixed probabilities of single operations corresponds to an influx of 17000 strands of possible replicators. This phase terminates at the moment, when the first replicator, which succeeds to reproduce, appears in the chemostat. After that, short-time expansion follows, which ends, when the replicator becomes the dominant molecule in the system. Then the second phase follows, characterized by a cyclic oscillation of concentration of the replicator, and by randomly occurring local "epidemics" of parasitic molecules. In the case of epidemics, short-lived spiral spatial structures appear in the chemostat, rotating around its center, though their appearance is strongly deformed by the high level of mutations, by influx of new strands, and the inherent instability induced by nonlinear replication rate. Such structures have been already described in other experiments with replicator + parasite systems.

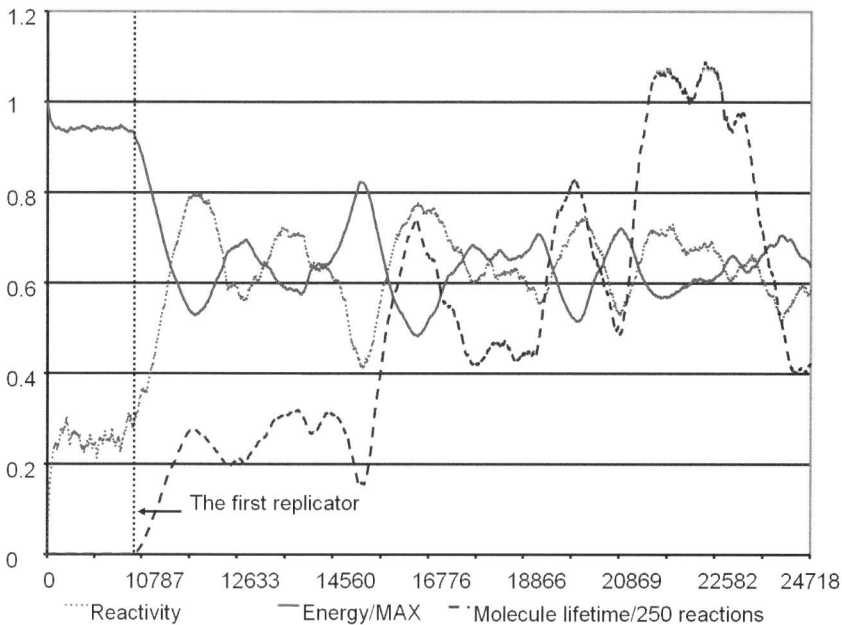

Fig. 15.21. The average values of energy, number of realized reactions per molecule, and average life-span of a molecule. Emergence of the first replicator is marked by a dotted vertical line. Prior to it is the abiotic phase characterized by energetic equilibrium, low reaction rates and short molecule lifetime to reaction number ratio. After the emergence of the replicator, and its initial spread, all values start fluctuate erratically, as dynamic spatial structure forms and persists.

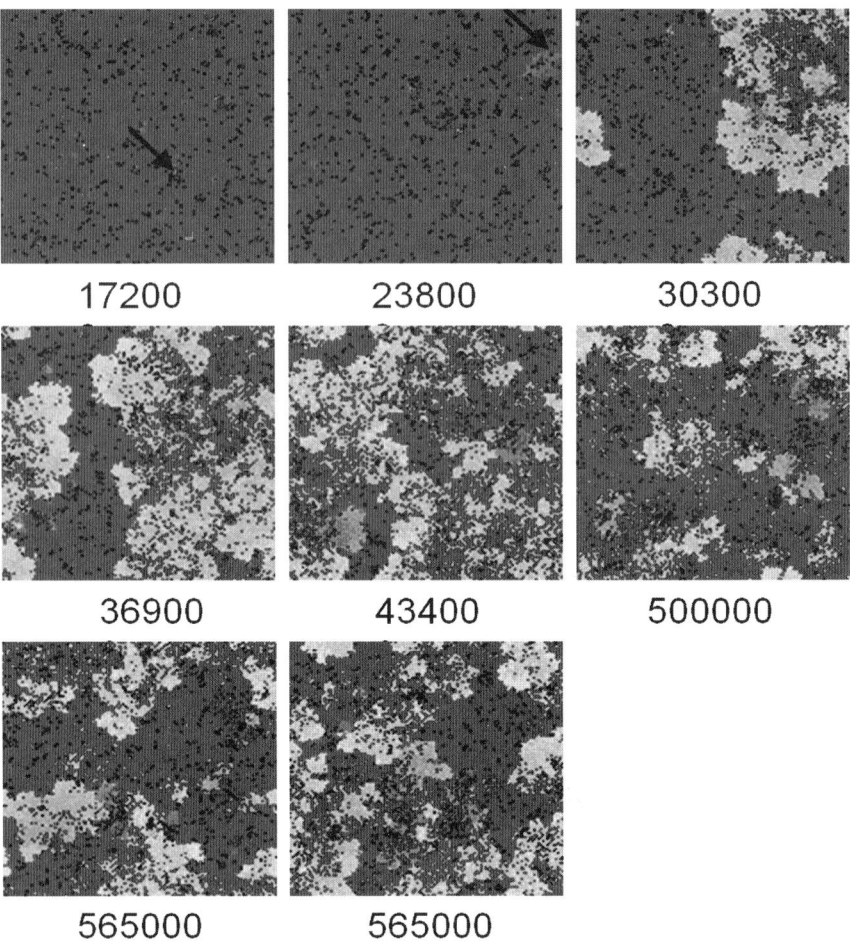

Fig. 15.22. The contents of the chemostat during the simulation. Blue are free cells with energy, cyan are molecules with energy that have undergone many replication cycles, green the same, but running out of energy, red are active molecules that had only a few reactions. And black are empty cells without energy.

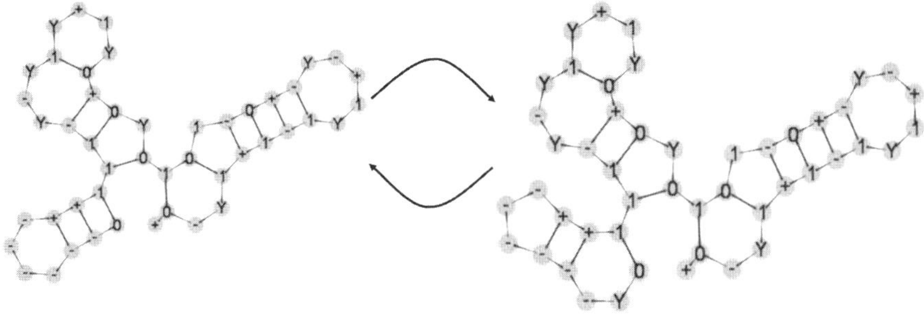

Fig. 15.23. Unstable hypercycle persisting only 10 cycles because running out of energy.

The average values of energy, reaction frequency, and lifespan of a molecule in Fig. 15.21 show, that during the initial phase the majority of molecules is either inert, or capable at most to carry out limited reactions with their neighboring molecules (see Fig. 15.23). An example can be seen in an unstable reaction marked by an arrow in the first square of the Fig. 15.22, which clung on in the chemostat for ten steps, and then expired. The second square of the Fig. 15.22 shows the initial appearance of the replicator, which eventually filled in the whole chemostat, but later on was superseded by more effective replicators, which endured till the end of simulation, i.e. till the 2^{21} = 2087152th step (see Fig. 15.24).

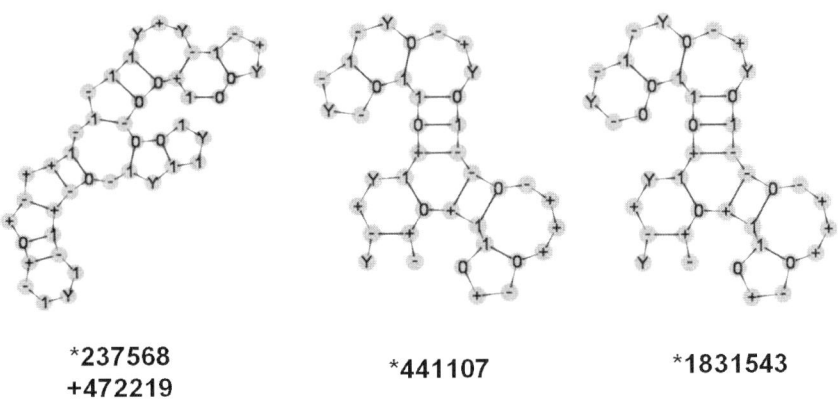

*237568
+472219

*441107

*1831543

Fig. 15.24. Three most numerous replicator swith a time of formation, and disappearance, if they did not last till the end of the run.

All of the simulations, which were carried out, had a similar course; the main difference between them was in the duration of the initial abiotic phase until the first formation of a replicator. Neither a stable hypercycle, nor other type of replicator than a "classic" replicator appeared during any of the simulations. Its formation would be very unexpected anyway, since the system was designed with a goal to facilitate a formation of a one-molecular replicator.

15.6.4 The Mechanism of Resistance against Parasites

In order to clarify the mechanism of resistance against parasites, we shall simplify again the system to contain only 2 kinds of molecules – replicator R and parasite P, and to their mutual interactions:

$R + R \Rightarrow R^- + 2R$ (replication)
$R + P \Rightarrow R^- + 2P$ (parasitism)
$R + R + P \Rightarrow R^- + 2R$ (replacement of parasite by replicator)
$R + R + P \Rightarrow R^- + 2P$ (replacement of replicator by parasite)
$P \Rightarrow P^-$ (degradation of parasite)
and another 2 reactions, equivalent to a degradation of replicator
$R + 2P \Rightarrow R^- + 2P$ (replacement of parasite by parasite)
$R + 2R \Rightarrow R^- + 2R$ (replacement of replicator by replicator)
$R + R \Rightarrow R^- + R + P$
$R + 2R \Rightarrow R^- + R + P$
$R + R + P \Rightarrow R^- + R + P$

The symbols R^-, resp. P^- signify consumption of energy.

The energy used for reactions $R + R$, $R + P$ and $P \Rightarrow P^-$ is set identical to the energy consumption of a replicator from the previous part, so that the behavior should be comparable. The random influx was restricted in this model only to energy, and the size of the chemostat was enlarged to 512×512. In order to keep the scale of the processes, the coefficient of diffusion was also enlarged four times.

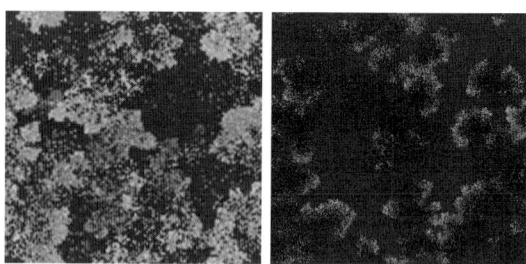

Fig. 15.25. (**Left**) a typical two-dimensional structure of the original system (**Right**) a typical two-dimensional structure of the approximation of the system with only replicator and parasite molecules (color coding is different).

It is apparent from Fig. 15.25, that the dynamics of the spatial structure remained practically untouched by this simplification to only 2 kinds of molecules. In both cases the activity is concentrated in unstable waves of "U" resp. "C" shape. At the outer edge of these waves are active replicators, which expand into empty space. In the opposite direction toward inside of the wave, the concentration of other molecules increases, and activity of replicators gradually decreases, until the process finishes by a local exhaustion of energy, and molecules are gradually erased by a process of adding energy to chemostat.

Since the replication is proportional to a square power of concentration of the replicator, the waves are unstable. When the wave spreads into the empty space, random fluctuations of concentration of a replicator at its outer edge are amplified faster than their diffusion can compensate, so that in the places with a lower concentration the replicator is soon entirely replaced, and their expansion stops, until the places with a higher concentration expand forward and sideways, and become the sources of the subsequent waves (see Fig. 15.28).

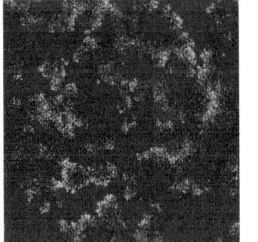
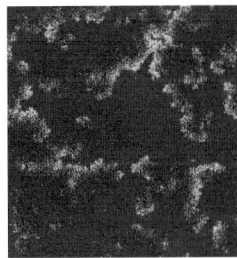
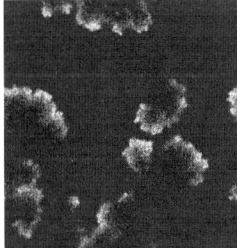

Fig. 15.26. The state of the chemostat for different values of probability of mutation of a replicator into a parasite.

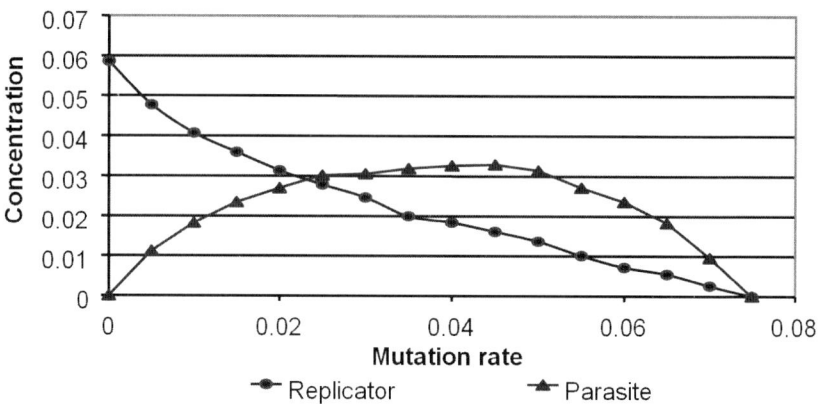

Fig. 15.27. Average concentrations of replicator and parasite plotted against probability of mutation of replicator into parasite.

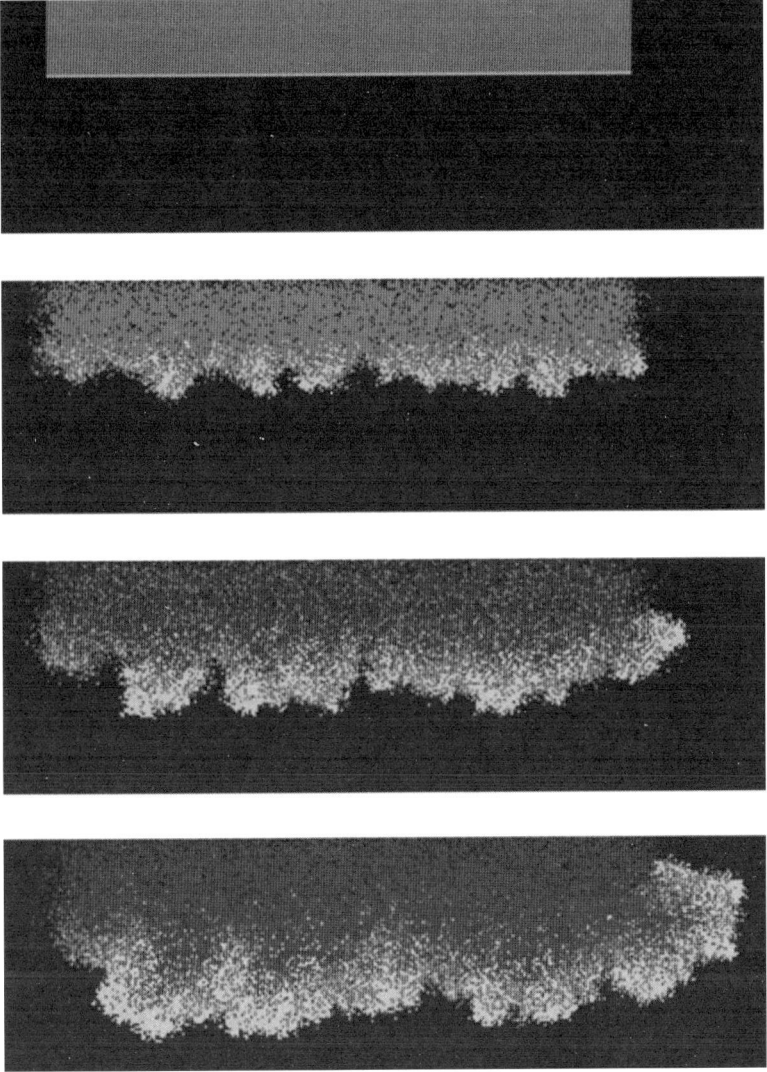

Fig. 15.28. The instability of the front of the wave of replicators. Replicators are green, parasites red; to increase contrast the squares with full energy load are black and squares with exhausted energy are blue (which is inverse to the coloring in the Fig. 15.25).

This phenomenon also limits a tolerance of replicators to parasites, since the probability of encountering parasites determines the limit, which must the density of replicator exceed in order to grow autocatalytically. This also determines a density of new sources of waves, and consequently the overall concentration of replicator in the chemostat (see Fig. 15.26 and Fig. 15.27).

The introduction of energy consumption within the chemostat proved necessary to maintain replicator presence in chemostat. It follows from the equation below, that locally the concentration $R/(R+P)$ of replicator can only decrease:

$$A = R(1-R-P)$$
$$\dot{R} = R(A - Out f) - mAR - \Delta R \simeq R(A - Out f' - rel) - mAR \qquad (15.5)$$
$$\dot{P} = P(A - Out f) + mAR - \Delta P \simeq P(A - Out f' - rel) - mAP$$

where *rel* is the relaxation constant. The variable A represents activity. After substitution $S = P + R$, and $f = R/(P+R)$ we get

$$\dot{S} = S(fS(1-S) - Out f - rel)$$
$$\dot{f} = -mf^2 S(1-S) \qquad (15.6)$$
$$\dot{f} \leqslant 0$$

So, the replicator would be replaced by parasites despite the introduction of the spatial structure. Without molecules running out of energy, parasites would not extinct in spots, where they are already in majority, their copying would not stop, and they would subsequently dominate the whole chemostat driving the actual replicator into extinction (see Fig. 15.29 and Fig. 15.30).

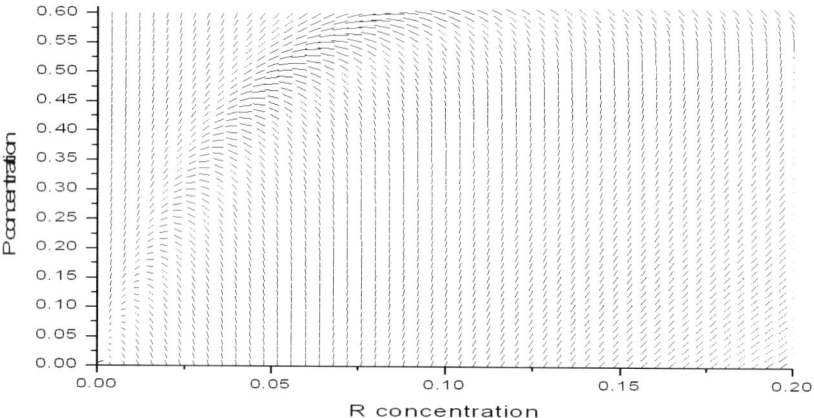

Fig. 15.29. Local phase portrait of the replicator+parasite system.

When the energy consumption is introduced into the model, its behavior is similar to the so called excitable systems [3], where an element first exists in an excitable state, then a wave of excitation hits it, and after some time it again returns to an excitable state, which enables a spread of another wave. The presented model differs from the basic model of the excitable system by having several states – each area proceeds through 5 states

- Zero concentration of both R and P, and maximum energy
- Expansion of a replicator from neighboring area, the concentration of replicators reaches maximum
- Expulsion of the replicator by parasites, concentration of the replicator quickly drops to zero, concentration of parasites reaches maximum
- Exhaustion of energy by parasites, their subsequent demise,
- Gradual accumulation of energy, up to the maximum, so that the cycle might start anew.

The state 1 corresponds to an excitable state, state 2 to excited state, and states 3 to 5 to a recovery state – the Fig. 15.28 shows, how all the 5 state cycle when the wave passes through.

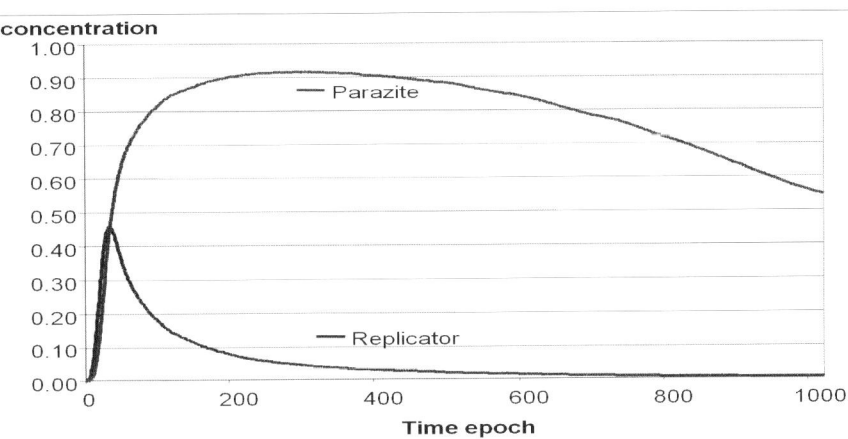

Fig. 15.30. Extinction of replicator without modeling energy consumption. After initial brief expansion, parasites build up, and sap the most of replicator capability, drive it to extinctions, and slowly extinct too.

15.7 Conclusions

New artificial life system was designed to combine (on an abstract level) function of catalytically active RNA, where their secondary and tertiary structure specifies their activity, with 'classical' artificial life systems based on linear instruction sequence.

By exploiting the fact, that the secondary structure of an RNA string can be represented in tree form, we can assign operations adapted from other artificial life system to its nodes, and interpret it as a program. We thus 'transplanted' the capability to produce functional self-replicators from random soup of programs, from one system, to another system more closely analogical to real biomacromolecules. Because RNA is supposed to be one of the first self-replicators (the RNA world scenario), this system can be used to model at least abstract aspects of the process of abiogenesis. For example, simulations in Section 15.5.2 concerning string splitting are analogous to experiments with real ribosomes.

The system was extended by a spatial interaction in a 2D environment with diffusion of the strings–molecules and with varied probability of collision and reaction, which is determined by their secondary structure. This system was then tested for ability to evolve of replicators, this time however without an explicit evaluation of the fitness, but with a duplication left solely to artificial molecules themselves. Apart from the evolved replicator, the chemostat contained in the end also a number of non-replicating sequences, which acted as parasites. Despite their presence, the replicator managed to keep its stable position of a dominant molecule in the system.

Even though the desired detailed similarity of behavior of simulated processes with real biological systems was not achieved yet, it was shown, that the proposed system is able to simulate an analogical process to the processes occurring in experiments with real biomacromolecules. The studied system can therefore serve to clarify (at least at the abstract level) the processes involved in the emergence of life.

References

[1] Adami C (1998) Introduction to Artificial Life. Springer, New York
[2] Ancel L, Fontana W (2000) Plasticity, Evolvability and Modularity in RNA. J. of Exp Zoology (Molecular and Developmental Evolution) 288: 242-283
[3] Barkley D, Kress M, Tucherman S (1990) Spiral-wave dynamics in a simple model of excitable media: transition from simple to compound rotation. Phys Rev A 42:2489-2491
[4] Boerlijst MC, Hogeweg P (1991) Spiral wave structure in pre-biotic evolution: Hypercycles stable against parasites. Physica D 48: 17-28
[5] Eigen M, Schuster P (1977) The Hypercycles: A Principle of Natural Evolution. Part A: Emergence of the Hypercycle. Naturwissenschaften 64: 541-565
[6] Eigen M, Schuster P (1978) The Hypercycles: A Principle of Natural Evolution. Part B: The Abstract Hypercycle. Naturwissenschaften 65: 7-41
[7] Eigen M, Schuster P (1978) The Hypercycles: A Principle of Natural Evolution. Part C: The Realistic Hypercycle. Naturwissenschaften 65: 341-369
[8] Evers DJ (2003) RNA Folding via Algebraic Dynamic Programming. Ph.D. Thesis, Bielefeld University
[9] Fernando C, Di Paolo EA (2004) The Chemoton: A model for the origin of long RNA templates. In: Pollack J, Bedau M, Husbands P, Ikegami T, Watson R (eds) Artificial Life IX. MIT Press, Cambridge, MA, pp 1-8
[10] Fontana W (1991) Algorithmic Chemistry. In: Langton CG (ed) Artificial Life II. Addison Wesley, Reading, MA, pp 159-210
[11] Hofacker IL (1994) The rules of the evolutionary game for RNA: A statistical characterization of the sequence to structure mapping in RNA. Ph.D. thesis, University of Vienna
[12] Hofstadter D (1979) Dialogues with Gödel, Escher, Bach: An Eternal Golden Braid. Basic Books, Inc, New York, Chapters XVI and XVII

[13] Ierymenko A (2005) Nanopond: The world's smallest and simplest evolvable instruction set virtual machine. Available at the Internet address http://www.greythumb.org/twiki/bin/view/GreyThumb/Nanopond
[14] Koza J (1992) Genetic programming. On the Programming of computers by Means of Natural Selection. MIT Press, Cambridge, MA
[15] Kvasnicka V (2000) An evolutionary model of symbiosis. In: Sincak P, Vascak J (eds) Quo Vadis Computational Intelligence? Physica-Verlag, Heidelberg, pp 293-304
[16] Kvasnicka V, Pospichal J (2003) Artificial Chemistry and Molecular Darwinian Evolution In Silico. Collection of Czechoslovak Chemical Communications 68: 139-177
[17] Lawrence M, Bartel DP (2005) New ligase-derived RNA polymerase ribozymes. RNA 11: 1173-1180
[18] Lenski RE, Ofria C, Pennock RT, Adami C (2003) The evolutionary origin of complex features. Nature, 423: 139-144
[19] Muller U (1993) Brainfuck: An Eight-Instruction Turing-Complete Programming Language. Available at the Internet address http://en.wikipedia.org/wiki/Brainfuck
[20] Newman MEJ, Engelhardt R (1998) Effects of neutral selection on the evolution of molecular species. Proc R Soc London, Ser B, 265: 1333-1338
[21] Pargellis AN (1996) The spontaneous generation of digital "life". Physica D 91: 86-96
[22] Ray TS (1992) An approach to the synthesis of life. In: Langton CG, Taylor C, Farmer JD, Rasmussen S (eds) Artificial Life II. Addison-Wesley, Redwood City, CA, pp 371-401
[23] Schuster P (1996) How does complexity arise in evolution. Complexity 2: 22-30
[24] Smith A, Turney PD, Ewaschuk R (2003) Self-replicating machines in continuous space with virtual physics. MIT Press, Cambridge, MA
[25] Snare AJ (2000) Typogenetics. B.Sci. Thesis, Monash Univesity, Australia
[26] Stephan-Otto Attolini C, Stadler P (2006) Evolving towards the hypercycle: A spatial model of molecular evolution. Physica D 217: 143-141
[27] Varetto L (1993) Typogenetics: An artificial genetic system. J Theor Biology 160: 185-205
[28] Varetto L (1998) Studying artificial life with a molecular automaton. J Theor Biology 193: 257-285
[29] Waterman MS, Smith TF (1978) RNA secondary structure: A complete mathematical analysis. Math Biosc 42: 257-266

Index

ρ-split function, 241
k-nearest neighbors query, 236
Caenorhabditis elegans, 26
Saccharomyces cerevisisae, 26
in-situ hybridization experiments, 23
'Database issue' of Nucleic Acids Research, 25

actin fibers, 269
actin fibres, 268
activator, 280
active learning, 37
agent, 222
aggregability, 69
algorithm, 277, 278
alignment
   algorithm, 152
   methods, 177
   scores, 153, 171
amino acid, 155, 156, 158, 159
   codes, 154
   distribution, 177
   properties, 177
   sequences, 152, 159, 163
   substitution, 170
annotation, 156, 167
approximate aggregability, 69
ARROWSMITH, 19
Artifial Intelligence, 19
artificial chemistry, 296, 298, 314, 337, 338
artificial life, 295, 307, 337, 338, 371

BAMS, 26
Bayesian network, 214

bibliographic databases, 18
biocurator, 25
BioCyc, 26
BioCyc family of databases, 25
BioGRID, 25, 26
biological sequences, 154–156, 159, 163, 168, 177
   quantification, 154
BLAST, 225
Block PCA, 118, 119, 125
BLOSUM, 155, 173–175
Boolean network, 213
bootstrapping, 34
brain, 222, 225
   disease, 231
   function, 223
   organization, 223
brain-gene ontology, 222

cell membranes, 269
cellular automata, 265, 266
cellular automaton, 274
cellular skeleton, 268
chemical, signalling, and metabolic paths, 268
chemicals, 265–269, 273, 274, 279
chemostat, 296, 303, 306
Chord routing protocol, 250
CMA-ES, 106
CoCoMac, 18, 26
CommmonKADS, 29
Common Logic, 19
complex systems, 266

compression
  biological sequences, 162
computational intelligence, 2, 5
Computational Neurogenetic Modelling, 225
conceptual biology, 19
conditional
  entropy, 169
  probability, 164
Conditional Random Field model, 35
Content Addressable Network (CAN), 248
conversed regions, 155
cosine similarity, 159
covariance matrix, 118
CRF, 35
cross-entropy, 164
curse of dimensionality, 191, 209

Darwinian evolution, 295, 298, 302, 316, 320, 326
database schema, 23
decomposability, 70
dependent variable, 20
depth of representation, 24
dictybase, 25
differential equations, 213, 296, 299
diffusion, 265, 267, 273, 274, 279
diffusion sub-step, 279
dimension reduction, 118
Directed Acyclic Graph, 156
Discriminant Analysis, 121
disease
  common, 2
  complex, 2
  mapping, 2
  multifactorial, 2
Distance index (D-index), 241
Distributed generalized hyperplane tree (GHT*), 246
Distributed vantage point tree (VPT*), 248
DNA, 265, 268
Document Classification, 33
double-labeling tract-tracing-experiments, 24
dynamic-programming, 323
dynamical system, 69

EANT, 99–104
EcoCyc, 25
efficient algorithm, VI, 69

Eigen genes, 189
Eigen theory of replicators, 298
Eigen's replicators, 306
Electronic Laboratory Notebook, 27
endocrinology, 18
entropy, 164, 169
epistasis, 2, 3
epithelium, 267, 273, 274, 280, 284, 292
EPNet, 104
Euclidean distance, 122, 211
Euclidian distance, 190
Event Characterization, 33
evolution strategies, 106
evolutionary algorithm, 69
evolutionary computing, 5
experimental models, 20
extracellular matrix, 268

F-Score, 40
FASTA, 225
finite element method (FEM), 291
fitness landscape, 295, 333
fitness surface, 295, 296
Fluoro Gold, 30
fly genetics, 18
FlyBase, 25
fuzzy k means algorithm, 217

Gaussian kernel estimator, 212
gene
  expression, 117, 185, 209, 224
  mutation, 231
  network, 209
  ontology, 222, 223
  profiling, 224
  regulatory network, 208
  regulatory networks, 209, 225
  selection, 186, 187
gene expression, 187
gene finding, 133
Gene Ontology, 20, 22, 26, 156, 177
gene regulatory network, 223, 265–267, 272, 273, 280
gene selection, 194
Generalized hyperplane tree (GHT), 246
Generic Model Organism Database, 25
GeneWays, 25, 26
Geneways, 18
GENIA, 26

Index   377

genome sequencing, 158
GMOD, 25
GNARL, 104
Google Scholar, 29
granular computing, 4

haplotype, 1, 3
Hapmap, 1
heuristic method, 215
hexamers, 134
Hidden Markov Models, 159, 177
high dimensionality, 117
Hilbert matrix, 122
homology, 152
hybridization, 187
hypercycle, 297, 298, 307–309, 319, 337, 339, 359, 366

incompressibility threshold, 275, 288
independent variables, 20
Index structure, 239, 244
information
    absolute, 160
    content, 157
    distance, 160
    heterogeneous, 4
    mutual, 169
    retrieval, 177
inhibitor, 280
injection site, 30
interaction
    gene-environment, 2, 3
    gene-gene, 2, 3
intermediate filaments, 268, 269
International Biocurator Meeting, 26
International Union of Basic and Clinical Pharmacology, 22
IUPHAR, 22

Journal of Comparative Neurology, 37

k-nearest neighbour, 190
kappa statistic, 39
KBs, 18
KDD challenge cup, 29
KEGG, 18, 25, 26
Knowledge Acquisition, 18
Knowledge Bases, 18
knowledge discovery, 187

Knowledge Representation, 18
knowledge representation, 222
Kolmogorov
    complexity, 160, 177
    conditional complexity, 160
Kronecker's delta, 317

language, 154
    engineering, 151, 176
    engineering techniques, 154
    model, 163, 164
    processing, 154, 155, 176
    techniques, 159
Latent Semantic Analysis, 158, 159, 177
linear programming, 192
linkage disequilibrium, 8
literature triage, 29
local alignment, 174, 175

macrovariable, 69
Mahalanobis distance, 118, 121, 122
MALLET CRF Toolkit, 35
mapping, 154
    of a protein sequence, 163
Markov chains, 163
maximum likelihood, 164, 168
mechanical, 265, 267–269, 271, 273, 274, 280, 292, 293
mechanical response, 265
MEDLINE, 27
Medline, 29
mesenchyme, 267, 273, 274, 279, 280, 292
meta-analysis, 28
MetaCyc, 25
metric, 161
Metric Chord (M-Chord), 250
Metric Content Addressable Network (MCAN), 248
Metric Grid (M-Grid), 244, 255
Metric space, 236
Metric tree (M-tree), 239
MGED, 22
MGI, 25
microarray, 185, 191, 209
    DNA, 117
Microarray Gene Expression Data Society, 22
microvariable, 69
minimum information, 24

missing data, 215
missing value, 191
model parts, 266
molecular automaton, 321
molecular Darwinian evolution, 296, 301
Monte Carlo, 196, 212
morphological development, 265, 266, 272, 273, 292
morphology, 265
multi-collinearity, 209
Multivalent, 37

n-grams, 159, 163–165
Named Entity Recognition, 33
National Center for Biomedical Ontology, 19
National Center for Biotechnology Information, 18
National Library of Medicine, 18
natural language processing, 18
natural languages, 154, 158, 163
NCBI, 18
NCBO, 19
NEAT, 104
NeuCom, 225
neural network, 134
neural networks, 93
neuroanatomical atlases, 27
neuroanatomy, 18
neurocomputing, 5
neuroinformatics, 18
NeuroScholar, 27
neuroscience, 18
Neuroscience Database Gateway, 25
neutral evolution, 354
neutral mutation, 357
neutral mutations, 330, 333, 334
NLP, 18
normalized
  compression distance, 161
  distance, 161
NP-hard, VI, 69

object-oriented model, 30
ontologies, 156
ontology, 221
Ontology engineering, 19
OntoViz, 32
Open Biomedical Ontology foundry, 19

open-access, 27
orthologous proteins, 174
OWL, 19

Parallel M-tree, 244
Part of Speech, 34
partial differential equations, 267, 291
pattern, 155, 159, 170
pattern-based approaches, 35
PDE, 267, 291
Pearson correlation, 193, 211, 212
Peer-to-peer network, 248, 250
Performance tuning, 254
Phaseolus Leuco-Agglutinin, 30
phylogenetic
  tree, 162, 171, 173, 177
physiology, 18
polygenic, 2
population genetics, 69
precision, 39
prediction
  of amino acids, 168
  of protein function, 152
  of secondary structure, 163
  structure, 156, 163
  protein family, 159
primary structure, 159
Principal Component Analysis, 118
Principal Components Analysis, 117
probability, 157
  density function, 164
Protégé, 22, 32
ProtComp, 169
protein, 151
  orthologous, 173
  similarity, 153, 171, 173
  structure, 159
proteins, 265, 268, 269, 274, 279
proteome, 169–171
  level, 173, 174
  sequences, 175
  similarity, 169, 170
pseudo-epithelium, 273, 292
PubMed, 18
PubMed Central, 18
PubMedCentral, 27

radioactive (tritiated) amino acids, 30
Range query, 236

ranking, 166
RDF, 19
recall, 39
regression, 191, 193
regulatory interactions, 210
regulatory path, 269
reinforcement learning, 96
Relation Extraction, 33
relative frequencies, 164
replication, 314
replicator, 302, 337, 339–342, 347, 348, 350, 351, 354, 357, 359, 361
research synthesis, 19, 28
RGD, 25
ribosomes, 268
RNA, 268

Scalability, 242, 244, 251
Scalable and Distributed Search Structures, 245
scientific facts, 20
scoring matrix, 153, 155
semantic
  distance, 156, 157
  meaning, 154, 163
  relations, 158
  similarity, 156, 157
sequence
  alignment, 152, 159, 168, 176
  similarity, 153, 168
SGD, 25
Siftware, 224
signal transduction, 18
Signal-Transduction Knowledge Environment, 26
signalling molecules, 265, 279, 280
signalling path, 269
signalling proteins, 273
similarity, 152
  analysis, 155
  measures, 153
Similarity hashing, 241
Similarity query, 236
Similarity searching, 236
Singular Value Decomposition, 158, 177
singular value decomposition, 189
Slim tree, 240
SNP, 1, 3

Spearman correlation, 211, 213, 217
statistical language modeling, 154, 163, 177
statistical significance analysis, 186
stochastic models, 163
strand, 297, 298, 307, 308, 343, 350, 351, 354, 357–362
structural design, 267
substitution matrix, 170, 174
SwissProt, 223

TAIR, 25
tensegrity models, 267
Textpresso, 25, 26, 34
Textspresso, 18
theoretic principles, 151, 154
theory
  algorithmic information, 160
  Kolmogorov, 160
Thyrotropin Releasing Factor, 20
TIGR, 25
tissues, 265–267, 271–273, 281
tool for the discovery of coding areas, 144
tracer chemical, 30
tract-tracing experiments, 23, 30
transneuronal labeling, 25
TREC, 29
tubulin, 268
Typogenetics, 296, 307, 316, 337

ultrastructure experiments, 24
UML, 32
UML notation, 30
UniProt, 18
University of Southern California, 27

Vantage point tree (VPT), 248
Vector Space Model, 158
Vex system, 38
visuo-motor control, 96
vocabulary, 154, 156, 158, 163

Weka, 224, 225
Wormbase, 25

XML, 32

yeast protein interaction networks, 18

ZFIN, 25

Printing: Krips bv, Meppel, The Netherlands
Binding: Stürtz, Würzburg, Germany